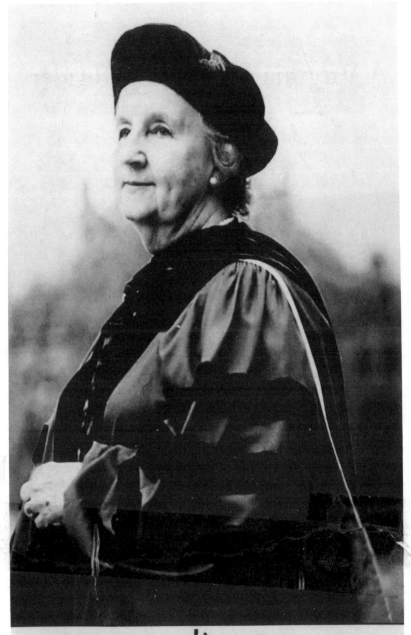

Virginia Henderson

A Virginia Henderson Reader

A VIRGINIA HENDERSON Reader

Excellence in Nursing

Edward J. Halloran, RN, PhD, FAAN

Editor

 Springer Publishing Company

Springer Publishing Company, Inc.
536 Broadway
New York, NY 10012-3955

Cover design by Tom Yabut
Production Editor: Pamela Ritzer
Second Printing

97 98 99 00 / 5 4 3 2

Library of Congress Cataloging-in-Publication Data

A Virginia Henderson reader: excellence in nursing / Edward J.
Halloran, editor.
    p. cm.
  Includes bibliographical references and index.
  ISBN 0-8261-8830-3
  1. Nursing. 2. Nursing—Philosophy. 3. Nursing—Study and
teaching. 4. Nursing—Research. I. Halloran, Edward Joseph.
II. Title.
  [DNLM: 1. Nursing Care—collected works. 2. Education,
Nursing—
collected works. 3. Nursing Research—collected works.
4. Nursing—collected works. WY 7 H497e 1995]
RT63.H46 1995
610.73 dc20
DNLM/DLC
for Library of Congress   94-42141

Printed in the United States of America

This work is dedicated to three families: the Hendersons, including their forebears in the Abbot and Minor clans, as well as their offspring in the Mark and Burdge house, the Houffs of Bellevue, the many Hallorans including the McMahons, the Kings, the Smiths, and their Plourde and Liskowsky relations, and my Yale family. Miss Henderson is present in the latter group, of course, as was John D. Thompson who introduced me to her. There are also three generations of Yale Deans, Florence Wald, Donna Diers, and Judy Krauss, and two Deans who have come from Yale, Angela McBride and Retaugh Dumas. My nature and nurture have emanated from these families.

E.J.H.

Contents

Foreword

In a world discombobulated by the quickened pace of change, the publication of this Virginia Henderson reader is particularly timely. The downsizing and reconfiguration of hospitals has left many professional nurses feeling dislocated and unsure of how they will fare in a health care delivery system seemingly more concerned about reimbursement policies than high-quality care. This reader is aptly subtitled "Excellence in Nursing" because the work of Virginia Henderson has been unfailingly concerned with excellence, particularly as applied to the essence of nursing. Like her own mentor, Annie Goodrich, Miss Henderson always criticized a mechanistic approach to patient care, so her words have added meaning when there are forces wishing to reduce nursing to a set of reimbursable procedures that might be just as well completed by other kinds of workers, too.

Miss Henderson's most meaningful contribution is that she provided the working definition of nursing adopted by the International Council of Nurses (ICN) and it was translated into dozens of languages. She envisioned nursing as a complex service that complements the patient by supplying what she or he needs to perform the activities of daily living. This view is one that can provide a sense of direction for our troubled times because of its emphasis on being patient centered and on maximizing functional ability. There is much in the readings brought together in this volume that has relevance for today—her outcomes orientation (i.e., decrease mortality, morbidity, symptoms, and dependency; increase a patient's sense of satisfaction and accomplishment), her urging of health promotion, continuity of care, patient advocacy, integration of the arts and sciences, and boundary spanning.

The readings also remind us of what a wonderful role model Virginia Henderson has been. Her thinking was shaped by the intellectual history of her times, and she did a great deal to compile that history through the *Nursing Studies Index*, *Inter-*

national Nursing Index, and her other writings. Her perceptions were data based, and she knew how to use findings to shape her field, most notably in shifting research away from studying nurses to studying the difference that nursing can make in people's lives. There were themes to her writings—for example, a clarity about the mission of nursing—and these themes were articulated with fresh insights in every decade of her prodigious career.

Free from formal institutional commitments, Miss Henderson used her "emeritus" years (from 1971 to the 1990s) to serve as nursing consultant to the world. As our at-large "wise woman," she questioned the direction of nursing research, the fashionable emphasis on nursing process, and society's unwillingness to confront death and dying. These writings now available in this reader remain relevant, but they also model the fresh eye that is the principal characteristic of excellent practitioners, educators, and researchers.

The last reading in this volume, with its thoughts on the health record, reminds me of a defining Henderson moment. It was June 1985 when the ICN presented her with the first Christianne Reimann Prize, acknowledging essentially that she was the foremost nurse of the world. She stood before the Congress in Tel Aviv and used the five minutes permitted her thank you to: (a) graciously acknowledge her appreciation for the honor bestowed; (b) recall her own links to the life and times of Christianne Reimann; and (c) challenge the assembly to take steps to encourage patients to be knowledgeable about their own health records. The impression conveyed was of a professional who knew how to use the moments available to her to advantage—a talent we must cultivate if we wish to make a difference.

Having been instrumental in getting her to agree in 1990 to lend her name to Sigma Theta Tau's International Nursing Library, I was surprised after the announcement was made to find that a number of my students and acquaintances were unfamiliar with her work. I had grown up in a world where Harmer and Henderson's *Principles and Practice of Nursing* was our bible; they had come of age at a time when you simply did not adopt required textbooks that were over 2000 pages in length. Edward Halloran has wisely decided to introduce new generations of nurses to the rich prose of Miss Henderson, for which we can all be very thankful.

ANGELA BARRON MCBRIDE, PHD, RN, FAAN
Distinguished Professor and University Dean
School of Nursing
Indiana University, IN

An Introduction to Virginia Henderson

It is with great pleasure that I introduce the reader to Miss Virginia Henderson. If you were to meet Miss Henderson in person as I have, you would have difficulty believing that this down-to-earth woman inquiring about your interests, exploring your perceptions of nursing, is a renowned nurse leader. Yet you would find traces of her genius in her insatiable curiosity—about where you came from, what name you were born with—in her grasp of nursing's history, and in her compelling vision for nursing's future.

Those of you who missed that personal acquaintanceship are still able to hear Miss Henderson's thoughts and ideas about nursing through her publications, a series of books and articles extending over a remarkable span of 50 years. This book is a sample of those writings. The conversational tone, the absence of medical and nursing jargon in all Henderson's works, allows the reader to imagine that (s)he is in Miss Henderson's presence, listening to this warm and gracious scholar, teacher, and nurse in an intimate setting.

Miss Virginia A. Henderson's texts and articles are used throughout the world. Indeed, she was one of the first nurses to emphasize the use of science, the need to seek out the opinions of experts, and certainly one of the first to define the unique functions of nurses. To my mind, she is the most influential nurse writer of the 20th century.

Perhaps Miss Henderson is best known for Harmer and Henderson's *Principles and Practice of Nursing*, taking over the project from Bertha Harmer, who wrote the first three editions in 1924, 1928, and 1935. Henderson went on to produce the fourth, fifth, and sixth editions (1939, 1955, and 1978), creating the thick tome that many nurses across the nation still remember. It was the chief nursing text used by students and nurse educators in hospital nursing schools for much of this century.

Henderson continued Harmer's emphasis on science and theory as the basis for nursing activity, replacing texts that emphasized the routine performance of nursing techniques and the strict following of physician's orders.

Miss Henderson made a lasting contribution to nursing theory by defining the function of nurses as;

> assisting individuals, sick or well, in the performance of those activities contributing to health, or its recovery (or to a peaceful death), that they would perform unaided if they had the necessary strength, will, or knowledge. And do this in such a way as to help them gain independence as rapidly as possible. (1955)

With the sole exception of her first revision of the Harmer text, Miss Henderson's description of nursing served as the philosophical and theoretical basis for all she was to write subsequently. This definition was widely promulgated in two books, *Basic Principles of Nursing Care* (1960, 1972), and *The Nature of Nursing* (1966). The International Council of Nurses continues to publish *Basic Principles of Nursing Care*, now available in twenty-seven languages and applicable to nursing in any setting, regardless of the state of technical development or the patient's disease.

Henderson's profession-defining contribution to nursing theory was soon to be joined by her contributions to nursing research. In 1953 she joined the Yale School of Nursing as a research associate and shortly thereafter began a review of the professional and scientific literature for a project entitled, *A Survey and Assessment of Research in Nursing* (1957). In her research she noted the dearth of studies about nursing care. Instead, she found that most reported studies were about the characteristics of nurses. It was then that she recognized the need for the profession to develop studies of nursing care, especially studies built on the results of previous research.

As a first step, she undertook a nineteen-year program to build the necessary access system, reviewing the nursing literature, cataloging and annotating reported studies, research in progress, research methods in use, and historical materials in periodicals, books, and pamphlets published in English. Five volumes resulted from this effort: *Nursing Research: Survey and Assessment* (with Leo Simmons, 1964) and the four-volume *Nursing Studies Index* (1963, 1966, 1970, and 1972).

Her sixth edition of *Principles and Practice of Nursing* (1978), written with Gladys Nite, benefited from this research, synthesizing the research findings and including expert opinions, creating an expansive view of nursing as a necessary human service capable of being delivered in and out of the existing health service delivery systems. As David L. Evans said in a review of the sixth edition, Miss Henderson treated every nurse as a researcher (1980).

In addition to her work in theory and research, Miss Henderson made known her views on the politics of health. She was a long-time proponent of publicly financed, universally accessible health services. She held that nurses should be both well-educated and more active as primary care service providers than they are in modern, Western society. She developed these views through her research and extensive travels throughout the world, observing the immense human need for nursing services, as well as the constraints (educational, economic, and political) placed on nurses. She particularly noted the constraints placed on nurses and society by gender issues and the ultimate inability of health service technology to cope with the modern culture's frenetic avoidance of the reality of death.

Miss Henderson was also a proponent of involving people in their own health care, advocating elimination of medical jargon from health records and giving the patient his/her records to read, contribute to, and retain in order to take to other health care providers.

Many of her advanced views can be traced to her personal biography. Virginia Avenel Henderson was born in Kansas City, Missouri on November 30th, 1897, named for the state to which her mother longed to return. That wish was granted when Virginia's father, an attorney for Native American Indians (he won a major case for the Klamath Indians against the U.S. Government in 1937), returned from the West to establish the family home at Trivium, near the Bellevue estate where her grandfather was principal of a boys' boarding school.

The fifth of eight children of Daniel B. and Lucy Minor (Abbot) Henderson, Virginia spent her school years at the Bellevue boarding school near Bedford, Virginia, where her grandfather, William Richardson Abbot, prepared boys for the University of Virginia. A former teacher at Bellevue, her father placed Virginia under the tutelage of teachers there—Mr. Abbot and especially an Aunt Anne Minor—during his extended absences.

The boarding school closed in 1909, and her schooling continued at home, at one point supervised by her sister Jane, a graduate of Sweet Briar College. All four Henderson sisters had professional careers, Lucy and Jane in education, Frances as a staff member of the American Federation of Arts.

During World War I, patriotic fervor drew Miss Henderson to the nursing profession. The U.S. Army School of Nursing, created to meet increased need for nurses during wartime, was headed by Miss Annie Warburton Goodrich, soon to be mentor to Miss Henderson and later to be the first Dean of Yale's School of Nursing. Miss Henderson completed nursing school in 1921 and said later that the students were treated with the same respect and courtesy as the cadets at the U.S. Military Academy.

Miss Henderson's early service was comprised of work in the Public Health Visiting Nurse Services in New York City and Washington, D.C. She assumed her role in education, the family tradition, with her first position as instructor at the Norfolk, Virginia Protestant Hospital School of Nursing. She returned to New York in 1929 to pursue further education at Teachers College, Columbia University, an education interrupted by a year serving as an outpatient instructor at the Strong Memorial Hospital in Rochester, New York. She completed her B.S. in 1932 and an M.A. in 1934.

Thereafter, Miss Henderson joined the nursing faculty at Teachers College and served as Instructor and Associate Professor of Nursing Education from 1934 until 1948. At Teachers College, she taught advanced clinical nursing to students affiliating in the New York Hospital, where she developed her philosophy of teaching nursing. Her philosophy entailed using advanced science and research, and collaboration with attending and resident physicians. She developed conferences with students, physicians, dietitians, family members, and sometimes patients in which the following questions were probed: What was done for the patient that worked? That didn't work? What should we have done that we didn't do? This case method system of education was used extensively for teaching patient care.

While still at Teachers College, Miss Henderson was asked to revise Miss Harmer's nursing textbook, a job she found easy because she felt the previous edition (the 3rd) needed little revision. Thus began a work commitment that would extend through much of her career. During this time period, Henderson served on a committee for the National League of Nursing Education that produced the influential *Curriculum Guide for Schools of Nursing* (1937) that adopted aspects of her teaching philosophy.

Leaving Teachers College in 1948, Miss Henderson spent the next five years on the fifth edition of *Principles and Practice of Nursing*, extensively revising it to incorporate scientific evidence and expert opinion in the selection of nursing techniques. (She had the help of her sister Lucy, a recently retired Richmond, VA English teacher, who retyped the manuscript.)

Bertha Harmer's name was retained through the fifth edition, in spite of her death in 1934, an event that prevented the two authors from ever meeting.

The fifth edition was used widely, helping to establish uniform standards for nursing practices. The book received awards for its design and illustrations. Many, if not most of the current generation of senior nursing leaders were taught nursing using this text. Like Nightingale's *Notes on Nursing* (1859), *Principles and Practice of Nursing* (5th ed.) was organized around a philosophy of nursing; all reference to specific diseases removed. When the book was nearly complete, Miss Henderson moved on to Yale.

Miss Henderson claimed that her work on the *Nursing Studies Index* project was her most important contribution to the nursing profession. Classifying, annotating, and indexing sixty years of literature for a profession as diverse as nursing was an immense undertaking. Although aided by a capable secretarial and library staff, and supported by Dean Florence Wald and the United States Public Health Service, the project was Miss Henderson's creation.

A new classification system was devised for the *Index*, but used medical subject headings so that the search for literature in medicine and nursing could more easily involve both disciplines. It was Miss Henderson's intention to seek greater cooperation between the two helping professions. As Dean Margaret Arnstein wrote about the project when it concluded:

> The staff and you have labored long
> For thirteen years unless I'm wrong
> The work you've done is quite immense
> To help us find that lost reference. (1972)[1]

The immediate impact of the project was the formation of nursing research teams at the Yale School of Nursing to redress the dearth of clinical nursing research. The theoretical underpinnings of nursing research were explored and the Yale school became the focal point for intellectual and practical advances in the nursing profession that continue to this day.

At age 76, Miss Henderson began her last major publishing project, a sixth edition of *Principles and Practice of Nursing*. Although the book was co-authored by Gladys Nite and included seventeen contributors, Miss Henderson co-wrote forty-nine of its fifty chapters. Five years were spent on the project which concluded in her eighty-second year.

Like Nightingale's establishment of modern nursing as separate from yet equal to the medical profession, Miss Henderson provides a compelling argument for the distinct nature of nursing. Sometimes complementing and sometimes competing with modern medicine, she emphasizes nurses as providing the strength, will, and knowledge (in conjunction with or in place of medicine, surgery, or institutionalization) to help others be independent, a perspective still timely in our era of the aging population, chronic disease, high medical costs, and marginal benefits from technology applied at life's end.

It is a tribute to Henderson's intellect that she could so clearly convey the human need for nurses and nurses' potential to meet that need. Moreover, much of what professional nursing organizations strive for today—autonomy and recognition for nurses—was already addressed in the sixth edition of *Principles and Practice of Nursing*. However, she insisted that nurses earn recognition through a scholarly and artistic approach to the care of individual patients. Knowledge is power and nowhere is the knowledge about nursing better expressed than in the sixth edition.

The sixth edition was not without its frustrations for her. It did not sell well in the United States. Some propose that the relocation of nursing education from hospitals to community colleges and universities was responsible; others say the book was too scholarly or simply too extensive for the needs of faculty teaching basic nursing. The book did sell well in foreign markets. For example, it was edited into four volumes and used extensively in Japan. Perhaps its success in foreign markets and its low sales in this country can be partially attributed to Henderson's lack of puffery. The book was written without reference to nursing process and without jargon, enabling educated people to use it in caring for themselves or others, operationalizing Henderson's concept of helping people to be independent.

Nor did Henderson sit on her laurels with the completion of the sixth edition of her textbook. She continued to write for professional periodicals, often arguing for a tax-supported health service and for patients' retention of their own health records. Until recently she continued her world travels, speaking on health care issues and receiving honors and awards.

Miss Henderson claimed that she hated to write, yet she wrote prolifically about every cause near to her heart and important to her profession. Those causes extended in a breadth of important directions: nursing theory, research, communication systems, education, and politics to name only a few. Like Nightingale, Miss Henderson is a reformer, possibly the only one who contends with Nightingale in her influence on nursing. It would not be unfair to say that Virginia Henderson is the 20th century's Florence Nightingale.

Notes

[1]Written by Margaret Arnstein, Dean of the Yale School of Nursing on the occasion of a party for Virginia Henderson at Yale, celebrating the completion of the *Index*, Summer, 1972.

References

Arnstein, M. (Summer, 1972). Untitled poem written in celebration of the completion of the Nursing Studies Index Project. New Haven, CT: Yale University School of Nursing (mimeo).

Evans, D. L. (1980). Every nurse as researcher. *Nursing Forum, XIX* 4:335–349.

Harmer, B. (1922, 1928, 1934). *The principles and practice of nursing* (1st, 2nd, 3rd eds.). New York: Macmillan.

Harmer, B., & Henderson, V. (1939). *Textbook of the principles and practice of nursing* (4th ed.). New York: Macmillan.

Harmer, B., & Henderson, V. (1955). *Textbook of the principles and practice of nursing* (5th ed.). New York: Macmillan.

Henderson, V. (1966). *The nature of nursing*, New York: Macmillan.

Henderson, V., & Nite, G. (1978). *Principles and practice of nursing* (6th ed.). New York: Macmillan.

Henderson, V., & Simmons, L. (1957). A survey and assessment of research in nursing. In: Cowan, M. C. (Ed.), *The Yearbook of Modern Nursing - 1956*. New York: G. P. Putnam's Sons, pp. 398–400.

Henderson, V., & the Yale University School of Nursing Index Staff (1963, 1966, 1970, 1972). *Nursing studies index*, (4 volumes; I-1900-29, II-1930-49, III-1950-56, IV-1957-59), Philadelphia: J. B. Lippincott.

Henderson, V. (1960, rev. 1969). *International Council of Nurses basic principles of nursing care*. Geneva, Switzerland: ICN.

National League for Nursing Education (1937). *A curriculum guide for schools of nursing*. New York: The League.

Nightingale, F. (1859). *Notes on nursing: What it is and what it is not*. London: Harrison.

Simmons, L., & Henderson, V (1964). *Nursing research: A survey and assessment*. New York: Appleton-Century-Crofts.

About the Editor

Edward J. Halloran, RN, PhD, FAAN, has been a professional nurse since 1964. Educated at the New Britain General Hospital School of Nursing, Southern Connecticut State College, Yale University, and the University of Illinois, he served for 25 years in nursing service settings. Since 1989 he has been a faculty member in the School of Nursing at the University of North Carolina at Chapel Hill. Dr. Halloran was formerly the chief nursing officer at University Hospitals of Cleveland (OH) and on the faculty of the Frances Payne Bolton School of Nursing at Case Western Reserve University. He also served as the chief nursing officer for Gottlieb (IL) and Winsted (CT) Memorial Hospitals.

Dr. Halloran has been an active participant in professional nursing organizations, having been elected to the Board of Directors of the National League for Nursing, the House of Delegates of the American Nurses Association, and the American Academy of Nursing. He also served as President of the American Assembly for Men in Nursing. He has written for professional journals as well as chapters for textbooks on nursing informatics, nursing administration, nursing theory, and men in the nursing profession. Dr. Halloran's current research activities include examining patient classification for cost, severity of illness, functional status and quality of life, as well as nursing history as it pertains to Florence Nightingale's effect on disease mortality in the American Civil War (1861–1865).

Dr. Halloran has consulted in North America, Europe, and Australia on the cost and quality of nursing services and speaks at professional meetings on the application of nursing theory, research, and history to meet contemporary professional challenges. He is married to Diane C. Halloran, RN, MPH, and they have collaborated on a number of publications. They are the parents of Jennifer A. Halloran of Chapel Hill and Alicia M. Halloran of New York City.

PART I

Patient Care

Introduction

In an anthology of Miss Virginia Henderson's writings, clinical care is apt to be given short shrift because of the impact of her work in theory and research. Yet two aspects of her writings on clinical care deserve special mention here. First, as the author of a standard nursing textbook Miss Henderson influenced several generations of nurses and helped standardize nursing care from 1940 to the present. Second, her textbooks, particularly *Principles and Practice of Nursing* (sixth edition), written with Gladys Nite and 17 contributors, thoroughly synthesized research and expert opinion on nursing, citing the nursing literature she had previously annotated for her four-volume *Nursing Studies Index*. This volume draws heavily on the *Principles and Practice of Nursing*, sixth edition.

The selections, along with the articles presented here, were chosen to illustrate the degree of esteem to which Miss Henderson held nurses, and to attest to the promise nurses hold in the reform of health care through their clinical work with their patients. No person who has ever experienced the care Miss Henderson describes, care that is provided day in and day out, around the clock, will ever deny nurses the professional credit and authority they deserve—for that care and for their ability to perpetuate their work through the education of the next generation of nurses and the development of new methods and techniques through research.

In her writings and talks about nursing care, Miss Henderson holds the most basic nursing care in the highest regard, befitting this intense and intimate human interaction. She considered no procedure too menial; to the contrary, anything a nurse could do to prevent or alleviate human malady was the noble task of the nurse. The nurses at Emory University Hospital and Nursing School presented Miss Henderson with a pair of gold-plated nail clippers in recognition of her admonition to them, "Cut their toenails." Cutting toenails is an aspect of foot care that prevents long and jagged nails from scratching the skin of the opposite leg. Such skin lesions are sometimes complicated by diminished circulation in older persons who lose the mobility to cut their own nails (*Principles and Practice of Nursing*, p. 792).

As in all her writings on nursing Miss Henderson advocates nurses to help people do what they would ordinarily do for themselves to maintain health, recover from illness, or die a peaceful death when persons lack the strength, will, or knowledge to take care of themselves. In *Principles and Practice of Nursing* (sixth edition) she says:

> Nurses must get inside the skin of each patient in order to know what help he or she needs from them. The nurse is temporarily the consciousness of the unconscious, the love of life for the suicidal, the leg of the amputee, the eyes of the newly blind, a means of confidence for the young mother, a voice for those too weak to speak, and so on. The activities people ordinarily perform without assistance are breathing, eating, eliminating, resting, sleeping and moving, cleaning the body and keeping it warm and properly clothed. Nurses also provide for those activities that make life more than a vegetative process, namely social intercourse, learning, occupations that are recreational and those that are productive in some way. (pp. 35–36)

Miss Henderson calls these the unique functions of nurses. In addition, nurses help persons identify and express their health needs, find and use community health resources, and carry out treatments prescribed by therapists or physicians when persons cannot perform them unaided. "And in the absence of physicians and other licensed therapists, nurses may function in these capacities. While nurses are not primarily therapists, nursing may include therapy, since everybody, in the absence of a physician, must necessarily treat themselves" (p. 36).

"It is this intimate, demanding, and yet inexpressibly rewarding service that nurses are best prepared to render. And because nurses are the most numerous of all health workers in most countries, and the nursing service in most agencies is the only 24-hour service, nursing is the only service organized to give this most essential help" (p. 36). Her ideas about clinical care and basic human needs matched with nurses' functions were summarized in a pamphlet, *Basic Principles of Nursing Care*, commissioned by the International Council of Nurses to reflect nursing care that could be provided regardless of the state of technological development where care is given and applicable no matter what disease the patient had.

The section on care of the dying person was written with Florence Wald, former Dean of the Yale School of Nursing and longtime friend of Miss Henderson. Mrs. Wald was one of the founding members of Connecticut Hospice and is an activist on the humane care of dying persons. Roberta O'Grady (Chapter 4), Gladys Nite and Catherine Temple (Chapter 6) also contributed to the patient care section.

Miss Virginia A. Henderson's career has involved a lifetime of practicing, teaching, researching, and writing about nursing. Her books progress as she studied and matured in her thinking about nursing and culminate in the 1978 edition of the *Principles and Practice of Nursing*. While it is unusual for a nurse in practice to return to such a text, I was compelled to do so because my practice in hospital nursing leadership required an understanding of the profession and its work for it to be translated to institutional policy. Hospital Board members, executives and medical staff needed to understand the nursing function in order to support it. *Principles and Practice of Nursing*, used as a reference, never failed to provide me insight into the functions, roles, and challenges for nurses and their profession in a language that could be readily interpreted to non-nurse members of society, patients included. The selections in the clinical care section of this book give only a hint at what can be gleaned in depth from *Principles and Practice of Nursing*, sixth edition. I recommend you obtain a copy of her text for reference.

References

Henderson, V. (1960). *International Council of Nurses basic principles of nursing care*. Geneva, ICN.

Henderson, V., & Nite, G. (1978). *Principles and practice of nursing* (sixth edition). New York: Macmillan.

Henderson, V., & the Yale University School of Nursing Index Staff. (1963, 1966, 1970, 1972). *Nursing studies index*, (4 volumes; I–1900–29, II–1930–49, III–1950–56, IV–1957–59). Philadelphia: J.B. Lippincott.

Chapter 1

Excellence in Nursing[1]

Being one of a large and vocal clan, I was brought up on discussions that lasted well into the night on such subjects as what is truth, beauty, charm, or goodness. In such arguments—for I fear they were more arguments than discussions—the theories advanced by those in our family who could make themselves heard were rarely acclaimed, nearly always attacked. No persons brought forward as exemplifying charm, beauty, or goodness were unanimously agreed upon by the others. In fact, it was dangerous to set up one's idol for it was sure to be knocked down.

I realize that the views I express here are likely to meet with the same kind of response. Some of us may see as most excellent the qualities we wish *we* had, the goals *we* have tried but failed to reach; or, to protect our egos, we may applaud the accomplishments that are nearest kin to our own. The topic of excellence might even be used as a psychoanalytic device, with anyone discussing it running the risk of an interpretive response.

Nevertheless, and despite the difficulty of being objective and the danger of revealing my limitations or biases, I would like to discuss my concept of excellence in nursing and to mention some of the nurses throughout history who, in my opinion, qualify as excellent.

The Nature of Excellence

Grading or judging the performance of students or co-workers is a difficult but an inescapable task for the teacher and the administrator. Hard as we may strive to put the burden of evaluation on the student or the worker, claiming rightly that self-evaluation is a means of developing self-knowledge and approaching self-imposed goals, there still comes a time when we must assume the responsibility for stating our own objectives for the student or worker and the extent to which we believe the person in question has reached them. This process of goal setting is at the root of curriculum building, of planning or evaluating nursing services, of ever-continuing efforts to improve patient care.

It has been said that to make a man healthy you have to begin with his grandfather. So, in discussing excellence in nursing, we must go back as far as it is practicable. If we seek to develop excellence in the graduate of an educational program, there must first be a potential for intellectual, emotional, or spiritual growth in the student. In other words, we must start with the selection of the promising candidate.

It is my opinion that the selection and preparation of individuals entering any of the health and welfare fields have much in common, and that in university centers there should be collaboration between these various disciplines or departments. Nursing school candidates, it seems to me, should have many of the same qualifications as those sought in candidates for schools of medicine, social work, the special therapies, or public health.

While I hope that the maternalistic and highly judgmental attitudes that characterized nursing schools in the early decades of this century are gone forever, I think that the personal integrity of the individual is inseparable from the quality of the service he or she gives. So, in the health professions, I believe we need sane minds in healthy bodies and persons with more than the average endowment of intelligence. What's more, since no one practices nursing except in relation to his or her times and in relation to the needs of a given society, I believe we should seek those persons who show promise of having a social conscience and civic interest. It seems hardly possible to me that an excellent nurse can be at the same time an indifferent or socially inexperienced citizen.

In other words, I think excellence in nursing is dependent upon what the candidate brings to it, and that it can be measured by the quality of the individual's personal life, by his or her contribution as a member of a community, as well as by the professional services he or she offers society. Excellence, to me, suggests the well-rounded, or complete, person.

Some universities collaborate on the identification of potential excellence in students of the health sciences. Some of these also collaborate on curriculum building and course offerings. If we believe that health personnel should work in a harmonious team relationship toward a common goal for the patients and families they serve—and we constantly say so—would not this unity of purpose be greatly fostered by having students of the health professions study together during their basic training? Not only would good working relationships be fostered but a broader point of view could be acquired than is possible when only one homogeneous group studies alone.

In order to set up a curriculum designed to produce an excellent nurse or other health worker we must know how to measure the competencies of the graduate. Among the measures that have been used in efforts to evaluate the nurse's clinical worth are the following:

1. Decreased mortality rates among those she serves
2. Decreased morbidity rates with respect to certain diseases or conditions such as impetigo in infants, rickets in children, or puerperal sepsis in mothers
3. Decrease in symptoms of nursing neglect such as pressure sores or incontinence
4. Decrease in psychological withdrawal symptoms, negativism, or mutism
5. Decrease in dependency with respect to daily activities or the degree of rehabilitation achieved
6. Favorable opinions of care given by the nurse as expressed by the patient, his family, other nurses, or associated medical personnel.

Clearly, some of these measures can also be used in evaluating the physician's work or that of related therapists. How can the effect of nursing be separated from the effect of medicine and vice versa? For example, the length of stay in psychiatric hospitals has markedly decreased in recent years. To what extent does this reflect better psychiatry and to what extent, better psychiatric nursing?

Similarly, the recovery rate from drastic surgery certainly reflects a great advance in the surgeon's knowledge and skill. But does it not also reflect a comparable advance in the knowledge and skill of the surgical nurse?

It is not possible to discuss every problem connected with this question of evaluation; many texts and articles deal with this subject in detail.[2] But I am firmly of the opinion that the published record of nursing does show that the excellence of specific nurses *has* affected the welfare of individuals or segments of the population.

Annie W. Goodrich (one of the most excellent of all nurses, in my opinion) used to refer to three stages in the development of nursing: the emotional, the technical, and the creative. Most nurses could probably identify each of these three phases in their own development.

Young students are motivated by compassion to help other human beings. But it is not until they have learned some techniques or skills that they can offer much more than sympathy and inept physical assistance. Then, as they learn the hundreds of procedures involved in practice, they may become temporarily engrossed in the technical (or second) phase of nursing. Unfortunately, some nurses—and some doctors, too—never seem to go much beyond this second phase.

The complete, mature, or excellent nurse, however, is the one who remains compassionate and sensitive to patients, who has thoroughly mastered nursing's technical skills, but who uses—and has the opportunity to use—her emotional and technical responses in a unique design that suits the peculiar needs of the person she serves and the situation in which she finds herself. This third phase is obviously a synthesis of the first and second, plus that intangible quality that makes work creative. But nursing offers so many ways of demonstrating creativity or excellence that we should avoid rigidity in selecting, preparing, and evaluating nurses.

The nurses who are presented here as my own candidates for "excellence" have demonstrated a wide range of accomplishments and confirm the danger of thinking that any one set of prerequisites, any one type of preparation, or any era has the final answer to the question of producing the creative nurse.

The Known

In Miss Nightingale, the first candidate, we see a largely self-taught, aristocratic woman who revolutionized army medical care, developed the science of health statistics, and created a genuine nursing school that produced the first example of the modern "trained nurse." Ethel Bedfore Fenwick, from the same social class in England, was the moving spirit in the formation of the International Council of Nurses, one of the first international health organizations. She also founded one of the early nursing journals and was largely instrumental in effecting nurse registration in England.

In this country, Annie W. Goodrich, a young woman with no college experience herself, upgraded nursing care in four of New York's largest hospitals and did more than any other person to introduce basic nursing education into colleges and universities. She established the first nursing program with a bachelor's degree as a prerequisite. In this struggle she was, of course, abetted by Lavinia M. Dock, M. Adelaide Nutting, Isabel M. Stewart, Effie J. Taylor, and a host of other enlightened nurses, as well as by some doctors, like Richard Olding Beard and William Welch, and by the great public health-leader C.-E. A. Winslow.

Another type of accomplishment was that of Lillian Wald, who fostered the settlement house or social center movement. In those days a district, or visiting, nurse service was a part of such centers. Actually, it is hard to name any welfare work of Miss Wald's era in which she failed to play some part. It was she, for instance, who suggested the creation of the Children's Bureau, taking an active role thereafter in protective legislation for women and children. She also promoted school nursing, particularly in New York City.

Alice G. Carr, a public health nurse with a preparation we would now consider entirely inadequate, directed a five-year health demonstration in Greece under the Near East Foundation following World War I. Faced with manifold health problems among the displaced persons she served, she realized that the largest returns would come from applying sanitary measures—more specifically, destroying mosquitoes—and she is credited with having eliminated malaria in the area. Dr. Haven Emerson used to refer to her work as one of the great public health accomplishments of that period.

Among other manifestations of excellence must be included the journalistic and historical achievement of Mary M. Roberts, the *American Journal of Nursing's* editor for 28 years; the order wrought in nursing legislation by such women as Elizabeth C. Burgess and Bernice Anderson; and the grasp Blanche Pfefferkorn demonstrated of certain kinds of research during the thirties, long before it became "fashionable." In this connection Lucile Petry Leone, Margaret Arnstein, Faye Abdellah, and others should be cited for their development not only of nursing studies within the federal government, but also of federal support for nursing research.

Another innovator, in still another field, was Mary Breckinridge, who brought British nurse-midwifery to this country, making an incomparable health record for her Frontier Nursing Service. Her work has been taken up, furthered, and made applicable to urban as well as rural communities by Hazel Corbin, Hattie Hempshmeyer, Ernestine Wiedenbach, Margaret Thomas, and Vera Keane, to mention a few clinically expert nurse midwives.

Dorothea Linde Dix, again a largely self-taught reformer, is credited with striking achievements in humanizing the care of the mentally ill. One of the first psychiatric nurses of our own day to demonstrate the therapeutic effect of a good nurse–patient relationship is Gwen Tudor Wills, who published what is possibly the first series of patient–nurse interactions. Hildegard Peplau, Ida Orlando, Rhetaugh Dumas, Jane Schmahl, June Mellow, Rachel Robinson, Florence Wald, and many others have added to the record of excellence in this clinical field.

In child care, Florence Blake in Chicago and Florence H. Erickson in Pittsburgh evolved a superior-type of nursing that utilizes or applies developmental psychology, the play therapy techniques of Carl Rogers, and much of what has been learned in recent years about working with parents. And, in the care of adults, Thelma Ingles' beautiful case studies and Gladys Nite's carefully documented work with cardiac patients are examples of excellent nursing described step by step.

In school or college health work Helene Fitzgerald and her associates at Yale University have demonstrated a uniquely successful type of interview or nurse–student interaction. This has proved to be as effective in identifying health problems of college students and encouraging their use of health facilities as the traditional health examination of the student by a physician.

Educationally, Mildred Montag has been an innovator or a creator. With the backing of Louise McManus and leaders in the junior college movement, she designed a program of basic nursing education on the junior or community college level that has made the resources of these institutions available for the preparation of nursing personnel. The rapid growth of these associate degree programs could free society from dependence on the hospital-controlled program.

Lydia Hall, another highly creative nurse and original thinker, designed and—until her recent death—directed a new type of health facility: the Loeb Nursing Center in New York City. Here nursing is the principal therapy. It is the nurse who helps the patient to understand and cope with his problems; the physician is called in as a consultant when, in the nurse's or patient's judgement, he is needed.

Dorothy Smith, of the University of Florida at Gainesville, started a new administrative pattern when she established the principle that every nursing faculty member, including the dean, should continue to care for patients. This assumption of a dual responsibility for nursing faculties is both old and new. It is original in its current form, however, since the traditional managerial role of the nurse that prevented her from nursing and teaching has been assigned to the non-nurse unit manager.

This marriage of education and nursing service is gaining wider and wider acceptance and is being studied at Case Western Reserve University by Rozella Schlotfeldt and her associates at the Frances Payne Bolton School of Nursing and University Hospitals of Cleveland. It is noteworthy that Luther Christman—another candidate for excellence on the basis of his clinical and nursing organization work in Michigan—has assumed responsibility for both nursing education and nursing care at Vanderbilt University.

While each person asked to identify nurses exemplifying excellence would probably produce a different list (and I could extend mine far beyond the practical limits of this paper) I believe that most nurses would gladly claim any of the persons I've mentioned as graduates of their school. It would be helpful if we could find the common denominators in their endowment, preparation, and experience. We need many more persons like these, who seem to have been free to exercise their talents and apply their natural gifts in dealing with some aspect of nursing.

If I left the discussion of excellence at this point at mentioning only recognized figures, I'd feel like a hypocrite and a traitor to nursing. I have deliberately chosen examples of accomplishments that are varied and often spectacular—more particularly, those accomplishments documented in nursing literature published in the English language. The record is there for anyone to read and to judge for himself whether or not I've exaggerated the social significance of these nurses' works. But the achievements of what might be called celebrated nurses represent only that small part of the iceberg that can be seen.

For every nurse who has made a record of excellence in the history of our calling there are thousands whose work is, I think, equally meritorious but who are completely unknown and who have received no public recognition. These nurses have worked *solely* for the inner satisfaction of knowing that they have helped one human being after another to get well, stay well, accept and adjust to the limitations of living, or to die with dignity and fortitude. All nurses who read this will at once think of some nurses they know who answer this description, and some readers who are not nurses must have been fortunate enough to experience care at the hands of such persons.

The Unknown

As a tribute to the *unknown excellent nurse* and to illustrate the combination of insight, compassion, skill, knowledge, and fidelity that characterizes all excellent nursing—this most personal and demanding service—I'd like to recount a personal experience.

About 1946 when I was a volunteer staff nurse for a few days a week in a large and famous hospital, I met a private duty nurse and her patient, both of whom interested me greatly. I came to know them because the nurse needed help from the floor nurses at certain times and I happened to give this help on several occasions. The patient was a young woman who, following the birth of her first child, had suffered an infection. In the course of six months it had progressed to the point where there were perhaps 20 to 30 abscesses or necrotic areas on the patient's emaciated body. The air in the room was filled with an uncontrollable stench.

This young woman, with the covers drawn up to her chin, was still beautiful and appealing. A devoted husband came to see her every night. He, her nurses, and the many doctors interested in her all hoped to conquer this condition, or at least behaved as if they did. There were always flowers in the tidy room and, except for the fearful odor, you would not have known that under the light covering lay a pitifully diseased body. The patient's dark hair was always carefully combed, with attractive yellow bows on each side of her head.

One day the nurse, a quiet woman in her early forties, asked me if I would take care of her patient on her (the nurse's) next free day. She had been on this case for five months with one day off a week. I knew I could not measure up to the demands of the task—but how could I refuse, especially as I was given to understand that the patient had asked for me?

The day came and I found it almost impossible to fit into it all that had to be done. In a desperate effort to save this doomed young woman, the doctors, after trying the available antibiotics, had finally resorted to immersion baths, an ordeal for the patient and the nurse that I hate to remember. Many other necessary but less dramatic aspects of her care, I can say without exaggeration, filled completely the hours I was with her.

The point of this story is that the next day, when I expressed to the nurse my great admiration for the care she was giving in this most distressing and difficult situation, her eyes filled with tears and she said, "Miss Henderson, this is the first word of praise I've had from another nurse since I graduated!" She—and others like her, I'm sure—must have felt that their excellence was unappreciated.

If nursing is essentially—as I believe it is—this sharing of another's burden freely, fully, ungrudgingly, and, when necessary, right up to the point of death, then excellence must take into consideration those qualities of endurance that enable a nurse to do this. Until the last disease is conquered, human beings are going to be made dependent by them; the very young and very old will always be dependent.

The nurse who complements the dependent—sick or well—by supplying him with the strength, knowledge, or will he needs for "wholeness" must be judged excellent if she can and will determine which and how much of each he needs, and if she can and will supply them for as long as he needs them. I call this "getting inside the other person's skin," even though I know this is impossible, literally and figuratively.

Most of us recognize this identification with another as a highly difficult task demanding unlimited knowledge, a large battery of skills, patience, tolerance, sensitivity, and a capacity for sustained effort that in old-fashioned parlance was called "character." The "flower children" and the modern Peace Corps and VISTA workers recognize it also as a capacity for loving and being willing to serve one's fellow man.

Nursing's True Significance

The essence of our problem in striving for excellence is to search out those with the capacity for developing it. Another aspect of the problem is to set up conditions that make it possible for the student of nursing to develop his or her full potential, to experiment, assess, and evaluate his or her work. Still another problem—and the one I think we have done the least to solve—is to provide working conditions that offer the nurse opportunity for creativity and growth as well as the satisfaction that should accompany the giving of excellent nursing care.

I know an eminent physician with a son and a daughter. The son went into medicine and the daughter into nursing; both graduated with honors. The young physician, his father tells me, is practicing enthusiastically; his daughter, he reports, is "disenchanted with nursing." This would be an incident hardly worth our notice except that we hear the same sort of thing so often. There are about half as many inactive as there are active registered nurses—or 300,000 nurses who are able to nurse but who for one reason or another do not choose to practice. Why?

The ANA has been reorganized to make provision for the clinical interests as well as the administrative, teaching, and research functions of the nurse. It works for adequate salaries for practitioners; in almost every measurable respect, working conditions for staff and private duty nurses have improved. What is still so wrong with clinical practice? Why does the practice of nursing so often disappoint the young graduate? Does the fault possibly lie within ourselves? Does the average nurse understand the complexity of her service, the extent to which she might help those she serves, the changes she might bring about in health care? Might we not persuade others if we were all as convinced of the *social and ethical significance of nursing* as was the author of the phrase, Annie W. Goodrich who gave this title to her collected works?

Note

---

[1]This chapter was adapted from an address given at the Alumnae College, University of West Virginia, May 1968.

[2]A brief summary of some of the published studies dealing with the evaluation of patient care can be found in Chapter 13 (pp. 376–389) of *Nursing Research: A Survey and Assessment*, by Simmons and Henderson, New York, Appleton-Century-Crofts, 1964.

Chapter 2

The Essence of Nursing in High Technology

What is Meant by High Technology in Nursing?

Some people believe that all hospital care is dependent on the complex machinery of high technology, especially the electronic communication of computers. The original cost of building, furnishing, equipping, and staffing modern hospitals has increased the average daily cost of hospital care in the United States so much that unless most individuals are very ill or their diagnosis and treatment depend on a hospital's technical resources, only the wealthy go to hospitals.[1]

Critical care units are increasingly found attached to most clinical services, reminders of the expression that the tail is wagging the dog. Nurses who staff intensive care units (ICUs) typify high technology in nursing and to nurses not assigned to ICUs, may be considered a breed apart. Often, experience with critical care nursing is limited to what is seen and heard during visits with friends and relatives who are patients in critical care units. This may mean 5 minutes of the hour with the friend or relative, and 55 minutes with other sorrowful people in the visitors' waiting room. A perception of not feeling welcomed by the nursing staff or not being impressed by their humane concern for patients or visitors may contribute to attitudes of prejudice against critical care nursing.

This prejudice can be considerably modified by efforts to become more informed about this branch of nursing. Several remarkably thorough texts discuss the subject. In an age where the psychosocial aspects of nursing have thrown into eclipse the physical aspects, it is gratifying to find some nurses who still think the latter as deserving of their attention as the former. One large, particularly useful text is edited by nurses and has nurse contributors.[2] The contributors also include physicians, and throughout a close collaboration between the two professions is implied.

While this work clarifies the wide range of knowledge of physiology, anatomy, physics, and chemistry demanded by critical care nursing, other books by nurse-authors on the subject are also useful.[3] Much can be learned by visiting several critical care units and listening to nurses staffing the units as they discuss the satisfactions and dissatisfactions of their work. The profession's dramatic, life-saving character is its most obvious appeal; the ethical questions it raises are a constant worry. For example, can the excessive cost of keeping a member of a needy family in the critical care unit be justified when it is believed by the staff that recovery is impossible? Or is it ethical to give families hope when the staff has none?

Listening to the papers presented at a recent London conference provided additional insight about the high technology involved in critical care nursing. A number of research reports focused on ethical and philosophical questions, although many dealt with high technology in assessing patients' conditions and with symptomatic treatment. Several physicians and surgeons were included among the speakers, in contrast to the one physician participating in the week-long program of a recent international congress.

The use of high technology, however, is not confined to those who work in critical care units. High technology is moving into home care and treatment. Partly to save as much as, or more than $200 daily, individuals and families are electing home rather than hospital care. Relatives or friends, taught and helped by nurses or technicians employed by the manufacturers of medical equipment, are providing home care for persons who require parenteral feeding, dressing and drainage of wounds, inhalation therapy, and comparable procedures. This development, described in numerous journal articles, suggests that differences among hospital, clinic, and home care may greatly diminish and that home care personnel and patients themselves must master many aspects of high technology.

Literature: A High Technology Learning Tool?

In his best seller, *Megatrends*, John Naisbitt lists "the ten new directions transforming our lives": The first is the trend from an industrial to "an information society and the second the movement from a forced technology to a high tech/high touch society."[4] An information society depends on rapid travel and electronic (nearly instant) communication, worldwide. J. David Bolter, in *Turing's Man—Western Culture in the Computer Age,*[5] says that tools epitomize the stages of human development. Clay pottery is the tool associated with ancient Greece; the clock and later the steam engine with the early stages of modern man, and the computer with contemporary man. Because the computer manipulates symbols electronically and so much more rapidly than humans can, Bolter thinks that all major intellectual efforts of the future will involve the use of computers.

Already, life in developed countries is dependent on computers. But now, only a hint of the help they can give in making and retrieving health records is evident. The disadvantages involved may also not be clear. If it ever is possible to develop an international medical or health record integrating the contribution of doctors, nurses, and others, and to give a copy of the record to the patient, computers will establish the information the person's health record should contain.

Suggested practices advocated in *Principles and Practice of Nursing* are based on a review of related research by nurses, physicians, and persons working in the physical, biological and social fields.[6] The ability to locate such research reports has been greatly facilitated by computerized retrieval systems. As editor of the four-volume retrospective *Nursing Studies Index*[7] to the nursing literature from 1900 through 1959, the author has been directly involved in developing information resources for nursing and the ability of nurses to use these resources effectively. This means knowing the indexes, abstracts, reviews, audiovisual listings and other library tools that are available, and how to use them.

Computerized data banks made it possible for the American Journal of Nursing Company, in collaboration with the National Library of Medicine, to begin publication in 1966 of *The International Nursing Index*[8] in line with *The Index Medicus.*[9] Every medical student must use *The Index Medicus*. Until the average practicing nurse learns how to use and will use indexes to retrieve information from data banks such as that of the National Library of Medicine, the nurse will not have taken the most elementary step to becoming part of a research-based profession—a claim nurses now like to make.

Any researcher who does not find, review, and build on related research is busy rediscovering the wheel—wasting time and usually someone else's money. Many nurses, even those in positions of authority, don't know anything about published nursing indexes or how to use them. Schools of nursing might well note a feature of the nursing diploma program at the Royal Victoria Hospital in London, Canada. In the seventies, this school was giving a one semester course to students who needed help in library skills. The students used an excellent workbook that enabled them to demonstrate and record their progress in finding information.

Technology: A Useful Tool to Provide Health Care Service?

One of the later books written by René Dubos (the great environmentalist, biologist, and humanist) stressed the limitations of science and technology in contributing to human happiness.[10] *The Harvard Magazine* article, "Needed: A New Way to Train Doctors," is Harvard President Derek Bok's way of reporting to the University's Board of Overseers for 1982 to 1983.[11] In the report he notes that despite miracle drugs, open heart surgery, kidney transplants, and computerized axial tomography (CAT) scanning, the United States has failed to achieve a comprehensive system of health care comparable to those achieved in other industrialized nations. He says, "To our shame, 28 million people are not yet covered either by federal programs or by private health insurance."[12]

Bok considers that the system of medical education is failing. He thinks its highly competitive nature is destructive; he thinks it overemphasizes the science of medicine and undervalues the art, often losing sight of society's needs.

There is a parallel in the variety of American nursing that claims to be research-based and that extols the science of nursing almost to the exclusion of its art. Nursing is so preoccupied with these concerns that it neglects to play a significant role in the development of an equitable health care system for the United States. Paul Starr's Pulitzer Prizewinning study, *The Social Transformation of American Medicine: The Rise of a Sovereign Profession and the Making of a Vast Industry*, is worth the attention of nurses. He reviews the efforts during this century of legislators and others concerned with the public's health to mandate access to health care by all citizens of the United States. Nursing is scarcely mentioned by Starr and never as a force for or against the proposed legislation that has nearly been enacted under several administrations.

High technology in health care is posing many philosophical, ethical, moral, and economic questions. It is encouraging that more and more health care providers, including nurses, are conducting conferences on ethics. But nursing must also come to grips with the economics of health care, or the question of how health dollars should be spent. Should money be spent on the extension of life by technology for the very rich or on the improvement of the quality of life for all?

The Economist for April 28, 1984 includes a startling report of the findings of Norman McCrae, who was asked by *The Economist's* editor to study international health care statistics.[13] Of the five countries reported on—the United States, West Germany, France, Japan, and Britain (ranked according to per capita expenditures on health)—the best results are shown by Japan, which, next to Britain, spends the least. According to this report, per capita health expenditures range from $1,500 in the United States to $400 in Britain. Good results from the five countries are measured by (1) life expectancy (the range is 73 to 77 years); (2) infant mortality (the range is 7 to 13 deaths per 1000 births); and (3) deaths from heart disease (the range is 266 to 584 per 100,000). Japan has the fewest doctors (128) per 100,000 of the population, and West Germany has the most (222). In McCrae's study, the ratio of nurses to a country's population is not reported or discussed as a significant statistic.

McCrae's study should be read critically and his estimates checked. But if the United States is spending more than twice as much on health care as is Japan and getting less for it, our distribution must be faulty, some of our workers may be overpaid, or perhaps money is being wasted on high technology to extend life for a few at great expense while basic needs of the general population, such as prevention of disease, are being neglected. Incidentally, this use of risky high technology influences the insurance rates our physicians and surgeons pay, in some cases more than $30,000 annually.[14]

It is also possible that Japanese nurses may be very successful in providing what may be the most constant and possibly the most important element in health care, what is reflected in the term "the essence of nursing."

What Is the Essence of Nursing?

The author's concept of nursing has been presented in books, pamphlets, and journal articles published over the last 40 years, with minor revisions. It is offered here again to clarify any misconceptions and to affirm its continuing validity.

The *unique* function of the nurse is to do for others what they would do for themselves if they had the strength, the will and the knowledge; and to do it in such a way that the recipient of the service acquires independence as soon as possible, or an ability to cope with a health handicap, or to die with dignity when death is inevitable.[15]

This concept is valid because nursing alone assumes responsibility for a 24-hour service. Other health workers, family members or friends may perform this function, but when they do they are said to be "nursing" the person who is helpless, sick, or injured.

To understand this concept, a nurse should try to "get inside the skin" of the client-patient and sense what help he/she wants and needs to perform the following daily activities:

- breathing;
- eating and drinking;
- eliminating;
- moving, maintaining normal posture, exercising;
- resting and sleeping;
- dressing and undressing;
- maintaining body temperature within a normal range;
- avoiding dangers in the environment (including infections) and protecting others;
- communicating with others in expressing emotions, needs, fears, questions, information, and ideas;
- worshipping according to one's faith;
- working at something that gives a sense of accomplishment;
- playing, or participating in some form of recreation; and
- learning, discovering, or satisfying one's curiosity so that normal development can proceed.

These activities include, but go beyond, those associated with the usual process of rehabilitation. They include physical, and psychosocial functions. This list makes it clear that the essence of nursing involves holistic health and care adjusted to the clients' perception of their needs. Sickness is threatening because it interferes with one or more of these aspects of life. Effective nursing can be measured by the extent to which this interference is minimized.

In addition to being responsible for these unique functions, nurses are also responsible for helping patients carry out the therapeutic regimen prescribed by physicians and, if no physician is available, for diagnosing and prescribing treatment. They have been doing both for decades in areas underserved by physicians. The roles of physicians and nurses overlap in every clinical field even as the roles of midwives and obstetricians overlap.

This concept or definition of nursing is so open that it might be interpreted to include overlapping of the nurse's function with many other health workers as well as with physicians. As noted, such overlapping occurs now when nurses work almost alone in the underserved areas and institutions of this and other countries. For differences in nurse–population ratios and functions, see *Nursing in the World*, edited by Nursing in the World Editorial Committee, published by the International Foundation of Japan, produced by Medical Friend Co., Ltd., Tokyo.

Is the Essence of Nursing Compatible with High Technology?

The essence of nursing is hard to preserve in high technology, but if the latter is to succeed, effective nursing in conjunction with it is essential. High technology has made it possible to treat successfully the most critically ill and to extend the life span of those who (in this country) can afford the cost.

This advance means that nursing has increased in complexity and demands increasingly mature clinical judgment from nurses, a development documented in Patricia Benner's investigation in five California hospitals.[16] In relating selected critical incidents, Benner, who directed the study, shows that nurses of this era, in order to save lives, must often respond almost instantly to changes in patients' conditions. And the nurses' responses may include cancellation of the physician's directives and initiation of such complex procedures as administration of blood, intubation, or other resuscitative measures.

Benner's study discusses the importance of experience in developing clinical judgment. The difference between nursing by rule (or with a prescribed process) and perceiving and meeting the needs of the client (patient) in each unique situation, is stressed. Benner and her associates believe that clinical judgment is so essential to excellence in practice that they have devoted years to studying its nature, stages in acquiring it, and a system of identifying and rewarding it.

The eminent physician Lewis Thomas, includes in his book *The Youngest Science: Notes of a Medicine Watcher,* an essay on nurses as perceived by a patient who has recently had heart surgery.[17] Stressing the importance of their role in the highly personal nurse–patient relationship, he worries over the adversarial relationship between medicine and nursing and the discrepancy between the material rewards of physicians and nurses. He says that nurses "hold the place (the hospital) together."[18] He ends this essay with the following:

> Knowing what I know, I am all for the nurse. If they continue their professional feud with the doctors, if they want their professional stature enhanced, and their pay increased, if they infuriate doctors by their claims to be equal professionals, if they ask for the moon, I am on their side.[19]

Nursing has never been more important than in this age when the comforting, caring presence and touch of the nurse enables the institutionalized patient to tolerate invasive, often frightening and sometimes painful technology. Now, as high technology invades home care, it is the nurse who teaches the patient and the family the uses and dangers of the machines involved and helps the patient and family carry out the prescribed regimen.

High technology has made the nurse's role simultaneously more important and more difficult and stressful. Nurses, especially those in hospitals, are faced daily with moral or ethical problems related to the use of high technology; they are faced with the public's fear and distrust. A growing tendency is to try noninvasive forms of therapy, folk medicine, and systems based on a belief in the body's restorative power—a return to the philosophy of Florence Nightingale, who said, "It is the nurse's function to put the patient in the best condition for nature to cure him . . ."[20]—and at life's end, to seek help from hospices where life is not prolonged beyond the stage when the critically ill person values it. In his book *Mortal Lessons: Notes on the Art of Surgery*, Richard Selzer, a surgeon, describes diagnoses and cures that have no recognized scientific explanation.[21] The most learned are among those who admit the mystery of life.

If misused, high technology can be self-defeating. Because nurses almost certainly know best how patients and their families feel about the treatment and care offered, nurses should be members of policy-making bodies in all health care agencies and institutions and should help develop constructive uses of technology.

Nurses have a critical role to play in the ethical use of technology. The Alfred P. Sloan Foundation has sponsored the publication of a series of books designed to inform the public and stimulate interest in the sciences that are determining the future of humanity. Freeman Dyson's *Disturbing the Universe* is the first in the series. (The previously cited work by Lewis Thomas is the book on medicine in this series.) Dyson[22] exemplifies those who have questioned the morality of creating the atomic bomb while commenting, at the same time, on the fascination of doing it. Researchers and providers in the health care service, so rightly called now "the health industry," might, with benefit to the human race, examine their motives as well as their competence.

References

1. Starr, P. *The Social Transformation of American Medicine: The Rise of a Sovereign Profession and the Making of a Vast Industry.* New York: Basic Books, 1982, p. 145-179.

2. Kinney, M.R., et al., eds. *AACN's Clinical Reference for Critical Care Nursing.* New York: McGraw-Hill, 1981.

3. Daly, B.J. *Intensive Care Nursing: Current Clinical Nursing Series.* Garden City: Medical Examination Publishing Co., 1980.

4. Naisbitt, J. *Megatrends: Ten New Directions Transforming Our Lives.* New York: Warner Books, 1982, Table of Contents.

5. Bolter, J.D. *Turing's Man: Western Culture in the Computer Age.* Chapel Hill, North Carolina: University of North Carolina Press, 1984.

6. Henderson, V., and Nite, G. *Principles and Practice of Nursing.* New York: Macmillan, 1978.

7. *Nursing Studies Index Annotated Guide to Report, Studies, Research in Progress in Periodicals, Books, and Pamphlets Published in English 1900–1959.* 4 vols. Edited by V. Henderson. New York: Garland Publishing, 1984.

8. American Journal of Nursing Company in Cooperation with the National Library of Medicine. *International Nursing Index.* New York: The Company, 1966.

9. *Index Medicus Including Bibliography of Medical Reviews.* Bethesda, Maryland: The Library, 1979.

10. Dubos, R. *So Human an Animal.* New York: Scribner's, 1968.

11. Bok, D. "A New Way to Train Doctors." *Harvard Magazine 86,* no. 5 (1984).

12. Ibid.

13. McCrae, N. "Health Care International." *The Economist* (London) (April 28, 1984): 19–32.

14. Ibid.

15. Henderson, V., and Nite, G. *Principles and Practice of Nursing,* 14, 95.

16. Benner, P. *From Novice to Expert: Excellence and Power in Clinical Practice.* Reading, MA: Addison-Wesley, 1984.

17. Thomas, L. *The Youngest Science: Notes of a Medicine Watcher.* New York: Viking Press, 1983.

18. Ibid., 66.

19. Ibid., 67.

20. Nightingale, F. *Notes on Nursing: What It Is and What It Is Not.* Philadelphia: Lippincott, 1946, p.7.

21. Selzer, R. *Mortal Lessons: Notes on the Art of Surgery.* New York: Simon and Schuster, 1974, p. 219.

22. Dyson, F. *Disturbing the Universe.* New York: Viking Press, 1979.

Chapter 3

The Art and Science of Health Assessment

Health Assessment is Everybody's Business

Universal greetings such as "How are you?" and "How do you do?" and farewells such as "Keep well" suggest a universal concern for the health of others which is expressed daily, even hourly. Those unduly preoccupied with their own health are called hypochondriacs, but knowledge of what constitutes health and the ability to use it characterize superior individuals and cultures. Certainly the "high-level wellness" described by Halbert R. Dunn[1] in his radio talks of 1961 (later published as a book) is a measure of superiority and can only be achieved by the knowledgeable and disciplined—those who develop the habit of consciously or unconsciously measuring their health behavior against demanding standards. They and persons whom Abraham H. Maslow[2] describes as "self-realized" would be prepared to know when such behavior (mental, emotional, and physical) is substandard, when they can modify it unaided, or when they need help from others. They would also know the kind of health worker to seek out.

But the concept "health" is also elusive. René Dubos[3] speaks of the "mirage of health." He thinks it is an ideal state we seek but never reach. Others say health is not freedom from disease but the ability to cope with life. Just as it is virtually impossible to find a "perfect" flower, a "perfect" leaf, or a flawless biologic specimen, just so is it impossible to find an anatomically and physiologically "perfect" human being, assuming that perfection can be defined.

If the above generalizations are true, health assessments can never be standardized, mechanized procedures, the sole responsibility of any one element of society, nor can they be divorced from the individual's concept of health, his attitudes toward life, his total being.

The Nature of Health Assessment as Discussed Here

While it is suggested that health assessment is a conscious or unconscious function of living for everybody, and an on-going process in all health care, this chapter describes only what is variously called "the health examination," "the health assessment," the medical examination," "the physical examination," and "the diagnostic process." This chapter focuses on the sessions and procedures devoted especially to mass screening programs, to initial and periodic health appraisals, and to diagnostic examinations. The difference in emphasis and in the methods used in assessing health, identifying hidden disease, and diagnosing, or discovering, the cause of symptoms from which a patient is suffering are discussed.

A Historical Note on Health Assessment: The Development of Current Practices

The art of health assessment is ancient and has existed in some form in all cultures; the science is newer and has been so highly developed in this age in Western countries that it has tended to diminish or obscure the art.

Since time immemorial, assessors, appraisers, or examiners have used their sense of sight, hearing, smell, and touch to measure the health status of clients. Today these senses have been extended and objective measurements substituted for subjective assessments by a wide variety of instruments or machines. The unaided senses are to some extent distrusted in this age.

In other ages health assessments tended to be estimates of the general state of the body or mind and this tendency persists in some cultures today. In primitive societies the "sick" person is usually thought to be made sick by forces outside the body. A man is ill because the gods are angry with him; a woman may be under a spell or curse; sickness might be attributed to "the dark of the moon" or to the change of seasons. The baleful force, whatever it is, must be bought off, or appeased. Medicine men, priests, and other assessors and healers are in some cultures appeasers or go-betweens; mystic powers are attributed to them. These concepts exist full-blown in certain primitive cultures today and some medical historians say that vestiges of them persist in all cultures.[4-6] For example, it is not unusual to find people in any country looking upon illness as punishment. They cry "O God, what did I do to deserve this?" And the practicing physician is thought to have almost magic powers. An obviously dying child is brought to a doctor and the parents say, "Doctor, *do* something!"

Another ancient, but more rational, approach to health assessment was taken by the Chinese at least 5000 years ago when they attributed sickness to an imbalance between the Yin-Yang[a] principle *within* the body rather than a force from without acting on it. This approach, although modified, is still used in China today. The editors of the *American Journal of Chinese Medicine* say, "Chinese medicine can . . . be seen as a nexus of ideas; the philosophical is inseparable from the physiological, myth from fact, theory from practice."[b]

Edith Hamilton[6a] and other classics scholars writing about Greece say that the Greeks made our (Western) world and so it is not surprising that Hippocrates is often called the father of Western medicine. Like the Chinese, he attributed health to an internal balance rather than to outside forces, but instead of Yin-Yang principles he sought a balance in the "humors" within the body.

Modern Western medicine has been, in this century, based largely on Claude Bernard's[7] dictum that health depends on the constancy of the intercellular fluid, or the cell's environment. Walter B. Cannon[8] in his much-quoted *Wisdom of the Body* elaborates on this concept and stresses homeostasis[c] as the physiological goal.

Psychiatrists and clinical psychologists tend to take the over-all view of health and disease. While most acknowledge the influence of the genetic endowment and recognize the physiologic basis of mental health, they also stress forces from without acting on the personality to change its structure. Sidney M. Jourard, for example, says he sees sickness "whether physical or mental" as "a form of protest against a way of life society seems to have demanded." He looks upon illness as "the last and loudest protest of a violated organism against the destructive way of life that he has lived."[d]

Also in this age are certain religious groups that look upon illness as a failure to think right. The Christian Science healer's assessment, for example, is general rather than specific and the "cure" is a metaphysical process.

Another approach to assessing health on an over-all basis, which is of this age, is the measurement of the electromagnetic field of the body. In Chapter 17 there is a brief description of a proposed interdisciplinary study along these lines to be directed by Dorothy Harrison, a nurse and anthropologist. It is based on the work of Harold Saxton Burr, his contemporary associates, and subsequent workers who have used his thesis. Electrometric study of the healing of wounds and of ovulation has demonstrated the clinical practicability of Burr's original investigations.[9-14] The philosophic implications of Burr's theory are discussed by Edward W. Russell, a journalist, in a popular work, *Design for Destiny: Science Reveals the Soul*. He calls it a "Layman's Guide to Harold S. Burr's Remarkable Discoveries and to Their Revolutionary Implications for Medicine and Psychiatry."[e] Burr himself relates his scientific work to philosophy and religion in his book *The Nature of Man and the Meaning of Existence*,[15] and earlier in an article with F. S. C. Northrop, a philosopher, "The Electro-Dynamic Theory of Life."[16] Leonard J. Ravitz[17] used Burr's theory and method in testing mood swings in psychiatric patients and he thought it an objective and reliable method as opposed to depending on what clients or patients say, since the latter are influenced by what they want the examiner to know.

It is interesting to speculate on the possibility that Burr's "scientific" approach to assessing the disease process by measuring the balance between positively charged and negatively charged particles (anodes and cathodes) with a voltmeter is close kin to the ancient Chinese medical concept of Yin-Yang balances. Burr presents a chart plotting the electromagnetic fields within the body; Chinese medicine that embodies the Yin-Yang concept and uses acupuncture as one of its principal diagnostic and therapeutic modes has traced "the loci and meridians of the body along which Ch'i or vital energy travels."[f] For example, Frederick F. Kao, discussing "the new Chinese medicine"—a marriage of ancient Eastern philosophy and Western science—says "Disease occurs when Ch'i is locally excessive or deficient. Acupuncture therapy is thought to correct energetic imbalances by removing obstructions or sedating excess and thereby restoring bodily function to its normal state."[g]

In contrast to these over-all concepts of health and the cause of "disease," there is the idea of specificity. The discovery in the nineteenth century that microorganisms caused many diseases, each with its characteristic group of symptoms, introduced a new medical era. The writings of Louis Pasteur, Robert Koch, Ignaz Semmelweis, and others were revolutionary. Since it was found that infectious disease could be prevented, controlled, or cured when the causative organism was isolated, and when a specific vaccine, toxin, antitoxin, or drug was developed that acted on the organism, specificity in diagnosis, prevention, and treatment came to be the goal. (Some chemicals effective in the treatment of diseases caused by microorganisms had, of course, been used pragmatically for centuries before microscopic life was demonstrated. Cinchona bark and its derivative quinine were, for example, used to treat malaria before the discovery of the plasmodium and its mode of transmission. No one, however, knew exactly how the drug acted.)

The importance attached to identifying the specific disease of microbial origin seems to have carried over into general medical practice. Medical education is still focused largely on the process of making *the* diagnosis, or treating "the chief complaint." Making *the* diagnosis is the major aim in taking the "medical history" and doing a physical examination.[18-20] Some believe that this is at least partially responsible for impersonalized health care and for categorizing, even segregating, patients according to diagnosis, or the body area or the body system receiving major attention. Treatment units still admit exclusively patients with tuberculosis, heart disease, or hemiplegia; or "chest cases," "head injuries," or "abdominal surgery"; or conditions of the skin, the urologic system, or the nervous system. In spite of the criticism of this practice, patients are still referred to as "the craniotomy in Ward B," "the pemphigus case in Room 221," or the "muscular dystrophy in Cubicle 3." Even people who are mentally ill are diagnosed as schizophrenics, manic-depressives, or involutional melancholics. In all but psychiatric practice, the laboratory tests or technologic aspects of health assessment are relied on heavily. In some mass-screening programs, physicians, or principal examiners, don't see patients until health measurements have been made by others and the laboratory findings are available. Then they discuss principally with the patient the meaning of test results. Some persons attach so much importance to computerized analysis of test data that they prophesy increasingly accurate diagnoses arrived at by computers in technologically developed countries.

But even in the most highly scientific circles there is a reaction to purely technologic and disease-centered medical care. There is currently an emphasis on the problem-oriented system of health care where an attempt is made to identify all the health problems of the patient, not just the "chief complaint;" there is emphasis on preventive care, or health maintenance, on health education, on public involvement in health care, and on comprehensive care. Patients in treatment units are now more likely to be segregated according to age, their need for care (self-help deficit), than on the basis of diagnosis, for example, people are assigned to intensive care units, intermediate ambulatory services, or half-way houses. In large psychiatric hospitals, patients may be assigned to cottages or wards, not according to diagnosis, but according to the city, town, or county in which they live. In such large state hospitals, health personnel are assigned on the same basis, the assumption being that a sense of community is therapeutic and that treatment is more likely under such circumstances to be comprehensive and family-centered than fragmented and technical.

The philosophy of care in the health agency or health practitioner's office influences the nature of the health examination and the roles played by patients, parents, physicians, and others. The numbers and availability of health workers in the area also determine the roles played by the various workers. If it were possible to review practices on an international basis it would be obvious that the dominant political philosophy influences the availability and nature of the process by which people enter the health care system; it also influences the numbers, distribution, or availability of health workers. These questions are discussed to some extent in this chapter but the particular practices described reflect chiefly those within the United States.

Roles of Patients, Parents, Physicians, Nurses, and Others in Assessing Health

The Health Examination as an Introduction to the Health Care System

Since the health examination in some form is part of the introduction to the health care system, it is essential that a way of conducting such examinations evolves that doesn't block admission to the system. Entry into the system is sometimes called *primary care*,[h] although other meanings are also assigned the term.

Supply of Health Manpower as It Affects the Conduct of Health Examinations

In the United States and many other countries, there aren't enough doctors to examine all those who want a health assessment, either as a basis for preventive care or for diagnosis and treatment of disease. Some persons suggest that the shortage of physicians can be overcome through their redistribution and reorganization; others think that many of the physician's current functions must be turned over to "intermediate-level" health practitioners; some writers suggest that machines, and the technicians who operate them, can provide computerized data that will sufficiently facilitate the physician's work to make it possible to keep health assessment and diagnosis in their hands; and others believe that the cost of medical care can only be brought within bounds by teaching the public to be more self-reliant in assessing and treating itself.[21-28] In the United States the incidence of disease goes down as the family income goes up.[29] Frances Storlie[30] and Nancy Milio[31] are nurses who have urged social action to prevent poverty as the most effective means of upgrading health.

Sidney R. Garfield, writing in 1970 on admission of people to the health care system and on delivery of health care, says: "Any realistic solution to the medical-care problem must . . . begin by facing up to the facts about the [inadequate] supply of physicians."[i] Garfield thinks the self-sustaining prepaid group practice, patterned after the Kaiser-Permanente program (which he started) is a step in the right direction but far from the entire answer. He believes that at the point of entry into the health care system clients must be divided into "(1) the well; (2) the worried well; (3) the early sick; and (4) the sick." He believes the fee for service keeps all but the sick away from the doctor since, as he puts it, nobody wants to pay for unneeded medical care. Garfield thinks health insurance, paid in a lump sum, induces "the well," "the worried well," and "the early sick" to seek treatment but it also overtaxes our present system. Garfield describes and illustrates a system of health testing designed to identify the categories of clients just itemized, to fully utilize technology and technicians, and to demand the minimum time of physicians.[j]

While Garfield's suggestions have been widely acclaimed, many persons believe that admission to the health care system should not depend solely on the availability of the physician for either maximum or minimum participation. They point out reasons why the physician has "guarded the entrance to the health care system" and why this concept is outmoded.

At the beginning of this century most persons with a physical or mental health problem, if they sought help, consulted a family doctor. Some might instead or in addition consult the clergy, a public health nurse, the corner druggist, or a neighbor. But traditionally and officially the physician guarded the entrance to health care services. Public health nurses, for instance, had the policy of paying only two or three visits to a family if there was no physician in attendance. Until recently only the dentist accepted patients for treatment without referral from the physician. The corner druggist, the bonesetter, the chiropractor, the faith healer, and others stepped into the breach left by an inadequate supply of physicians, but their advice and treatment was given outside the pale of *the* medical care system. To this day medical practice acts to make diagnosis and treatment by persons other than physicians (and dentists) illegal. Many persons recognize the necessity of modifying these acts, for the picture is changing and many physicians realize that they cannot supply all the primary care needed, or all "first contacts with the health care system."

The categories and numbers of health workers prepared under the auspices of higher education and qualifying as "professionals" have multiplied. Clinical psychologists, psychotherapists, social workers, nutritionists, physical, occupational and speech therapists, health educators, nurse-midwives and other nurse practitioners qualify as professionals under most accepted criteria. And while the public still recognizes the physician's preeminence in the diagnosis and treatment of disease, it is relying more and more on its own knowledge and it recognizes the special competence of other health workers. For example, the public often turns to nutritionists for advice on the selection and preparation of food; to marriage counsellors for advice on sex; to the physical culturist for help in muscular development; to the speech therapist for advice on language development; and to the nurse for help with a wide range of health problems including, for example, infant and child feeding, obesity, skin care, postural defects, fatigue, insomnia, constipation, depression, contraception, and family planning. Health workers with preparations that qualify them as "professionals" are effectively promoting legislation that enables them to serve the public without referral from physicians.

Actually health workers with less than professional preparation and people not classified as health workers but with special life experiences may be able to give certain kinds of help that most physicians and nurses either cannot give or are not interested in giving. Recovered alcoholics and other rehabilitated drug abusers staff and operate highly effective treatment centers. Alcoholics Anonymous, Synanon, Reach for Recovery, and Weight Watchers are examples of nonmedical agencies that have been uniquely successful in helping individuals and groups of "patients," or clients, with stubborn health problems.[k]

Physicians themselves are questioning their traditional roles, alerting the public to iatrogenic disease (disease resulting from treatment), and urging everyone to accept more responsibility for their own health. Works in this category are Halbert R. Dunn's *High-Level Wellness*,[32] Michael Crichton's *Five Patients. The Hospital Explained*,[33] Mike Samuels' and Hal Bennett's *The Well Body Book*,[34] and Andrew Malleson's *Need Your Doctor Be So Useless?*[35]

Outside the United States, Canada, and the other countries where typically "Western medicine" is practiced, there are different kinds of health care "systems," and ways of entering them. The preparation and function of feldshers in Russia are discussed in Chapter 19, as are the roles of "barefoot" and "Red Guard" doctors in China. The latter outnumber physicians (whose preparation is comparable to medical education in the United States) and they examine and treat certain categories of patients in certain situations. Kao says:

> Common recurrent diseases, e.g., common cold, respiratory infections, skin diseases and gastrointestinal disorders are . . . treated by barefoot doctors in the commune, red guard doctors in the factories and health officers in the PLA and the hospitals. Propaganda teams are efficient in educating the public. . . . As a mater of fact, the emphasis in the treatment of disease is on prevention. . . .[1]

In any successful national, state, provincial, or local health planning, who does what in assessing health and treating disease must depend on the numbers and types of workers available, the effective use made of them, the way society sees their functions, the customary and legal scope of their practice, and how much money the people of the area elect to spend on health care.

The Client's or Patient's Role in Health Examinations

In health examinations, as in most aspects of health care, the client's or patient's role is the most important; or in the case of infants and small children the parent's role. They decide when to seek help; whether to use primary preventive measures such as immunization, or whether to wait for alarming symptoms before consulting a health worker. Samuels and Bennett wrote *The Well Body Book* as a "tool" to help youths and adults examine their own bodies and develop their own "practical system of healing and preventive medicine using the physician as a consultant." They say "Your body is a three million year healer."[m] They think most people know far too little about the structure and function of the body but could learn enough about anatomy and physiology, about normal health values, to examine their own body or that of a friend. Malleson, author of *Need Your Doctor Be So Useless?*[36] thinks that people are increasingly knowledgeable and that only when they do assume optimum responsibility for preventing illness and treating minor ailments can the "cancer" of spiraling health care costs be controlled. He notes legislation in the United States that requires physicians to have "informed consent" from the patient for treatment. This means that the physician must explain the prescribed treatment, the benefits, risks, and alternatives. We believe, however, that there are even now people like the Victorian lady who said to her doctor as he tried to explain the nature of constipation "Oh, don't tell me, doctor, I like to think of myself as lined with pink crepe de chine!"

Arlene and Howard Eisenberg,[37] two journalists, describe a course in "self-help preventive medicine" in Reston, VA., said to be the first of its kind in the United States. It is sponsored by Georgetown University Community Health Plan's Department of Community Medicine and is taught by nine physicians who are said to encourage people to save money by attending to minor problems or by becoming "activated" patients. Those taking the course are referred by one doctor to a 1734 text by Dr. John Tennent, *Everyman His Own Doctor or The Poor Planter's Physician*.[38] Students are taught to use the sphygmomanometer, to take temperature, pulse, and respiration, to look at eardrums with otoscopes, what to do in emergencies, and how to treat some less serious ailments. While this course has much in common with those taught for many years under Red Cross auspices, the significant feature of it, as related to this chapter, is that doctors are now teaching the public certain skills of health evaluation, diagnosis, and treatment that have until recently been reserved for the physician's use.

Beside the importance of the subject's role in knowing how his or her body should function, how to deal with minor ailments, and when to seek help, a great deal depends upon the ability of patients to give a clear and accurate account of their health practices and the signs and symptoms of disease. With babies and young children, the health worker, of course, depends on the ability of parents or guardians to do this. Some autobiographies describe the subject's feelings and behavior so accurately that physicians reading the descriptions centuries later can say with assurance that they suffered from such and such a disease. Health examiners depend heavily on what patients tell them, how honestly they answer the questions put to them, and on how highly motivated they are to be healthy, to correct defects, and to eliminate disease.

Roles of Physicians, Nurses, and Other Health Workers in Conducting Health Examinations

The roles of various types of health examiners depend on the setting, the type of examination, and the personnel available. *Physicians* in their private offices may conduct the entire examination with minimum help from nurses or other attendants although they seldom take simple measurements such as the temperature, pulse, and respiration or make the laboratory tests or take x-rays that are a part of the health examination. Some physicians have professional nurses associated with them in their private practice who may conduct most health examinations or most aspects of the examination. Pediatricians especially are turning over the health assessments of well infants and children to professional nurses, and obstetricians who have professional nurses and nurse-midwives working with them may ask these nurses and nurse-midwives to carry out the initial health examination.

In health screening units and agencies with optimum technologic facilities and processes, physicians may not see patients until a series of health measurements and tests have been made and until patients themselves have answered an extensive questionnaire. If physicians practice as a group or offer a comprehensive health service, several may meet with the patient or patients and their families, after the initial screening process to discuss the health problems identified during the examination and to suggest a corrective program or treatment regimen.

In large hospitals—especially those with medical schools—residents, interns, and medical students usually examine the patient and discuss their findings with the attending physician. The latter may then repeat certain aspects of or the whole examination. When patients are very ill or when the cause of the illness is obscure, not only one but several physicians may examine them.

Professional nurses in independent practice examine their patients, or clients, in the nurse's office with or without assistance from other workers. Nurse-midwives and public health nurses in clinics conduct health examinations on certain categories of patients, and health examinations are made by community nurses in patients' homes. Professional nurses in ambulatory services of hospitals are more and more frequently conducting health examinations. This is particularly true in services for children, the chronically ill, and the elderly. Most nurses conducting health examinations have had post-basic preparation and acquire differentiating titles.[n] It is, however, increasingly common in the United States to include training for and experience in physical diagnosis in basic collegiate nursing programs.

It is recognized that nurses have, actually for many years in certain geographical areas and in certain agencies, made health assessments.[39-44] Community nurses ("public health nurses") have throughout this century assumed considerable responsibility for health assessment. Nurses examined immigrants to the United States as they went through the Health Service on Ellis Island (New York City) in the first decade of this century. Canadian nurses in the Indian Health Service, nurses on certain islands where there are no physicians, and nurses of the Frontier Nursing Service in Kentucky are other examples. The relative unavailability of medical care in the latter areas has obliged them to make assessments and institute treatment, using physicians as consultants when necessary, and arranging for transportation to large treatment centers for the most seriously ill and injured.

In all settings where there are physicians and nurses, both may be cast in their "traditional" roles—physicians carrying out most steps in the physical examination and discussing their findings with the patient; nurses helping patients get ready for the examination, explaining the procedure to those who are unfamiliar with it, adjusting positions, clothing, and covering, and giving such reassurance as seems needed. In most settings, nursing personnel make certain measurements such as body temperature, pulse and respiratory rates, weight and height, and see that a specimen of urine is available for analysis. These are the usual procedures, but they may make other measurements and get other specimens. Nurses may stay with the patient and physician throughout the examination, providing as much comfort for the patient as is possible, often holding an infant if the mother is not present. If the patient and doctor are of the same sex, the nurse may not be present during the entire examination, but in the case of a female patient and male physician, the presence of a woman nurse during the pelvic examination is a protection for both the patient and the physician. After the examination, nurses answer patients' questions, reinforce the physician's directions for follow-up, and carry out any other forms of health teaching that are indicated.

Physician's assistants may conduct health examinations under (almost) the same circumstances as do professional nurses. *Feldshers* in Russia are surrogates for the physician and examine patients just as physicians do.

They are more likely to be found in satellite hospitals, ambulatory services, and mobile units than in the large teaching hospitals,[45,46] Barefoot and Red Guard doctors in the People's Republic of China have comparable responsibilities.[47]

In the United States *clinical psychologists* and other specialists, as, for instance, the *physical therapist*, may conduct special aspects of the health examination. The psychologist may administer psychometric tests and the physical therapist tests for motor power and motor skills. The *vocational guidance expert* in a rehabilitation center may administer a battery of tests to measure potentialities for employment; the *speech therapist* in such a center or in the stroke program of a hospital may give a series of tests to determine the nature of the speech impairment and the possibility of improving or restoring normal speech.

With the improvement of health services, which must come if the needs of the people are to be met, the health examination will vary according to the problems presented by the patient and the examination will be made by a team of workers, the composition of which is determined by the patient's needs, the purpose of the examination, and the available health manpower.

Notes

---

[a]Yin = shady side, earth, moon, night, female, negative, death, destroying, etc. Yang = sunny side, heaven, sun, day, male, life-creating, hot, etc.

[b](Editorial), *Am. J. Chinese Med., 1*:viii, (Jan.) 1973.

[c]Homeostasis is the condition in which the circulatory system is supplying the cells with necessary nutrients and is removing cell secretions and excretions, all of which maintain the constancy of inter- and intracellular fluids.

[d]Jourard, Sidney M.: *Disclosing Man to Himself.* Van Nostrand & Reinhold Co., New York, 1968, p. 38.

[e]Russell, Edward W.: *Design for Destiny: Science Reveals the Soul.* Ballantine Books, New York, 1971.

[f]Kao, Frederick F.: "Part III—The New Chinese Medicine 'Chung Kuo I Hsueh' (1949 to Present)." *Am. J. Chinese Med., 1*:26, (Jan.) 1973.

[g]ibid.

[h]The report of the U.S. Department of Health, Education, and Welfare Secre-

tary's Committee to Study Extended Roles for Nurses gives the following definition of primary care:

(a) a person's first contact in any given episode of illness with the health care system that leads to a decision of [on] what must be done to help resolve his problem; and

(b) the responsibility for the continuum of care—that is, maintenance of health, evaluation and management of symptoms, and appropriate referrals. (U.S. Department of Health, Education, and Welfare: *Extending the Scope of Nursing Practice. A Report of the Secretary's Committee to Study Extended Roles for Nurses*. U.S. Government Printing Office, Washington, D.C., 1972; "Extending the Scope of Nursing Practice," *Nurs. Outlook, 20*:46, [Jan] 1972).

The Canadian Nurses' Association and the Canadian Medical Association have agreed jointly on the following description of primary care:

> . . . all of those health services which are provided for individuals mainly on an ambulatory basis in the community or in their homes . . . preventive and health maintenance services in the community; diagnostic and therapeutic services offered in physicians' offices, in clinics, or in health centers; home care services for those who are ill; and rehabilitative services. ("Extended Role of Nurse and Preparation for it as Defined in Canadian R.N. and M.D. Statement," *Am. J. Nurs., 73*:964, [June] 1973.)

[i]Garfield, Sidney R.: "Delivery of Medical Care," *Sci. Am., 225*:15, (Apr.) 1970.

[j]Ivan Illich (a nonmedical critic of health care systems) thinks the routine health assessment harmful. He maintains that periodic health examinations make every person a patient and turn the well into the worried well. He says: "Effective health care depends on self-care: this fact is currently heralded as if it were a discovery. . . . The medicalization of early diagnosis not only hampers and discourages preventative health care but it also trains the patient-to-be to function in the meantime as an acolyte to his doctor. He learns to depend on the physician in sickness and in health. He turns into a lifelong patient." (Illich, Ivan: *Medical nemesis. The Expropriation of Health*. McClelland & Stewart, Ltd., Toronto, 1975, p. 50.)

Lewis Thomas, a physician, agrees with Illich on some but not all points. Discussing "your very good health," he decries the terms "health industry" and "health maintenance organizations," and the implication that if adequately "maintained" enough is known to prevent all disease. On the other hand, he thinks too little emphasis is put on the capacity of the body to resist disease. He says, "Meanwhile, we are paying too little attention, and respect, to the built-in durability and sheer power of the human organism. Its surest tendency is toward stability and balance. It is a distortion, with something profoundly disloyal about it, to picture the human being as a teetering, fallible contraption, always needing watching and patching, always on the verge of flapping to pieces; this is the doctrine that people hear most often, and most eloquently, on all our information media. We ought to be developing a much better system for general education about human health, with more curricular time for acknowledgment, and even some celebration, of the absolute marvel of good health that is the real lot of most of us, most of the time."

Thomas says that none of his internist friends have routine physical examinations, that "almost all have resisted surgery," and that "laboratory tests for anyone in the family are extremely rare." He thinks doctors' families "seem a normal, generally healthy lot, with a remarkably low incidence of iatrogenic illness." (Thomas, Lewis: *The Lives of a Cell. Notes of a Biology Watcher*. Viking Press, New York, 1974, pp. 83, 84, 85.)

[k]Many groups of former hospital patients are organizing themselves to help each other, as, for example, psychiatric and neurotic patients, and people who have had colostomies or laryngectomies.

[l]Kao, Frederick F.: "China, Chinese Medicine and the Chinese Medical System," *Am. J. Chinese Med., 1*:1, (Jan.) 1973.

[m]Samuels, Mike, and Bennett, Hal: *The Well Body Book*. Random House, New York, 1973, pp. x, 1.

[n]In the United States the terminology is confusing. Nurses prepared to assume an "expanded role" may be called variously "family nurse practitioners," "primary care nurses," "pediatric nurse practitioners," "pediatric associates," clinical specialists," or by other titles.

References

1. Dunn, Halbert, R.: *High-Level Wellness*. Mt. Vernon Publishing Co., Washington, D.C., 1961.

2. Maslow, Abraham H.: *Religions, Values, and Peak Experiences*. Ohio State University Press, Columbus, 1964.

3. Dubos, René: *Mirage of Health*. Doubleday Anchor Books, Garden City, N.Y., 1961.

4. Haggard, Howard W.: *The Doctor in History*. Yale University Press, New Haven, Conn., 1934.

5. Haggard, Howard W.: *Devils, Drugs and Doctors*. Harper & Row, New York, 1929.

6. Sigerist, Henry E.: *A History of Medicine*. Oxford University Press, New York, 1951.

6a. Hamilton, Edith: *The Echo of Greece*. W. W. Norton & Co., New York, 1957.

7. Bernard, Claude: *Introduction to the Study of Experimental Medicine*. Macmillan Publishing Co., Inc., New York, 1927.

8. Cannon, Walter B.: *The Wisdom of the Body*. W. W. Norton & Co., New York, 1939.

9. Burr, Harold Saxton: *The Electric Fields of Life*. Ballantine Books, New York, 1972. (Originally published by Neville Spearman, London, 1935).

10. Burr, Harold Saxton, and Northrop, F. S. C.: "The Electro-Dynamic Theory of Life," *Q. Rev. Biol., 10*:322, (Sept.) 1935.

11. Burr, Harold Saxton, et al.: "An Electrometric Study of the Healing of Wounds in Man," *Yale J. Biol. Med., 12*:483, (May) 1939.

12. Burr, Harold Saxton, et al.: "A Bioelectric Record of Human Ovulation," *Science, 86*:312, (Oct.) 1937.

13. Geddes, L. A., et al.: "Continuous Measurement of Ventricular Stroke Volume by Electrical Impedance," *Cardiovasc. Res. Cent. Bull., 4*:118 (Apr.–June) 1966.

14. Pressman, A.: *The Electromagnetic Fields of Life*. Plenum Press, New York, 1970.

15. Burr, H. S.: *The Nature of Man and the Meaning of Existence*. Charles C Thomas, Publisher, Springfield, Ill., 1962.

16. Burr, Harold Saxton, and Northrop, F. S. C.: *op. cit.*

17. Ravitz, Leonard J.: "Electrodynamic Field Theory in Psychiatry," *South. Med. J., 46*:650, (July) 1953.

18. Carnegie Commission on Higher Education: *Higher Education and the Nation's Health—Policies for Medical and Dental Education*. McGraw-Hill Book Co., New York, 1970.

19. Lynaugh, Joan E., and Bates, Barbara: "The Two Languages of Nursing and Medicine," *Am. J. Nurs., 73*:66, (Jan.) 1973.

20. Weed, Lawrence L.: *Medical Records: Medical Education and Patient Care*. Press of Case-Western Reserve University, Cleveland, 1970.

21. Carnegie Commission on Higher Education: *op. cit.*

22. Dillon, John B.: "How Did It Happen?" *Calif. Med., 113*:86, (Aug.) 1970.

23. Dunn, Halbert R.: *op. cit.*

24. Engel, George L.: "A Unified Concept of Health and Disease," *Perspect. Biol. Med.*, 3:459, (Summer) 1960.

25. The Royal Society of Medicine and the Josiah Macy, Jr. Foundation: *The Greater Medical Profession*. The Foundation, New York, 1973.

26. Samuels, Mike, and Bennett, Hal: *The Well Body Book*. Random House, New York, 1973.

27. Kao, Frederick F.: "China, Chinese Medicine and the Chinese Medical System" *Am. J. Chinese Med., 1*:1, (Jan.) 1973.

28. Malleson, Andrew: *Need Your Doctor Be So Useless?* George Allen & Unwin, Ltd., London, 1973.

29. U.S. Department of Health, Education, and Welfare: *Human Investment Program. Delivery of Health Services for the Poor*. U.S. Government Printing Office, Washington, D.C., 1968.

30. Storlie, Frances: *Nursing and the Social Conscience*. Appleton-Century-Crofts, New York, 1970.

31. Milio, Nancy: *9226 Kercheval. The Storefront That Did Not Burn*. University of Michigan Press, Ann Arbor, 1970.

32. Dunn, Halbert R.: *op. cit.*

33. Crichton, Michael: *Five Patients. The Hospital Explained*. Alfred A. Knopf, New York, 1970.

34. Samuels, Mike, and Bennett, Hal: *op. cit.*

35. Malleson, Andrew: *op. cit.*

36. *Ibid.*

37. Eisenberg, Arlene, and Eisenberg, Howard: "A New Teaching Program. How to Be Your Own Doctor—Sometimes," *New Haven Register*, (Feb. 24) 1974, p. 11.

38. Tennent, John: *Everyman His Own Doctor or The Poor Planter's Physician* [1734].

39. Gregg, Elinor D.: *The Indians and the Nurse*. University of Oklahoma Press, Norman, 1965.

40. McNicholas, Ellen L.: "International Nurse-Practitioner Committees," *Int. Nurse Rev., 16*:279, (No. 3) 1969.

41. Quinn, S.: "The Immediate Past, the Urgent Present, and Focus on the Future," *Niger Nurse, 2*:6, (July) 1970.

42. Thomas, B.: "Mountaineering with Nursing,"*AORN J., 12*:11, (Oct.) 1970.

43. US Public Health Service, Health Services and Mental Health Administration: *Nursing Careers in the Indian Health Service.* U.S. Government Printing Office, Washington, D.C., 1971.

44. Weber, C. V.: "The Value of the Nurse's Role in Innovation of Care," in *Continuity of Care—Can or Should the Nurse Innovate Change.* Papers presented at the Nursing Sessions of the National Tuberculosis and Respiratory Disease Association 1970 Annual Meeting. National League for Nursing, New York, 1970.

45. Andreoli, Kathleen G.: "A Look at the Physician's Assistant," *Am. J. Nurs., 72*:710, (Apr.) 1972.

46. World Health Organization: *Report of the Travelling Seminar on Nursing in the U.S.S.R..* The Organization, Geneva, 1967.

47. Kao, Frederick F.: *op. cit.*

Chapter 4

The Importance of Observation

Observation is described by Abraham Kaplan[1] as a deliberate search, carried out with care and forethought. People observe their surroundings constantly, but these acts are largely passive, rather than deliberate or planned. Often they cannot be recalled or communicated to others. It is the deliberation and control of the process of observation that is distinctive of science in general and health sciences in particular. The aim of observation is to get information that will play a part in subsequent phases of inquiry or diagnosis, to order the observations, to formulate a problem, to intervene or institute therapy, and to evaluate the intervention.

R. D. Judge and G. D. Zuidema list three major sources of inaccurate observation and ways to overcome them:

> . . . the three major sources of inaccurate observation are (1) oversight, (2) forgetting, (3) bias. Oversights are minimized by habituation to method and by fractionating observations into logical, sequential small units. Forgetting is minimized by jotting down immediate notes . . . and by transferring the information to the permanent record as promptly as possible. Bias is a life-long challenge. It may be lessened by understanding how it distorts. By repeated self analysis . . . you may minimize the tendency, but . . . you will fall prey to your prejudices. We all do, unfortunately.[a]

Many of the problems inherent in the observation of people, which is a major activity of nurses, stem from what Kaplan calls the "shared humanity of the scientist and his subject matter."[b] In other words, the act of observation affects both the observer and the person observed. Behavior has meaning to the person engaging in it as well as to the observer, and the two meanings may not necessarily coincide. Ida Jean Orlando describes this duality as it affects the process of patient care:

> It is . . . exceedingly important for the nurse to distinguish between her understanding of general principles and the meanings which she must discover in the immediate nursing situation in order to help the patient. In making the distinction, the nurse first attempts to understand the meaning to the patient in a time and place context of what she observes and how she can exercise her professional function in relation to it. She also becomes aware of how the patient is affected by what she says or does.[c]

Responsibility of the Nurse

All those who contribute to the care of patients develop the ability to learn about them by listening to them and studying their appearance and actions. The sum total of their findings and the continuous analysis of their observations are the basis for the initial and evolving plan of care. Diagnosis, prognosis, and therapy are steps in the process of giving care which the physician, nurse, psychologist, social worker, and special therapist all employ. Definitions of these acts in relation to specific professionals are found in every American jurisdiction in the practice acts for a specific professional group. The *International Digest of Health Legislation* is published quarterly by the World Health Organization in two editions, English and French, and contains a selection of health laws and regulations and studies in comparative health legislation. This journal is a valuable resource for the study of practice acts and educational programs for specific health workers.[d]

The beginning practitioner will note that there is a continual realignment of professional functions of physician, nurse, and others. The statutes governing the practice of nursing define professional nursing in general terms that permit practice to advance into areas of increasing complexity. It need only be shown that the newly assumed nursing function is predicated on the practitioner's ability to draw on knowledge of physical, biologic, and social sciences.[2]

There can be no question that nurses observe symptoms and reactions and interpret these observations. Only then are they able to take intelligent and humane action with or on behalf of their patients.

Florence Nightingale, who probably saw the nurse's function more clearly than had any one before her, said that without the habit of ready and correct observation nurses are useless, no matter how devoted. She also pointed out that otherwise nursing becomes a mechanical routine often inimical to the patient's interests.[3] It is of interest to note in the *Nursing Studies Index, Vol. 1 (1900–1929),*[4] that there are nine titles listed referring to articles on the responsibility of the nurse to observe, interpret, and record signs and symptoms of illness. More recently, Katherine Kelly states:

> The observational function is now conceived to be a process that includes three specific operations:
> 1. Observation—the recognition of signs and symptoms presented by the patient.
> 2. Inference—making a judgment about the state of the patient and/or the nursing needs of the patient.
> 3. Decision-making—determining the action which should be taken that will be of optimal benefit to the patient.[e]

Throughout the discussion in this chapter of observation, reporting, and recording, one must keep in mind the ways in which the nurse's observational function varies according to the education and experience of the nurse, the needs of patients, and the settings in which care is provided in health and illness. Institutional nurses may corroborate or correct their judgment with other members of the medical team continuously, because of the proximity of various professionals in the institutional setting. Nurses working in homes have to depend more completely on their own observations. A great deal of the success of a community health program is the result of the nurse's ability to detect early signs of disease. Community nurses need specific knowledge of "norms" in all ages so that they can recognize deviations. They should also be able to observe environmental conditions adversely affecting health, since correction by a health agency is often in response to a request from the nurse.[f]

Medical and nursing research is dependent on observations accurately made and recorded. Such sciences as physiology, medicine, and nursing are built on observations. Observing, recording, analyzing, and making deductions are the essential steps in scientific inquiry.

Of all the patients' medical attendants, nurses are with them most constantly. For this reason the quality of their observations and reports, written and oral, are of utmost importance. Their observations guide them primarily in assessing the patients' temporary and permanent limitations so that they may give adequate nursing care, but because nurses are in touch with the institutionalized patients around the clock, all other medical attendants have come to depend upon their observations. It is they who watch patients in danger of hemorrhage, checking the pulse and blood pressure at brief intervals; they note the signs and symptoms during labor, and it is they who get the obstetrician when needed; it is their vigilance and judgment that prevent self-destruction in the suicidal; it is they who watch the heavily anesthetized postoperative patient. These examples suggest crises of a more or less exceptional nature; it is, on the other hand, impossible to enumerate the kinds of observations nurses must make, nor can any limit be set to their value in the role of observer. Two nurses may be equally skillful with their hands; yet the first is outstanding in clinical judgment and the other is a technician who, when she or he looks at the patient, notices only a small fraction of what the first nurse sees. The beginning practitioner must realize that *there is no substitute for continuing education and experience in actual nursing*. The capacity for detecting disabilities and perceiving slight changes in the patient's physical or emotional state, the ability to discriminate between the significant and inconsequential remark, and the art of reporting accurately and succinctly are built up gradually and increase with every year of nursing experience. Nurses can add to the value of experience by listening to what their patients tell them about the impact of illness, by going to medical and nursing clinics, when they can see highly trained and experienced observers at work, and by comparing their observations with those of veteran nurses and doctors. Signe S. Cooper[5] describes the need for continuing education in nursing and the variety of educational opportunities available to practicing nurses. She says, however, that "self-directed learning is the most significant aspect of continuing education."

Nurses must be guided in everything they do for patients by what they believe to be their needs; the estimate of patients' needs is, of course, based on observation. Nurses cannot carry out prescribed treatments effectively unless they observe intelligently. They do not, for example, continue ruthlessly to apply cold applications when they see signs of a circulatory stasis in the area, nor do they continue to give a prescribed drug when toxic symptoms appear. Nurses who can most nearly distinguish between normal and abnormal behavior—physical, emotional, and mental—and can describe such behavior contribute in largest measure to determining patients' diagnoses. Obviously, this capacity knows no bounds. The physician is particularly dependent upon the nurse in treating infants and children, the irrational and unconscious, but the observations of an able nurse contribute toward effective medical care in any case.

Nurses learn to observe gradually and unconsciously. The technique of observation, like others used in nursing, is based on knowledge, interest, attention, and the empathy that enables nurses to put themselves in the position of the patient. The trained mind is essential. Louis Pasteur said: "In the field of observation, chance favors only the mind that is prepared." A patient often will tell the nurse important facts which he or she "did not like to tell the doctor," "did not want to bother the doctor with," or "did not think it important enough" to tell the doctor. Such symptoms should always be listened to attentively, and, if important, reported in the words of the patient as far as possible.

Symptoms may be misleading in various ways. They may be exaggerated by the patient's imagination, or minimized by shyness and dislike of giving trouble. Often patients are unable to describe symptoms, or they may report those having little bearing on their condition and neglect to mention those most important. Patients may be too ill to concentrate on what the doctors or nurses are saying, or they may be confused by the questions asked and give answers that they know to be misleading. Skillful questioning on the part of the professional is always necessary to draw from patients the subjective symptoms bearing on the case, and the answers must be supplemented by their observations.

Moreover, symptoms may be misleading because they frequently manifest themselves in some part of the body remote, or seemingly not connected, with the seat of the disease; for instance, such symptoms as difficult breathing or coughing and spitting may be caused not by disease of the lungs but of the heart; a cough may be the result of an abscess in the ear that is pressing on a nerve connected with that supplying the lungs, and so giving rise to a "reflex cough." Pain is often a misleading symptom, because it may be "referred" or felt in a spot far from the seat of trouble. Physical signs must frequently be relied on in making a correct diagnosis. The fact that certain symptoms may be misleading is all the more reason that they should be reported fully, accurately, and at the time of their occurrence; a symptom by itself may seem to be of no importance, but when associated with others, a group of symptoms may be very significant indeed.

Directed observations made by the patients or their families, as well as those by nurses, contribute to making the diagnosis. For example, nurses may ask patients in their homes to take their temperature once or twice a day and keep a record of it for a period of a week or more. Patients are sometimes taught to make estimates and records of their blood pressure. The American Cancer Society recommends that women make a monthly self-examination of the breasts. The Society says: "The nurse should encourage women to examine their breasts once a month just after the menstrual period and, equally important, at regular monthly intervals after the cessation of menses."[8] This society is teaching every one the "seven danger signals of cancer": (1) Any sore that does not heal; (2) a lump or thickening in the breasts or elsewhere; (3) unusual bleeding or discharge; (4) any change in a wart or mole; (5) persistent indigestion or difficulty in swallowing; (6) persistent hoarseness or cough; and (7) any change in normal bowel habits. Likewise the National Tuberculosis and Respiratory Disease Association, the American Heart Association, and other health agencies are educating the public to recognize signs of disease and to seek immediate medical advice. Nurses must be alert to the patient's particular need for guidance in making effective observations. Busy physicians rarely give full explanations or complete demonstrations of the procedures involved. In both hospitals and homes, nurses must assume the responsibility for teaching patients and their families to make certain health estimates.

To summarize: nurses are responsible for observations that (1) guide them in constant adaptation of nursing care to meet the patient's changing needs; (2) serve as a basis for diagnosis, prognosis, and treatment; (3) guide others, such as social workers or rehabilitation officers, in their services to the patient; (4) contribute toward their own knowledge and the accumulation of data on which the development of medical science depends; and (5) assist patients or their families to make effective observations.

How and What the Nurse Observes

While observation usually means what one sees, the term as used in medicine includes the discoveries made with all the senses. Certainly the nurse, like the physician, looks, listens, feels, and smells in making a continuous estimate of the patient's condition. Any impairment in the sense of sight, sound, touch, or smell would seriously handicap either a physician or a nurse.

Symptoms are usually divided into the subjective—those felt or experienced by patients, of which they may or may not complain, such as pain or itching; and the objective—those that may be seen, felt, heard, or smelled by others, as, for example, pallor, swelling, coughing, or fetid breath. Although the terms "physical sign" and "symptom" are often used interchangeably, the former is more properly used for objective symptoms detected by such special methods of examination as listening with a stethoscope, manipulating a part, or measuring body temperature with a thermometer.

The most effective nurses observe the patient in every aspect of his or her being. They realize that "mind," "spirit," "intellect," and body of the person are interdependent and inseparable, even if disease is put by some persons into categories of mental, functional, and organic, as if "mind" might be separated from the body and an organ from its function. The experienced observer tries first to estimate the temperament, or the habitual pattern of moods, and the general appearance; in other words to get an over-all picture. No accurate idea of the patient's condition can be formed, however, without a long period of observation and study; even then our knowledge of others is always relatively incomplete. The necessity for continued observation cannot be overstressed.

Observation in nursing is inseparable from the development and application of questions or hypotheses about events. All observations are made within a set of basic assumptions that delimit and determine that which is to be observed. This set of assumptions is modified as the constant interplay of observing, asking, and resolving questions in nursing care proceeds. Basic assumptions in nursing practice come from many sources and are often a synthesis from related social and physical sciences. With the continued reporting of case studies in nursing and research in clinical practice, one can expect a synthesis of old concepts and a discovery of new relationships for understanding and explaining what takes place in patient care.

The following is intended to suggest the scope of the nurse's observations and to serve as a limited guide in the terminology of reporting. This chapter should be read in conjunction with Chapter 3 on the health examination, and texts on psychiatric and physical diagnosis should be consulted for more detailed help. It is intentional that no separation is made here between psychic and physical behavior. By observation, nurses attempt to assess the general physical and emotional make-up. They try to determine how normally people function in expressing their interests, needs, desires, and affection; how normally they function in working, playing, learning, breathing, eating, excreting, regulating body temperature, moving, maintaining muscle tone and normal posture, resting and sleeping. Nurses also try to recognize indications that are, but may not seem, part of the abnormality of the functions just listed. Examples of such symptoms are pain, tenderness, itching, burning, tingling, swelling, hypertrophy, atrophy, discoloration of any visible tissues, the presence of a discharge from a normally moist or dry area, the presence of a growth, a lesion, and a rash.

General Appearance

It is natural to make an over-all estimate of a person by noting his or her physical make-up. Common terms used in describing a physique are tall, medium height, short, emaciated, thin, well-nourished, fat, and obese. The description may indicate whether the person is symmetrically and normally developed for his or her age or the opposite. The observer notes any missing members, prostheses (artificial parts), or obvious blemishes. The muscle tone, posture, and gait contribute to the general impression of personality and state of health. They may express excitement, vigor, interest, lassitude, acute fatigue, dejection, depression, anxiety, and other emotions.

Levels of consciousness are also indicated by posture and muscle tone. Facial expression is no less a part of the general appearance. One may note signs of cheerfulness, anxiety, exhaustion, or anger. The symmetry of the face is important. Long-standing effects of happiness or unhappiness, productivity or frustration may be reflected in the facial lines, as well as chronologic age and apparent age.[6] Throughout their association with patients nurses should be acutely aware of their general appearance.

Temperament, Mental or Emotional Life, Feeling, "Affect," or Psychic Condition

Temperament is the characteristic phenomenon of a person's emotional nature, including susceptibility to emotional stimulation, customary strength and speed of response, the quality of his or her prevailing mood, and fluctuations and intensity of mood. A person may be described as habitually interested in others and expressing interest and affection, or as withdrawn, or self-centered. When a person's moods are of normal intensity but usually under control and when his or her behavior is consistent, he or she is said to be "well-balanced" or "well-adjusted." To form any reasonably accurate estimate of temperament, it is necessary to study a person's relationship to family, friends, acquaintances, and strangers; to note behavior in work and play; and to take account of participation in the activities of their immediate environment and those of the larger community. Nurses can learn a great deal about peoples' interests, occupation and education, and family and social life from the medical history, but everything they do for, or with, patients gives them additional opportunity to study the personality. Nursing care and treatment are affected by the nurse's ability to recognize varying states of alertness, interest, enthusiasm, excitement, apathy, aggressiveness, passivity, irritability, anxiety, fear, resignation, and acceptance.

Gender Identity and Sexuality

The health status cannot be fully understood without knowledge of the individual's gender, his or her sexual identity, and its pattern of expression. Observations can be made to determine the relative degree to which an individual's sexual impulses are integrated with the realities of the environment and the relative degree of acceptance of responsibility for their own sexuality.

There are many illnesses that result in changes of physical capacity for sexual expression or in which the individual perceives that his or her sexual identity and behavior will be changed. Cynthia Scalzi[7] describes aggressive sexual behavior in the cardiac patient and the meaning it may have in the total situation. Milton J. Senn and Albert J. Solnit[8] describe the young child's awareness of sexuality and sex differences. The anxious feelings that children have when undergoing intrusive and operative procedures in the hospital can often be attributed to their concern about their bodies and fear of genital injury.

Sexuality is expressed not only through heterosexual and homosexual intercourse but also through friendship, ideals, parent–child affection, love of abstractions, and self-love. A lack of knowledge about the patient's view of his or her sexuality makes it impossible to meet the total needs for care. George Griffith[9] makes an urgent appeal that health care practitioners know more about the meaning of sexual behavior in the lives of patients who must change their sexual behavior to achieve a healthy state or learn about their sexual capacities following severe illness. As in all caregiving activities, understanding of one's own sexuality is essential to helping another individual whose sexuality and sexual function are a source of stress.

Relationships to Other Persons, Places, and Things

To find meaning and significance as a person is to mean something to someone else, to be acknowledged by someone, to have life in the thoughts and feelings of another, and to be reflected in another's existence in an understanding and affectionate way. There is a human need to belong and to participate in a unit thought greater than the self.

Nurses will learn from individuals in their care what other persons and activities are important to them—in what situations they enjoy a sense of well-being and in what situations they lose the feeling of self-worth. Most persons wish to be of service to another, a group, or a cause. They seek an experience of mutuality in interaction with persons or things. They are accustomed to a certain role or reciprocal modes of behavior between themselves and others. The experience of illness can temporarily or permanently change a person's role within the family or community. Symptoms of disrupted relationships may be persistent feelings of separateness and isolation, inability to trust a professional person, inability to communicate needs, and failure to respond appropriately, both physically and psychologically, to treatment.

Seeing that persons who seek care have the companionship of those people who are most important to them and those objects they treasure will promote their sense of identity and self-worth.

Consciousness, Awareness of Surroundings, Sleep

Since the help patients must have from nurses is so dependent on their state of consciousness and their interpretation of time, place, and people, it is especially important that the nurse be able to make an accurate estimate of the patient's orientation.

The condition of normal persons when fully awake is such that they are responsive to psychological stimuli and indicate by their behavior and speech that they are aware of themselves and their environment. Sleep is a state of physical and mental inactivity from which the person may be aroused to normal consciousness. Sleeping persons give little evidence of being aware of themselves or their environment, yet they differ from comatose patients in that they may still respond to unaccustomed stimuli and be capable of mental activity in the form of dreams. Observation of sleep should indicate the time of day or night and the duration. This is so important in some cases that a graphic sleep chart is kept in order that the physician can see the sleep pattern at a glance. The depth or soundness of the sleep should be noted.

Inattentiveness or confusion implies that the individual does not take into account all the elements of the immediate environment. He or she is usually unable to do more than carry out a few simple instructions; capacity for speech may be limited to a few words or phrases, and there is little awareness of the surrounding activity.

Reduced states of consciousness are described as stupor—a state in which the person can still be aroused—and coma—a state in which he or she cannot be aroused. Reporting certain signs and their change gives a more exact description of the level of consciousness. The signs that are reported are the predominant posture of the body, the posture of the head and eyes, the rate, depth, and rhythm of respiration, the pulse, and the temperature. The state of responsiveness is the reaction when the name is called and the ability to execute simple directions or to respond to painful stimuli. By grading these responses, both the degree of coma and the changes from hour to hour can be evaluated.

Loss or Impairment of Special Senses

The patient who is handicapped in speaking or hearing, seeing, maintaining equilibrium, or interpreting tactile sensations requires special help from the nurse; the loss of the sense of smell, or ability to differentiate common odors, is less serious but should be noted.

The condition of the eyes is particularly significant. Signs of disease may be evident in the face and eyelids, the prominence of the eyes, and their expression.[10] The pupils may fail to respond to light or distance; there may be *photophobia* (sensitiveness to moderate light) and abnormal eye movements. *Nystagmus* is an example of the latter. Failure to interpret objects correctly should be reported. This may be a defect of vision or a misinterpretation.

Speech is affected by normal moods and almost always reflects the mental, if not the physical, condition. What the person says and how he or she says it should be noted. Some disease conditions produce aphasia (inability to arrange words into a meaningful sentence); others produce mutism, tremulous speech, subspeech (grunts), blocking (pausing), irrelevancy, echolalia (repetition of what others say), incoherency, and speech that is explosive, slurring, whispering, or hoarse. The mentally ill may go from one subject to another so rapidly and disconnectedly that they are said to have a "flight of ideas." In reporting the content of a patient's speech, samples of exact words should be given.

Indications of deafness should be reported as they occur. Inattention to what is said may or may not be the result of deafness. Ringing in the ears or any tenderness in or around the ears should be noted. Impairment of equilibrium is often not apparent when the person can compensate by sight. Dizziness, swaying, and falling when the eyes are closed are serious symptoms.

Disease may affect the nerve endings in the skin or the centers in the brain that interpret sensation of touch or heat and cold. Complete failure to respond or failure to respond normally to such stimuli should be reported.

Abnormalities in Sensation or Interpretation of Stimuli; Abnormality in the Realm of Thought

The systematic examination of intelligence, mood, memory, and judgment, which are affective and cognitive functions, permits the observer to reach certain conclusions about the mental status of the patient.[11] Without these data, errors will be made in evaluating the reliability of the patient's history or in diagnosing neurologic or psychiatric disease.

People are said to be confused when there is a general reduction in alertness, attentiveness, and perception of environmental stimuli. They may also be slow and inefficient in thinking and fail to remember.

Loss of memory should always be noted, and a differentiation made between loss of memory for the immediate and distant past.

Fabrication is a term used to describe the practice of making statements contrary to fact if there is reason to believe that the memory is intact.

Delirium describes a disorder of consciousness characterized by excessive alertness, sleeplessness, and frenzied excitement.

A person is said to have an illusion when an object in his or her environment is incorrectly interpreted—a sick man may think his wife is sitting in a chair when it is only a coat thrown over the chair. When a woman with a high fever hears nonexistent voices or feels rats running over her while nothing is touching her but her own bedding or clothing, she is said to have hallucinations—sensations without external stimuli. Delusions are common symptoms of psychoses. Deluded persons hold a belief that has no basis in fact. They have what might be called pathological experiences in thought. They often think they are someone they are not, rich when they are poor, a holder of high office when they hold none; or they may believe they are being persecuted and that their friends, family, or the medical personnel are menacing them. Often these ideas are systematically worked out, and in describing the grandiose position or persecution, they will be very convincing. It is important for the nurse to report *exactly what they say*.

Phobias—unreasonable fears and compulsions resulting in acts the person feels compelled to perform—are not uncommon, nor are obsessions—thoughts from which the person cannot rid himself or herself. Sometimes the mentally ill will say they feel unreal or that an outside force controls their actions.

Thinking may be defined as selective ordering of symbols for problem-solving and the capacity to reason and form sound judgments. In a general way, the thinking processes may be examined for speed and efficiency, conceptual content, coherence and logical relationship of ideas, quantity and quality of association to a given idea, and appropriateness of feeling and behavior in relation to the idea.[12]

These features of the thought process may be examined by analyzing the person's spontaneous speech and by engaging him or her in conversation. Disorders of thought are frequent in delirium and in degenerative and other types of cerebral disease. Fragmentation, repetition, and perseverance may characterize the organization of thoughts. Criticizing and rationalizing is a type of thinking seen in depressive psychoses. The flight of ideas, in which a person moves from one idea to another, with numerous and loosely linked associations, is a common feature of hypomanic and manic states. A poverty of ideas combined with gloomy thoughts is found in depression.[13]

Motor Activity—Posture and Symptoms of Impaired Motor Function

The activity of the neuromuscular system may be studied by inspection, by touch, and by moving parts of the body to determine range-of-motion. The physician and nurse are particularly interested in muscle tone as a health index.

Posture is studied for signs of weakness, such as continuously slipping down from an erect sitting posture. Posture may indicate pain, as when the legs are flexed to relax muscles over a distended abdomen or when a side-lying position is assumed to limit the expansion of the chest, as in pleurisy. When any position is assumed habitually it should be noted, as should any unusual position.

The condition of the muscles of the eyes, of swallowing, and of respiration and that of the urethral and rectal sphincters are studied in order to determine the normality of specific body areas. Disease, including highly emotional states, may produce hyperactivity or hypoactivity. The normal amount of activity differs with the personality so that the nurse should describe the behavior rather than designate it as a hyper- or hypoactive. The gait should be noted in terms such as rapid, slow, hesitant, dragging, rolling, rocking, running, tottering, or staggering. Any rigidity, or tension of the whole body or part thereof, is significant, as are paralysis and difficulty or discomfort in moving an extremity, eyes, or eyelids, in speaking, swallowing, breathing, defecating, or voiding. Rhythmic, stereotyped, or automatic motions, tremors, convulsions, and unnatural flexibility are motor symptoms that should be reported.

Breathing

Respiration is an automatic function, but its rate and depth are nevertheless affected by emotional states, exercise, drugs, and anything that alters the body's need of oxygen. Mechanical interference with respiration also affects the rate and depth. The nurse should note the character of the respiration; the symmetry of structure and movements of the chest, abdomen, and nose; the sounds accompanying respiration; the patient's position, expression, and change in color; and actual complaints indicating difficult breathing.

Through auscultation the nurse learns the normal sounds of air moving through the nose, throat, and lungs, as well as abnormal respiratory murmurs arising from disease. Considerable experience in listening to the wide range of normal breath sounds is necessary before abnormal sounds can be distinguished. Some characteristics of abnormal breathing are noisy or musical sounds (rhonchi). These are caused by movement of exudate in the bronchial tubes or inflammation or narrowing of the bronchial tubes. There may be a grating sound from the rub of an inflamed serous surface or a crackling sound (rale) which indicates the presence of fluid or inflammation within the respiratory tract. Judge and Zuidema[14] present a useful classification of breath sounds and methods of listening to the chest. Variations in respiration are characterized by the following descriptions and may indicate physical disease or emotional stress: sensation of difficulty breathing or shortness of breath is called *dyspnea*, and increased depth of respiration is called *hyperpnea*. A more common term to describe increased depth of respiration is *hyperventilation*. Inability to breathe comfortably while lying down is *orthopnea*, and an increased rate of respiration is *tachypnea*. *Stridor* is difficult respiration characterized by high-pitched crowing sounds in inspiration. *Apnea* is a temporary suspension of breathing. *Cyanosis* is the term used to describe the blush tint of the lips, nail beds, or skin resulting from inadequate oxygenation of the blood. Breathing with the mouth open habitually is abnormal and should be reported.

Eating and Drinking

Reva Rubin[15] describes food not only as a source of nutrition and physical sustenance but also as the source of nurturance, the interactive and interpersonal matrix in which we learn about ourselves and others. M. F. K. Fisher takes the same position in a book titled *The Gastronomical Me*:

> It seems to me that our three basic needs, for food and security and love, are so mixed and mingled and entwined that we cannot straightly think of one without the others.[h]

Food has many symbolic meanings and one's response to offered food is influenced by how one feels about oneself in the situation or relationship.[16] In helping the person who is seeking health care or being treated for illness, the social and cultural significance of food and ways of eating must be considered before attempts at feeding or teaching nutritional needs can succeed. Food intake is usually balanced with the caloric demands of the body. As a rule, people eat what they need and no more. Nevertheless, habits of eating continue beyond the necessity for them and appetite becomes related to desire more than need.[17] Overeating may be a response to a nonspecific emotional tension, a substitute gratification, or a symptom of emotional illness. Undernutrition, or a progressive weight loss without obvious explanation, should be treated as a symptom of illness and receive serious consideration in the over-all assessment of the person.[18]

It is obvious that health and recovery from disease are dependent on food intake. Unless patients are aware of their nutritional needs and are able and willing to meet them, the burden of seeing that they get adequate nourishment rests largely upon nurses. They should observe signs of appetite or its lack, food likes, cravings, dislikes, idiosyncrasies, and phobias. If patients do not enjoy their meals, nurses should try to discover the cause. Actually they may be hungry, but eating may be for some reason painful or uncomfortable. Sore mouth, ill-fitting dentures, difficulty in swallowing, or weakness may interfere with the satisfaction of eating. The mentally ill may think themselves unworthy of food, they may believe the food is poisoned, or it may represent an object that is unfit for consumption.

Elimination

Individuals defecate, urinate, and dispose of excreta in ways that meet physiological demands of their bodies, are satisfying to them, and are compatible with cultural expectations. Acts of elimination are invested with feelings about control of self and environment. In Western cultures the prevalent attitudes toward excreta are ones of distaste, if not revulsion. The odors are considered unpleasant, and it is expected that body parts associated with elimination be covered. Self-care during elimination is highly valued and is taught to the child in Western cultures at an early age, often with little regard for the physiologic readiness to urinate and defecate voluntarily.

Cultural values vested in elimination are those of regularity, cleanliness, conformity, obedience, privacy, and modesty. An individual is interested in elimination as a subjective index of the integrity of the body. For the adult and child, the acts of elimination can be a vehicle for the expression of emotions. For example, a child may develop constipation as a way of expressing his or her feelings about events that he or she cannot understand, such as a new place in the family when a brother or sister is born.

Reports on the amount, frequency, and nature of elimination are included in all patient observations. If people are rational and ambulatory, they may assume the responsibility for reporting to the nurse or doctor any irregularity in defecation, urination, and sweating; if they are not able to assume this responsibility, nurses note the character of the excretions and the frequency of defecation and urination. If pain or discomfort accompanies these acts, this should be noted. Attention should be called at once to cessation of these functions. Sweating or abnormal dryness of the skin and the body areas affected should be reported. If the sweat has an unusual odor, as of urine, it should be noted. The balance between fluid taken in and eliminated cannot be too greatly upset without serious consequence. A record is therefore kept as a basis for estimating how nearly intake and output tally. Sunken eyes, dry mouth, loose skin, and concentrated urine are characteristic of dehydration and are danger signs. Any indication that fluid is held in the tissues is also significant. Puffy eyes, clubbed fingers, swollen hands and feet (edema), or accumulation of fluid in the tissues of the back when the patient is sitting should be noted. *Ascites* is the term used when free fluid distends the abdominal cavity. Occasionally, with the use of certain drugs, or in the case of poisoning, excretions are discolored or have an unusual odor. Drugs may be deposited in the tissues and give the mucous membranes, skin, or the sclera of the eye an unnatural appearance that should be noted and described.

Regulation of Body Temperature

Maintenance of body temperature within the normal range is accomplished by a number of physiologic processes involving both chemical and physical transfer of heat. The operation of these mechanisms is mediated by the central nervous system.

The principal source of body heat is combustion of food in the body. Heat produced by muscular activity maintains a uniform body temperature, the activity readily increasing or decreasing according to need. Heat is eliminated by the processes of radiation, vaporization, and convection. Fever is an elevation of temperature due to disease or exposure to high environmental temperatures. Evaluation of the significance of fever requires knowledge of temperature control and the various ways in which the control can be disturbed.[19]

The oral or rectal glass and mercury thermometer is available to anybody who wants to measure his or her body temperature. This is the most common instrument for measuring body temperature in homes and in ambulatory and inpatient services. A portable electronic thermometer will measure oral or rectal temperature within seconds, as against minutes with the traditional instrument, and displays the temperature reading simultaneously on a screen on the instrument. The electronic thermometer has disposable covers for the temperature probe. This instrument is the most practical to use where there are large groups of individuals who need periodic measurement of their temperature.

The measurement of body temperature differs depending on the area of the body where the measurement is taken.[20] For example, oral temperature is not considered to be the best reflection of deep body temperature. Knowing the deep body temperature is important in critical illness and certain surgical procedures. Therefore, in critical care hospital units various devices for the continuous measurement of body temperature are available which are introduced into the rectum or esophagus to measure deep body temperature.

Abdominal skin temperature is monitored in the premature or sick infant, as the temperature at this site most closely approximates the deep body temperature.[21] Failure to provide an optimal environment (thermoneutral) for newborn infants will subject them to such metabolic difficulties as oxygen deprivation and metabolic acidosis.[22] The thermoneutral environment for newborns is that environment in which they can maintain abdominal skin temperature or axillary temperature between 36.6° and 37.5°C (97° and 99°F).

The measurement and control of body temperature will undoubtedly become more convenient and comfortable for the individual and more precise for the collection of data on health and disease processes than they are today. Nevertheless, close observation of other signs of disturbance in body temperature will never be negated by technologic developments in equipment. The condition of the skin may be described as hot, flushed, cold, or clammy. There may be an obvious chill or a sensation of which the person complains. If the patient has a dry nose and mouth, which makes swallowing difficult, the lips get cracked and parched and the tongue appears coated and discolored. All of these are signs of dehydration accompanying fever that the nurse can see and should record.

Noting Gross Disease Processes

Abnormal functioning of the body constitutes disease, but there are pathologic processes the nurse should note that have not been emphasized under the functional headings just used. For example, any signs of inflammation—redness, heat, swelling, discomfort, or pain—should be reported. Note and report any discoloration of the skin or mucous membranes, swelling, hypertrophy, any sign of a growth, break in the tissues, discharges from body orifices or lesions, abnormal odors, tenderness as the body is manipulated, and all subjective symptoms of which the patient complains. Examples are pain, tenderness, itching, burning, tingling, prickling, numbness, throbbing, chilliness or a sensation of being overheated, headache, nausea, dizziness, spots before the eyes, ringing in the ears (tinnitus), deafness, a sense of fullness, pressure, or a "gone" or weak feeling. All of these should be reported in the patient's own words with the sensation localized when it is local and characterized as the patient describes it. Patients may say that they have a "gnawing pain that comes and goes" in the stomach and that "it is relieved by food," or they "feel as if there is a heavy weight" on the chest, or they "can't get their breath." Since such comments may have a different significance for any two medical attendants, a verbatim report is desirable.

Feelings or emotions are expressed in such questions or statements as "Isn't the doctor coming soon?" "Does the doctor think my condition is serious?" "I know it isn't cancer." "There's no danger in a blood pressure of 180, is there?" or "Do you think I'll get well?" When the nurse thinks that a question indicates any emotional state that markedly affects the patient's diagnosis, prognosis, or treatment, it is wise to record it in the patient's words. All symptoms are important, though not equally so; therefore, a selection must be made from the patient's acts, including speech, that seem significant. Anything a patient does is an indication of what concerns him or her, of the effectiveness or ineffectiveness of the care given, and of the nature of the illness.

Methods of Reporting and Recording

Observation of the patient is continuous, as has been said repeatedly, and serves as a basis for the hourly and daily modification of nursing care. Since it is obviously impossible for nurses to record all their observations, some guide is necessary in making a selection of items that may be helpful to patients, nurses, physicians, social workers, and special therapists.

Nurses should report any signs of disorientation, unconsciousness, anxiety, fear, or any strong emotion and particularly instability of mood, deterioration of the patient's relationship with others, or any marked change in the personality. They should report any handicap or limitation of function as soon as it is noted. In general, symptoms should be reported that have any of the following characteristics:

1. are intense or severe in character, as severe pain;
2. are prolonged, even though not severe;
3. are a departure from normal, as an increase or decrease in pulse rate;
4. tend to recur, as pain between meals;
5. show progressive development, as loss of weight;
6. are known danger signals, as a sharp abdominal pain in perforated peptic ulcer;
7. indicate a complication, as coughing following an operation;
8. point to the onset of a disease, as a rash;
9. cannot be relieved by nursing measures, as failure to eat or sleep, void, or defecate;

10. show faulty hygiene or health habits that cannot be corrected by nursing care, as neglected teeth, the need of eyeglasses, or a more balanced diet;
11. indicate a disturbance in function of any organ or part of the body; and
12. show a change for the better or for the worse.

Reports are made orally, by notation on the patient's chart, or both ways. Anything that is serious or that requires immediate attention should be reported promptly, both orally and on the medical record—the patient's chart. The written report must never be omitted, for this helps to ensure notice of the condition and to protect medical personnel from accusations of negligence. Patient-centered conferences among nurses, doctors, nutritionists, social workers, rehabilitation officers, and special therapists offer an invaluable opportunity to exchange such observations and opinions as are difficult to report fully in writing. The beginning practitioner of nursing should err on the side of being overzealous in reporting to the nurse in charge of the service or to the physician responsible for the patient's medical program any observation that he or she thinks may even possibly have serious consequences. Ninety-nine times the caution may be unnecessary, the nurse's judgment questioned, but the hundredth time he or she may save a life.

The patient's record, or chart, is still the most commonly used medium for reporting observations (signs and symptoms of patient behavior). The value of nurses' notations is a fairly good index of their nursing ability. Gradually nurses build up a technique of observing and recording. Before going to the patient, they regularly review what others have written on the record and the treatment prescribed by the physician. Nurses get whatever oral reports they can from others, they welcome the opinions of the patient's family and friends; then, after observation made while they care for the patient, they report and record whatever they think is significant. Such records are made daily, hourly, or at less frequent intervals, according to the patient's needs and the time available for nursing care.

Notes

---

[a]Judge, R. D., and Zuidema, G. D. (eds.): *Physical Diagnosis: A Physiological Approach to the Clinical Examination*, 2nd ed. Little, Brown & Co., Boston, 1968, p. 38.

[b]Kaplan, Abraham: *The Conduct of Inquiry.* Chandler Publishing Co., San Francisco, 1964, p. 126.

[c]Orlando, Ida Jean: *The Dynamic Nurse Patient Relationship: Functions, Process, and Principles.* G. P. Putnam's Sons, New York, 1961, p. 1.

[d]For example, see the following issues of the *International Digest of Health Legislation,* published by the World Health Organization, Geneva: "Nursing: A Survey of Recent Legislation," *4*:463–497, 1952–1953; "Midwives: A Survey of Recent Legislation," *5*:433–480, 1954; "Auxiliary Personnel in Nursing," *17*:198–229, 1966; "Medical, Dental and Pharmaceutical Auxiliaries," *19*:4–129, 1968.

[e]Kelly, Katherine: "Clinical Inference in Nursing. I. A Nurse's Viewpoint," *Nurs. Res., 15*:23 (Winter) 1966.

[f]Nervi Ahla, studying the cooperation between the visiting nurse and the social caseworker, calls attention to the strategic position of the nurse in observing and reporting "family social disintegrations." She concludes that when many different nurses are assigned to one family, the referral of the family to social case workers is likely to be delayed. ("Briefs," *Nurs. Res., 1*:37, [June] 1952.)

[g]American Cancer Society: *A Breast Check—So Simple . . . So Important.* The Society, New York, 1973.

[h]Fisher, M. F. K.: *The Gastronomical Me,* Duell, Sloan & Pearce, New York, 1943, p. vii.

References

---

1. Kaplan, Abraham: *The Conduct of Inquiry.* Chandler Publishing Co., San Francisco, 1964, p. 126.

2. Murchison, Irene A., and Nichols, Thomas S.: *Legal Foundations of Nursing Practice.* Macmillan Publishing Co., New York, 1970, p. 82.

3. Nightingale, Florence: *Notes on Nursing: What It Is, and What It Is Not* (facsimile of 1859 ed.). J. B. Lippincott Co., Philadelphia, 1946.

4. *Nursing Studies Index, Vol. I (1900–1920).* Prepared by Yale University School of Nursing Index Staff under the direction of Virginia Henderson. J. B. Lippincott Co., Philadelphia, 1972.

5. Cooper, Signe S.: "Why Continuing Education in Nursing," *Cardiovasc. Nurs., 9*:13, (May–June) 1973.

6. Judge, R. C., and Zuidema, G. D. (eds.): *Physical Diagnosis: A Physio-*

logic Approach to the Clinical Examination. 2nd ed. Little, Brown & Co., Boston, 1968.

7. Scalzi, Cynthia: "Nursing Management of Behavioral Responses Following an Acute Myocardial Infarction," *Heart Lung, 2*:62, (Jan–Feb.) 1973.

8. Senn, Milton J., and Solnit, Albert J.: *Problems in Child Behavior and Development*. Lea & Febiger, Philadelphia, 1968, p. 65.

9. Griffith, George: "Sexuality and the Cardiac Patient," *Heart Lung, 2*:70, (Jan.–Feb.) 1973.

10. Judge, R. D., and Zuidema, G. D. (eds.): *op. cit.*, p. 81.

11. Wintrobe, Maxwell M., et al. (eds.): *Harrison's Principles of Internal Medicine*, 6th ed. McGraw-Hill Book Co., New York, 1970, p. 185.

12. *Ibid.*, p. 187.

13. *Ibid.*, p. 187.

14. Judge, R. D., and Zuidema, G. D. (eds.): *op. cit.*, p. 131.

15. Rubin, Reva: "Food and Feeding. A Matrix of Relationships," *Nurs. Forum, 6*:195, (No. 2) 1967.

16. *Ibid.*

17. MacBryde, Cyril M., and Blacklow, Robert S. (eds.): *Signs and Symptoms: Applied Pathologic Physiology and Clinical Interpretation*, 5th ed. J. B. Lippincott Co., Philadelphia, 1970 p. 864.

18. *Ibid.*, p. 874.

19. *Ibid.*, p. 451.

20. *Ibid.*, p. 454.

21. Korones, Sheldon B., et al.: *High Risk Newborn Infants: The Basis for Intensive Nursing Care*. C. V. Mosby Co., St. Louis, 1972, p. 61.

22. *Ibid.*, p. 61.

Chapter 5

On Diagnosis, Decision-Making, and Autonomy

Definition, Various Meanings of Diagnosis

Diagnosis is a word that can be used specifically or generally. It is a Greek word derived from verbs meaning to distinguish and to know. Webster gives the first meaning of diagnosis as "the art or act" of recognizing disease from its symptoms and also "the decision reached"; its second meaning as "scientific determination, critical scrutiny or its resulting judgment." If "scientific determination" and "critical scrutiny" are accepted as legitimate meanings, clearly the term can be used not only in the specific sense of recognizing disease from its symptoms, but in the very general sense of critical scrutiny and scientific determination in solving any problem, whether or not it is in the field of health.

Role of Patient, Family, and Friends in Diagnosis and Decision-Making in Matters of Health

Usually when people think that they are functioning abnormally, or, most particularly, if they have pain or discomfort, they want to know why, or "what's wrong." Sometimes, as in the case of infants or small children, it is the parent or guardian who notices malfunction or signs of pain and wants to know "what's wrong." Occasionally a change in function may be so gradual that it is unrecognized by the subject; he or she is shocked to have a relative or friend say, "Why are you so short of breath?" or "When did you get so deaf?" But usually those affected realize they are sick or disabled and by the time they take the problem to someone who they believe more knowledgeable than themselves—be it the corner druggist, the tribal medicine man, the physician, the nurse, or some other health worker—they have one or more "diagnoses" in mind. They may, in fact, have been quietly treating themselves on the assumption that they did know what was wrong. Many a person, for example, has attributed pain in the area of the stomach to "too much acid" and has used bicarbonate of soda to cure their "dyspepsia," or "acid-indigestion," only to find, after being correctly diagnosed as having pernicious anemia, that their indigestion could be relieved by taking an acid (hydrochloric) after each meal instead of the alkaline salt they thought they needed. On the other hand, a man with an alcoholic wife may know subconsciously that his indigestion has an emotional origin but, not wanting to admit his problem to himself or to a doctor, may never be correctly diagnosed or treated.

Effective treatment depends, therefore, on many things, including an accurate health history, a thorough examination (physical and mental or psychologic), a correct diagnosis, and upon the acceptance of the diagnosis and treatment by patients and families. So it is important for health workers to begin the diagnostic process by identifying what patients and families believe to be the health problem or problems and what steps they have taken to solve it or them. With the "neurotic" and "hypochondriac," self-knowledge is essential to improvement; for everyone, understanding of the problem, participation in solving it, or decision-making, is most important.

There is a present-day legal stress on "informed consent" from the patient before instituting treatment. But this is only the beginning. The patient's participation in decision-making is almost necessary if he or she is to be fully rehabilitated or regain independence.

Some physicians clearly recognize the necessity of self-diagnosis and self-treatment and have written many home remedy texts designed to help the layman recognize and treat common diseases. A 1973 publication, *The Well Body Book,*[1] by Mike Samuels (a physician) and Hal Bennett (an educator) tells laymen how to examine their own or a friend's body and how to recognize and treat conditions such as acne, scabies, impacted ear wax, influenza, hay fever, hemorrhoids, lower back pain, varicose veins, and infectious mononucleosis. The authors tell the layman how to use the doctor as a "consultant" and in some cases what tests the patient might ask the doctor to make, or what drugs or type of drug the doctor might be asked to prescribe. Obviously, the authors expect the patient to play a leading role in preventing, diagnosing, and treating disease.

References in this and other chapters have been made to the role of nurses and other health workers in diagnostic and decision-making processes. Practice varies greatly from country to country, from state to state (or province), and from one institution to another. The following discussion is an attempt to identify trends in varied and rapidly changing roles.

Role of the Physician

Of all health workers, physicians are best prepared to diagnose disease. Diagnosis and treatment of disease are the functions that organized medicine values most, although some physicians spend their professional lives in preventing disease while others specialize in research. The wording of medical practice acts limits the right to diagnose and treat disease to physicians (and dentists). This has been and still is a road-block in the delivery of health care in those countries with so few, such poorly distributed, or such specialized physicians that they cannot provide primary medical care for the entire population. Organized medicine in many countries is moving toward compromise, toward changes in medical practice acts that enable physicians to share with other health workers the responsibility for diagnosis and treatment. State medical associations have endorsed nurse practice acts that include "diagnosis" and "decision-making" as nursing functions. Eliot Friedson,[2] in his monograph, *Professional Dominance*, expresses the opinion that the competition doctors are now experiencing is "healthy"; Barbara Bates,[3-8] a physician, who has worked for years with nurses as colleagues, expresses the opinion that doctors must accept the fact that as other health professionals assume some of their traditional functions, they must necessarily compete for "the health dollar," for working space, and for institutional privileges. She and her colleagues make a strong plea for colleague relationships and shared responsibility, presenting diagrams that show the overlapping functions of doctors and nurses. Lynaugh and Bates[9] point out differences in medical and nursing emphases and terminology, suggesting that a doctor and a nurse looking at the same problem can suggest a better solution than either might suggest working alone.

Western medicine has, until very recently, concentrated on diagnosis of disease rather than assessment of health and disease prevention. DeGowin and DeGowin give the following meanings of diagnosis:

> The name of the patient's disease or state of altered function is termed *the diagnosis* or *a diagnosis*. . . . But the act of searching for or determining the patient's disease is commonly referred to as *diagnosis* (without the article). . . .[a]

Judge and Zuidema say the elements of diagnostic logic may be identified as observation, description, interpretation, verification, diagnosis, and action. They say, "diagnosis . . . involves applying the final label. *The decision*: which disease or diseases account for the illness." Under action, they say that "This involves determining a course based on the diagnosis. *The decision*: selecting the proper treatment, whether it be surgical or nonsurgical."[b] Engel and Morgan say "The diagnostic process is the mental operation through which *the disease* [italics ours] is identified and the illness evaluated."[c] Engel[10] in 1960 had called for a unified concept of health and disease.

Alvin R. Feinstein,[11] *in Clinical Judgment*, urges doctors to make diagnoses more "patient centered," saying that the care of the patient is the ultimate specific act that characterizes a clinician, but he says diagnosis is that "which gives the disease a name and tells what is wrong."

Recently Weed[12] has led a movement away from the kind of diagnostic process that focuses on *the* diagnosis; that is, naming *the* disease or condition from which the patient suffers and is to be treated. Under this plan of medical management many problems may be identified by physicians and others. The patient may get help with some or all of them but all problems are recorded and progress in solving them assessed.

The problem-oriented system of medical management is receiving wide attention and support from many quarters. It is in line with the observation of the Carnegie Commission on Higher Education[13] that emphasis in medical education is changing from naming the disease to helping families with health problems and recognizing that assessing behavior is as important as seeing physical symptoms. John B. Dillon,[14] a physician, in an article decrying the overemphasis on technologic research in medical education, entitled "How Did It Happen?" pointed out that Abraham Flexner, whose report of 1910 "reformed" medical education, actually considered preventive medicine and teaching the patient essential aspects of medical practice.

Medicine has invested an inordinate amount of time in identifying and categorizing diseases, as evidenced by many publications.[15,16] Several hundred years of effort have culminated in an *International Classification of Diseases*[17] prepared under the auspices of, and published by, the World Health Organization. The tabulation of diseases and surgical operations in the following categories fills a volume of 671 pages in its 8th edition (1963).

Tabular List of Inclusions and Fourth-Digit Subcategories

Infective and Parasitic Diseases; Neoplasms; Endocrine, Nutritional, and Metabolic Diseases; Diseases of the Blood and Blood-Forming Organs; Mental Disorders; Diseases of the Nervous System and Sense Organs, Diseases of the Circulation System; Diseases of the Respiratory System; Diseases of the Digestive System; Diseases of the Genitourinary System; Complications of Pregnancy, Childbirth, and the Puerperium; Diseases of the Skin and Subcutaneous Tissue; Diseases of the Musculoskeletal System and Connective Tissue; Congenital Anomalies; Certain Causes of Perinatal Morbidity and Mortality; Symptoms and Ill-Defined Conditions; Accidents, Poisonings, and Violence (External Cause).

Surgical Operations, Diagnostic and Other Therapeutic Procedures

Neurosurgery; Ophthalmology; Otorhinolaryngology; Operations on Thyroid, Parathyroid, Thymus, and Adrenals; Vascular and Cardiac Surgery; Thoracic Surgery; Abdominal Surgery; Proctologic Surgery; Urologic Surgery; Breast Surgery; Gynecologic Surgery; Obstetric Procedures; Orthopedic Surgery; Plastic Surgery; Oral and Maxillofacial Surgery; Dental Surgery; Biopsy; Diagnostic Endoscopy; Diagnostic Radiography; Radiotherapy and Related Therapies; Physical Medicine and Rehabilitation; Other Nonsurgical Procedures.

Uniform nomenclature is essential for morbidity and mortality statistics—international, national, state or province, county, city, and institutional.

Physicians who see the diagnostic and decision-making process as a matter of deciding on *the* disease or condition from which the patient is suffering and *the* treatment for it are more likely to think of the doctor's role as *the* diagnostician; physicians who see diagnosis and decision-making as a matter of identifying the health problems of individuals and families and helping them cope with them are more likely to see diagnosis and decision-making as a collaborative procedure. Bates[18,19] and Aradine and Pridham[20] are among the physicians who have tried to show, in some cases writing with nurses, just how collaboration with nurses works.

In hospitals and clinics with medical students, interns, and residents and highly qualified nurses, the physical examination is very often made by one of them with attending physicians repeating the whole, parts of, or no parts of the procedure but discussing the findings with the examiner; in hospitals and nursing homes where there is no resident medical personnel, the patient's physician has usually made some sort of examination before asking that the patient be admitted. In schools and industries, practices vary greatly in the quality of the health services they provide, but in most, if not all of them, nurses and other health workers conserve the physicians' time by carrying out such aspects of the physical examination as the physicians do not elect to carry out themselves.[21-25] This is also true in the health screening processes in military recruitment centers, health maintenance units, and comparable services. As has been described by Garfield,[26] health screening services depend heavily on technology, with the physician's role being that of an analyzer of data collected by technicians and machines, an interpreter of the findings to the client, and a consultant to him or her on following up or correcting defects identified during the health assessment.

Role of the Nurse

The circumstances under which nurses practice have always affected their roles in diagnosis and decision-making. Nurses working on islands and in remote rural areas where there are no doctors have been forced by the urgent needs of those they served to take histories, do physical examinations, analyze their findings, "diagnose" or label the "presenting problem" or problems, and institute action or "treatment," and they have often been very effective. For example, the success of nurse-midwives working independently of physicians most of the time in the Kentucky mountains is relatively well-documented.[27-29] The effectiveness of nurses working with minimal recourse to medical collaboration in the health services for Eskimos and Native Americans in Canada and the United States has been recognized.[30-34] Nurses in schools, in industry, in corrective institutions (and in many hospitals where doctors are not readily available at night) must of necessity make "diagnoses" and decide on courses of action. J.J.A. Reid, a British medical officer of health, says there is still an argument as to whether the nurse should have a role in diagnosis, but he thinks much depends on what is meant by the term. He says:

> District nurses have for many years been accustomed to . . . the public consulting them about minor ailments and . . . being asked for advice on whether the condition is serious enough to warrant consulting a doctor. In the hospital . . . the ward sister or night superintendent has always had to decide on whether a doctor should be called because of some change in a patient's condition. Similarly the . . . occupational health nurse has long been used to assessing whether a patient . . . with a minor ailment or injury should be treated on the spot or whether he should be referred to his general practitioner or to the hospital . . . emergency department. There is ample precedent for involvement of nurses in the diagnostic process.[d]

Jane Henderson, A Canadian nurse, is quoted as follows in a news item: " . . . as we broaden the definition of care from one centered on pathology to one concerned with life style and environment we simultaneously broaden the definition of diagnosis."[e] J. Fry makes a similar point that most health problems are not brought to the physician or a surrogate for solution but are actually "diagnosed" by the person who has the symptoms, or by the family.

While people intimately associated with health services know that nurses everywhere have been forced by circumstances to fill the role of diagnostician and decision-maker the function has never been written into nurse practice acts until this decade, nor have history-taking and methods of physical (or clinical) assessment been taught in basic nursing curricula. They have been taught, however, in some form in graduate programs.

Since 1972, when the New York State Nurse Practice Act was amended to include the following description of nursing practice, other states have followed suit or have committees working on amendments to their practice acts:

> The practice of the profession of nursing as a registered professional nurse is defined as diagnosing and treating human responses to actual or potential health problems through such services as casefinding, health teaching, health counseling, and provision of care supportive to or restorative of life

and well-being, and executing medical regimens prescribed by a licensed or otherwise legally authorized physician or dentist. A nursing regimen shall be consistent with and not vary any existing medical regime.[f]

A Bill to amend Sections 2725 and 2726 of the Business and Professions Code relating to nurses was referred to the Committee on Health of the California legislature in February 1974. It reads, in part, as follows:

> The practice of nursing means those functions helping people cope with difficulties in daily living which are associated with their actual or potential health or illness problems or the treatment thereof which require a substantial amount of scientific knowledge or technical skill, and includes all of the following:
> (a) Direct and indirect patient care services that insure the safety, comfort, personal hygiene, and protection of patients; and the performance of disease prevention and restorative measures.
> (b) Direct and indirect patient care services, including, but not limited to, the administration of medications and therapeutic agents, necessary to implement a treatment, disease prevention, or rehabilitative regimen prescribed by a physician, dentist, or podiatrist.
> (c) The performance of basic health care, testing, and prevention procedures, including, but not limited to, skin tests, immunization techniques, and the withdrawal of human blood from veins and arteries.
> (d) Observation of signs and symptoms of illness, reactions to treatment, general behavior, or general physical condition, and (1) determination of whether such signs, symptoms, reactions, behavior, or general appearance exhibit abnormal characteristics; and (2) implementation, based on observed abnormalities, of appropriate reporting, or referral, or standardized procedures, or changes, in treatment regimen in accordance with standardized procedures, or the initiation of emergency procedures.

Using the words "diagnosis" or "diagnose" and "treatment" in proposed nurse practice acts seems to delay enactment and to elicit opposition from organized medicine. However, if modifying terms that limit the nurse's role in diagnosis and treatment are used, the opposition is overcome. Eileen M. Jacobi, analyzing nurse practice acts in 1973 and responses to a questionnaire on the expanded role of the nurse, noted that "In two states, the definition of nursing practice has been modified (1) to permit diagnosis and treatment under emergency or special conditions, including special training, and (2) by rules and regulations promulgated jointly by the board of nursing and the board of medicine.[8] Jacobi questioned whether definitions of nursing practice in the laws of the United States were flexible enough to allow nurses to expand their role. She noted that definitions in 18 states restricted the right of nurses to diagnose and prescribe treatment. In Chapter 1, the study for the National Joint Practice Commission by Virginia C. Hall, *Statutory Regulation of the Scope of Nursing Practice—A Critical Survey*, was cited. She made the following observation:

> The only way to permit expansion of the independent practice of nursing into medicine, and at the same time retain in the law the traditional notion of the distinct nature of the independent practice of the two, is to adopt a theory that whatever is nursing cannot, by definition, *because* it is nursing, fall within the scope of what is medical, even if it includes acts which if performed by a physician would concededly be medical—in other words, that the nature of the practitioner determines the nature of the act. This theory seems much too metaphysical to be credible. In addition, it proves too much, because in effect it obliterates any exclusive province of medicine and by its terms would permit the expansion of nursing into all of medicine. Any express or implicit statutory prohibition against acts of medical diagnosis or other medical acts would simply be irrelevant as applied to nursing.
>
> Even in the unlikely event that some such theory of interpretation is judicially accepted in some States, it would still amount to a highly circuitous and unnecessarily complex way to achieve the desired result. There is no reason why the traditional medicine/nursing dichotomy should be retained where it is no longer realistic. Therefore, except where political realities dictate otherwise, it should be discarded entirely and, optimally, be replaced by an explicit recognition of the overlap of the independent practice of the professions of nursing and medicine.[h]

Hall thinks that exempting nurses from the prohibition against the practice of medicine in medical practice acts the simplest way to solve the legal problems involved in the expanded role of the nurse.

Lucie Young Kelly, also studying nurse practice acts, said in 1974:

> The silent conspiracy among hospital administrators, nurses, and physicians to allow nurses to perform services that were desired by and convenient to all concerned, under the guise of overall physician supervision and medical protocol, continued as it had for a hundred years, although in a more sophisticated manner. It was obvious that nurses practiced effectively in ICUs and saved countless lives. What else could anyone ask?[i]

Fowkes and Hunn,[35] discussing "legal considerations" in clinical assessment for the nurse practitioner in 1973, express the opinion that proposed revision in state nurse practice acts will define "areas of responsibility" and "provide legal coverage."

In Canada, a joint statement of the Canadian Nurses' Association and the Canadian Medical Association on the expanded role of the nurse included the following:

> . . . priority should be given to expanding the role of nurses who work in direct and close association with physicians in the field of primary health care. . . .
>
> . . . primary health care . . . refers to . . . services . . . provided for individuals mainly on an ambulatory basis in the community or in their homes and includes . . . diagnostic and therapeutic services offered in physicians' offices, in clinics or in health centers. . . .

The Joint Committee concluded that the roles of nurses and physicians are "interdependent," that the associative role is an "evolving one," and that the "mix of professionals working in a setting will influence what a nurse would regularly do." The Joint Committee said that the "ultimate responsibility for diagnosis and establishment of a medical therapeutic plan will remain with the physician." The Canadian report seemed to suggest that with special preparation, graduates of 2-year or 3-year basic nursing programs might take over "selected responsibilities now tending to be handled by physicians" if the nurse is working "in association with the physician."[j]

In a period of rapid social change—and no one questions that this is one of them—it is understandable that roles of the doctors and nurses change and that change alters their relationship. As nurses take over in certain institutions and agencies the function of health assessment for all or groups of patients, it may be expected that they will bring to it the emphasis of nursing, which has been on how people cope with life, or the daily activities of living, rather than on the existence within them of a particular disease.[k] For this reason, nursing has welcomed Weed's approach to medical management, since it emphasizes identification of patients' problems rather than the identification of a particular disease or *the* diagnosis.[36,37,38] Mack Lipkin, whose text *The Care of Patients, Concepts and Tactics* (Oxford University Press, New York, 1974) is as helpful to nurses as to physicians, makes the following comment on the Weed system:

> Its advantages are numerous and important. Properly used, it produces better data, better organized. It encourages a clearer appreciation of the pa-

tient's problems and their logical evaluation. It has been a powerful stimulus to changing the existing pattern of devoting more teaching time to pathophysiology than to the needs of the patient. (p. 108)

Because certain nurses have thought that they needed something more than the medical diagnosis to guide them in giving nursing care, they propose that nurses make a "nursing diagnosis" for each patient. They see the nurse's diagnosis as something apart from the physician's diagnosis.

Kristine Gebbie and Mary Ann Lavin, in a report of the First National Conference on the Classification of Nursing Diagnoses held at St. Louis University, October 1973, gave the following "Tentative List of [34] Nursing Diagnoses,"[1] which are listed alphabetically because the conference participants couldn't agree on a classification system:

Alterations in faith

Altered relationships with self and others

Altered self-concept

Anxiety

Body fluids, depletion of

Bowel function, irregular

Cognitive functioning, alteration in the level of

Comfort level, alterations in

Confusion (disorientation)

Deprivation

Digestion, impairment of

Family's adjustment to illness, impairment of

Family process, inadequate

Fear

Grieving

Lack of understanding

Level of consciousness, alterations in

Malnutrition

Manipulation

Mobility, impaired

Motor incoordination

Noncompliance

Pain

Regulatory function of the skin, impairment of

Respiration, impairment of

Respiratory distress

Self-care activities, altered ability to perform

Sensory disturbances

Skin integrity, impairment of

Sleep–rest pattern, ineffective

Susceptibility to hazards

Thought process, impaired

Urinary elimination, impairment of

Verbal communication, impairment of

Most of these diagnoses are psychosocial problems in coping with which the patient presumably needs help from nurses. Gebbie and Lavin note that it has taken the medical profession 300 years to develop the "sophisticated" *International Classification of Diseases and Systematized Nomenclature of Pathology*: they suggest that nursing should "learn from other disciplines" but they imply that it should develop a parallel list of nursing diagnoses. It may be that nursing will take this direction or it may be that nursing and medicine will develop a thoroughly collaborative role in which the patient will benefit from the medical emphasis on specific pathology and the nurse's sensitivity to the psychosocial needs of the patient. The latter approach has been taken in this text and seems to be suggested by the writings of Weed and other physicians, who say that all professional health workers may identify patient problems, and by Bates and her associates, who call attention to the improvement of patient care through "nurse-physician teamwork."[38-40]

Just as diagnosis or patient problems may be identified collaboratively by the patient, the physician, the nurse (and other health professionals), the decision-making, treatment, or course of action is most likely to be effective if it is arrived at jointly.

In the report of a study of the nurse's role made by Evelyn R. Anderson for the Royal College of Nursing and the National Council of Nurses of the United Kingdom, it is noted that "the doctor is most concerned with the technical aspects of the nurse's work," but later Anderson says, "Nurses must not stress technical competence at the expense of continuing to give emotional support that is so strongly needed, as *evidenced by patient comments*. Therefore the training of doctors and nurses should include methods of dealing with the emotional problems of hospitalized patients." In another context Anderson says "Doctor/nurse partnerships in the form of health teams in the community are being advanced. The nurse in 1980 may be moving freely between home and hospital, being responsible for family groups in a role similar to that of the family [medical] practitioner. This changing role will require much adaptation from the nursing profession."[m]

The role of the nurse in health assessment, diagnosis, and decision-making is under discussion around the world, as evidenced by programs at the 1973 International Council of Nurses' Quadrennial Meeting in Mexico. The Josiah Macy, Jr. Foundation sponsored two conferences on the roles of various health workers in delivering health care in various countries.[41,42] The National Science Foundation in the United States sponsored the preparation of a critical annotated bibliography of research on new health practitioners [nurse practitioners, physician's assistants, and others]. By 1974, about 200 studies had been identified.[43]

There is general agreement that the nurse's actual role has, throughout this century, often been a more independent one than is reflected in nurse practice acts; that nurse practice acts should be amended to enable nurses to legally practice more independently and to be accountable for their acts. It is also believed by many that nursing education must regularly prepare professional nurses for independent practice—most especially for clinical assessment, diagnosis, and decision-making.

As indicated throughout this chapter, the decision or plan of care, is always, in the final analysis, the right of the adult, or, for the infant or child, the right of the parents or guardian. The "decision" of the health worker can take the form of health counseling or prescribing treatment but either can be accepted or rejected by the patient or the parents or guardian.

If prevention of disease is really more important than its cure, and many writers say that more "health dollars" should be spent on prevention than on cure, it follows that health counseling is more important than treatment. Malleson,[44] in his critique of medical care titled *Need Your Doctor Be So Useless?* seems to come to this conclusion. He believes no system yet devised is really effective; he thinks "treatment can be lethal," and he believes drugs are overused by doctors. He cited studies indicating that doctors spend so little time with patients that they can't possibly know enough about patients' conditions to prescribe drugs, particularly dangerous drugs and ones that demand close medical supervision. Malleson attributes much of the abuse of drugs to the fact that the public expects, even demands, drug prescriptions from the doctor. Whatever treatment medical workers give, Malleson makes the over-all judgment that it tends to produce dependency rather than self-reliance, which should be the goal of therapy. Like Samuels and Bennett,[45] Ivan Illich,[46a] and Rick J. Carlson[46b] Malleson sees the concerned, educated, independent patient as the only hope for reversing the unfortunate consequences of much of the present-day spiraling medical care and its spiraling cost.

Health counseling begins with population control—preventing the birth of unwanted children and diseased or defective children. The increasing incidence of "the battered child syndrome" is, according to some writers, a symptom of overpopulation. Preventing the birth of unwanted children is certainly one effective approach to abolishing child abuse. Another way of attacking the problem is to prevent the birth of defective infants by genetic counseling,[n] for defective children are most likely to be abused.

Genetics is a rapidly developing science and the significance of DNA (deoxyribonucleic acid) has received wide attention in professional and popular journals. As everyone knows, this global subject involves controversy. The very titles of recent works on the subject suggest it: *Brave New Baby; Promise and Peril of the Biological Revolution* (David M. Rorwik, 1971)[47]; *Fabricated Man; The Ethics of Genetic Control* (Paul Ramsey, 1970)[48]; *Early Diagnosis of Human Genetic Defects; Scientific and Ethical Considerations* (M. Harris, ed., 1971)[49]; and *Moral Dilemmas in Contraceptive Developments* (R. F. R. Gardner, 1973).[50] There are general texts on genetics such as *The Genetics of Human Populations* (L. L. Cavalli-Sforza and L. L. Bodmer, 1971)[51]; *Principles of Genetics* (E. J. Gardner, 1971)[52]; and general works on genetic counseling such as that by Alan C. Stevenson and his associates[53] and James R. Sorenson[54]; and genetics in medical practice by M. Bartolos.[55] In some general works on nursing, as for example *Advanced Concepts in Clinical Nursing* by Kay Corman Kintzel, there is a chapter on genetics and the nurse.[56] Since 1966 articles have been appearing in nursing journals that point out opportunities nurses have for genetic counseling.[57-60]

In 1971, Theodore Friedmann[61] published, in *Scientific American*, an article, "Prenatal Diagnosis of Genetic Disease," in which he said that over 1600 diseases are known to be genetically determined. Examples are cystic fibrosis, sickle cell anemia, and phenylketonuria. (The last condition has had, perhaps, most attention.)[62-64] Forty diseases, according to Friedmann, can be diagnosed prenatally from samples of amniotic fluid. Pregnant women over 35, many persons believe, should have genetic evaluations and be counseled according to the findings.

Claire O. Leonard and associates[65] evaluated the effectiveness of genetic counseling by physicians, giving "the consumer's view." Their findings reinforce the conclusion that this is a complex problem with which few health professionals are prepared to help people effectively and it is a problem few parents will face. Nursing education programs should provide opportunities for nurses who assume the role of genetic counselors to make a special study of the subject. Nurses may be employed in genetic clinics and specialize in this field. Considering the improvement in plants and animals that has resulted from the application of genetic principles, it seems as if humans might learn how to apply genetic principles to the improvement of the human race.

Actually, all health counseling is as specialized as clinical practice, and while all nurses might be expected to give generalized help, the most effective counseling on child care comes from pediatric nurses and counseling on problems of the aged from geriatric nurses. Following examinations in which disease is diagnosed, the patient with cancer, for example, should get the best help from the oncologic nurse; the patient with heart disease from the cardiac nurse; and the patient with tuberculosis from the nurse who has specialized in chest disease.

The nurse's role in diagnosis and decision-making always involves patients and families; most often nurses are members of a team of health workers. They participate in these processes with other professionals in helping the client or patient. In some cases, when other health workers are unavailable or when nurses assume responsibility for giving primary care, act as principal therapists or as private practitioners, they may play as independent a role as the physician, the dentist, the clinical psychologist, or the marriage counselor. There are hundreds of articles that might be cited dealing with this old but newly articulated function of the nurse. Reference has been made to published bibliographies and to those in preparation and to specific reports.[66-74]

Notes

---

[a]DeGowin, E. L., & DeGowin, R. L.: *Bedside Diagnostic Examination*, 3rd ed. Macmillan Publishing Co., Inc. New York, 1976.

[b]Judge, Richard D., and Zuidema, George D.: *Physical Diagnosis, A Physiologic Approach to the Clinical Examination*, 2nd ed. Little, Brown & Co., Boston, 1968, p. 9.

[c]Engel, George L., and Morgan, William L.: *Interviewing the Patient*. W. B. Saunders Co., Philadelphia, 1973, p. 16.

[d]Reid, J. J. A.: "Preventive Medicine. In Great Britain," in the Royal Society of Medicine and the Josiah Macy, Jr. Foundation: *The Greater Medical Profession.* The Foundation, New York, 1973, p. 111.

[e]"Basic Health Care Changes Needed, Nurse Tells Physicians' Meeting," *Can. Nurse,* 69:7, (Nov.) 1973.

[f]New York State, Senate-Assembly: *An Act to Amend the Law in Relation to the Practice of Nursing, 1972.* N.Y. Ed. Law Section 6902.

[g]Jacobi, Eileen M.: "Accountability of the Nurse." "Are There Legal Barriers to Assuming Full Professional Responsibility?" (Speeches presented during the 48th Convention of the American Nurses' Association.) The Association, Kansas City, Mo., 1973, p. 1.

[h]Hall, Virginia C.: *Statutory Regulation of the Scope of Nursing Practice—A Critical Survey.* National Joint Practice Commission, Chicago, 1975, pp. 21–22.

[i]Kelly, Lucie Young: "Nursing Practice Acts," *Am. J. Nurs.,* 74:1310, (July) 1974.

[j]"The Expanded Role of the Nurse: A Joint Statement of CNA/CMA," *Can. Nurse,* 69:23, (May) 1973; "Extended Role of the Nurse and Preparation for It as Defined in Canadian RN–MD Statement," *Am. J. Nurs.,* 73:964, (June) 1973.

[k]Joan E. Lynaugh and Barbara Bates, a nurse and physician, discussing "The Two Languages of Nursing and Medicine," (*Am. J. Nurs.,* 73:66, [Jan.] 1973) note that, among the contrasting emphases, nurses talk about patients' problems and how nurses can help them deal with them; physicians talk about the diagnosis and treatment.

[l]Gebbie, Kristine, and Lavin, Mary Ann: "Classifying Nursing Diagnoses," *Am. J. Nurs.,* 74:250 (Feb.) 1974.

[m]Anderson, Evelyn R.: *The Role of the Nurse. Views of the Patient, Nurse and Doctor in some General Hospitals in England.* The Study of Nursing Care Project Reports, Series 2. Number 1. Royal College of Nursing, London, 1973.

[n]In genetic counseling, someone with special knowledge of genetics (physician, nurse, physiologist, or other) discusses the inheritance of defects and diseases with parents, or potential partners, and its implications for birth control, abortion, treatment during pregnancy, and family planning.

References

1. Samuels, Mike, and Bennett, Hal: *The Well Body Book*. Random House, New York, 1973.

2. Friedson, Eliot: *Professional Dominance: The Social Structure of Medical Care*. Aldine-Atherton, Inc., Chicago, 1970.

3. Bates, Barbara: "Comprehensive Medicine; a Conference Approach With Inpatient Emphasis," *J. Med. Educ., 40*:778, (Apr.) 1986.

4. _____: "Nurse-Physician Teamwork," *Med. Care, 4*:69, (Apr.–June) 1966.

5. _____, and Kern, M. Sue: "Doctor-Nurse Teamwork: What Helps? What Hinders?" *Am. J. Nurs., 67*:2066, (Oct.) 1967.

6. _____: "Doctor and Nurse: Changing Roles and Relations," *N Engl. J. Med., 283*:129, (July 16) 1970.

7. _____, and Chamberlin, Robert W.: "Physician Leadership as Perceived by Nurses," *Nurs. Res., 19*:534, (Dec.) 1970.

8. "Nursing in a Health Maintenance Organization. Report on the Harvard Community Health Plan," *Am. J. Public Health, 62*:991, (July) 1972.

9. Lynaugh, Joan E., and Bates, Barbara: *op. cit.*

10. Engel, George L.: "A Unified Concept of Health and Disease." *Perspectives on Biology and Medicine 3*:459, (Summer) 1960.

11. Feinstein, Alvin R.: *Clinical Judgment*. Williams & Wilkins Co., Baltimore, 1967, p. 25.

12. Weed, Lawrence L.: "Medical Records That Guide and Teach, Parts 1 and 2," *N. Engl. J. Med., 278*:593, (March 14); :652, (March 21) 1968.

13. Carnegie Commission on Higher Education: *Higher Education and the Nation's Health—Policies for Medical and Dental Education*. McGraw-Hill Book Company, New York, 1970.

14. Dillon, John B.: "How Did It Happen?" *Calif. Med. 113*:86, (Aug.) 1970.

15. U.S. Department of Health, Education, and Welfare; Regional Council for International Education: *The Dynamics of Interinstitutional Cooperation in International Education*. U.S. Government Printing Office, Washington, D.C., 1971.

16. Surawicz, Frida, and Sandifer, M. G.: "Cross Cultural Diagnosis: A Study of Psychiatric Diagnosis Comparing Switzerland, the United States and the United Kingdom," *Int. J. Soc. Psychiatry, 16*:232, (Summer) 1970.

17. World Health Organization: *International Classification of Diseases*, 8th ed. The Organization, Geneva, 1963, Vol. 1.

18. Bates, Barbara, and Kern, M. Sue: *op. cit.*

19. Bates, Barbara: "Doctor and Nurse: Changing Roles and Relations," *N. Engl J. Med., 283*:129, (July 16) 1970.

20. Aradine, Carolyn R., and Pridham, Karen F.: "Model for Collaboration," *Nurs. Outlook, 21*:655, (Oct.) 1973.

21. Silver, Henry K., et al.: "Pediatric Nurse-Practitioner Program; Expanding the Role of the Nurse to Provide Increased Health Care for Children," *J.A.M.A., 204*:298, (Apr. 22) 1968.

22. deCastro, Fernando J., and Rolfe, Ursula T.: *The Pediatric Nurse Practitioner*, 2nd ed. C. V. Mosby Co., St. Louis, 1976.

23. Pinder, J. E.: "A Reply to the Role Conflicts of the New Breed Health Visitor." *Health Visitor, 44*:188, (June) 1971.

24. O'Boyle, Catherine: "A New Era in Emergency Service," *Am. J. Nurs., 72*:1392. (Aug.) 1972.

25. Sheedy, Susan Gerberding: "Medical Nurse Practitioner in a Neighborhood Clinic." *Am. J. Nurs., 72*:1416, (Aug.) 1972.

26. Garfield, Sidney R.: "Delivery of Medical Care" *Sci. Am. 222*:15 (Apr.) 1970.

27. Poole, Ernest: *Nurses on Horseback.* Macmillan Publishing Co., Inc., New York, 1932.

28. "Family Nurse Practitioner Program," *Frontier Nurs. Serv. Q. Bull., 47*:31, (Summer) 1971.

29. Schutt, Barbara G.: "Frontier's Family Nurses," *Am. J. Nurs., 72*:903, (May) 1972.

30. Bain, H. W., and Goldthorpe, Garey: "The University of Toronto Sioux Lookout Project: A Model of Health Care Delivery." *Can. Med. Assoc. J., 107*:523, (Sept. 23) 1972.

31. DeMarsh, Kathleen G.: "Red Cross Outpost Nursing in New Brunswick," *Can. Nurse, 69*:24, (June) 1973.

32. Hazlett, C. B.: "Task Analysis of the Clinically Trained Nurse (C.T.N.)," *Nurs. Clin. North Am., 10*:699, (Dec.) 1975.

33. Keith, Catharine W.: *Role and Preparation of the Outpost Nurse (Canada).* (Paper prepared for Pan American Conference on Health Manpower Planning, Ottawa, Sept. 1973). Processed.

34. Sutherland, Ruth, and Besner, Jeanne: "Community Nursing in a Northern Setting," *Nurs. Clin. North Am., 10*:731, (Dec.) 1975.

35. Fowkes, William C., Jr., and Hunn, Virginia K., *Clinical Assessment for the Nurse Practitioner.* C. V. Mosby Co., St. Louis, 1973, p. 5.

36. Weed, Lawrence L.: "Medical Records That Guide and Teach, Parts 1 and 2." *N. Engl. J. Med., 278*:593, (March. 14); 278:652, (Mar. 21) 1968.

37. _____: *Medical Records; Medical Education and Patient Care.* Press of Case-Western Reserve University, Cleveland, 1970.

37a. _____: *Your Health Care and How to Manage It.* Promise Laboratory, University of Vermont, Burlington, 1975.

38. Bjorn, J. C., and Cross, H. D.: *Problem-Oriented Private Practice of Medicine: System for Comprehensive Health Care.* Modern Hospital Press, McGraw-Hill Publications Co., New York, 1970.

39. Bates, Barbara: "Nurse-Physician Teamwork," *Med. Care, 4*:69, (Apr.–June) 1966.

40. _____, and Kern, M. Sue: *op cit.*

41. The Royal Society of Medicine and the Josiah Macy, Jr. Foundation: *The Greater Medical Profession.* The Foundation, New York, 1973.

42. Lippard, Vernon W., and Purcell, Elizabeth R. (eds.): *Intermediate-Level Health Practitioners.* Josiah Macy, Jr. Foundation, New York, 1973.

43. Cohen, Eva D. (ed.): *Evaluation of Research on New Health Practitioners.* (Under a grant from the National Science Foundation, Office of Regional Activities and Continuing Education.) Yale University School of Medicine, New Haven, Conn., 1974.

44. Malleson, Andrew: *op. cit.*

45. Samuels, Mike, and Bennett, Hal: *op. cit.*

46a. Illich, Ivan: *Medical Nemesis. The Expropriation of Health.* McClelland & Stewart, Ltd., Toronto, 1975.

46b. Carlson, Rick J.: *The End of Medicine.* John Wiley & Sons, New York, 1975.

47. Rorwik, David M.: *Brave New Baby; Promise and Peril of the Biological Revolution.* Doubleday & Co., Garden City, N.Y., 1971.

48. Ramsey, Paul: *Fabricated Man. The Ethics of Genetic Control.* Yale University Press, New Haven, Conn., 1970.

49. Harris, M. (ed.): *Early Diagnosis of Human Genetic Defects; Scientific and Ethical Considerations.* U.S. Government Printing Office, Washington, D.C., 1971.

50. Gardner, R. F. R.: *Moral Dilemmas in Contraceptive Developments.* CMF Publications, London, [1973].

51. Cavalli-Sforza, L. L., and Bodmer, L. L.: *The Genetics of Human Populations.* W. H. Freeman, San Francisco, 1971.

52. Gardner, E. J.: *Principles of Genetics*, 4th ed. John Wiley & Sons, New York, [1971].

53. Stevenson, Alan C., et al.: *Genetic Counseling*. J. B. Lippincott Co., Philadelphia, 1970.

54. Sorensen, James R.: *Genetic Counseling*. Princeton University, Princeton, N.J., 1971.

55. Bartolos, M. (ed.): *Genetics in Medical Practice*. J. B. Lippincott Co., Philadelphia, 1968.

56. Kintzel, Kay Corman, and Lake, Dolores: "Medical Genetics and the Nurse," in Kintzel, Kay Corman (ed.): *Advanced Concepts in Clinical Nursing*. J. B. Lippincott Co., Philadelphia, 1971.

57. Forbes, N.: "The Nurse and Genetic Counseling," *Nurs. Clin. North Am., 1*:679, (Dec.) 1966.

58. Hillman, G. M.: "Genetics and the Nurse," *Nurs. Outlook, 14*:34, (Jan.) 1966.

59. Nitowsky, Harold M.: "Prenatal Diagnosis of Genetic Abnormality," *Am. J. Nurs., 71*:1551, (Oct.) 1971.

60. Ragsdale, N., and Koch, R.: "Phenylketonuria: Detection and Therapy," *Am. J. Nurs., 64*:90, (Jan.) 1964.

61. Friedmann, Theodore: "Prenatal Diagnosis of Genetic Disease," *Sci. Am., 225*:34, (Nov.) 1971.

62. Lake, D.: "Nursing Implications from an Investigation of Mothering, Diet and Development in Two Groups of Children with Phenylketonuria," in *ANA Clinical Sessions, 1968*. Appleton-Century-Crofts, New York, 1968.

63. U.S. Health Services and Mental Health Administration, Maternal and Child Health Service: *State Laws Pertaining to Phenylketonuria as of November 1970*. U.S. Government Printing Office, Washington, D.C., 1971.

64. _____: *What Do You Know About PKU?* U. S. Government Printing Office, Washington, D.C., 1972.

65. Leonard, Claire O., et al.: "Genetic Counseling: A Consumer's View," *N. Engl. J. Med., 287*:443, (Aug. 31) 1972.

66. Mundinger, Mary O'Neill: "Primary Nurse—Role Evaluation," *Nurs. Outlook, 21*:642, (Oct.) 1973.

67. Mussallem, Helen K.: "The Changing Role of the Nurse," *Am. J. Nurs., 69*:514, (Mar.) 1969.

68. National Commission for the Study of Nursing and Nursing Education: *Nurse Clinician and Physician's Assistant: The Relationship Between two Emerging Practitioner Concepts*. The Commission, Rochester, [1971].

69. Perry, Lesley: *The Nurse as a Primary Health Provider and the Nurse*

Practitioner: An Annotated Bibliography. Genesee Valley Nurses' Association, Rochester, N.Y., 1971.

70. Pranulis, Maryann F., and Roth, Oscar: "Medical and Legal Aspects of the Role of the Nurse in Coronary Care," in *Yearbook of Legal Medicine.* Appleton-Century-Crofts, New York, 1972.

71. Reed, D. E., et al.: "Acceptability of an Expanded Nurse Role to Nurses and Physicians," *Med. Care, 9*:372, (July–Aug.) 1971.

72. Sheedy, Susan Gerberding: *op. cit.*

73. Sheldon, Alan, and Hope, Penelope K.: "Developing Role of the Nurse in a Community Mental Health Program," *Perspect. Psychiatr. Care, 5*:272, (Nov.–Dec.) 1967.

74. Stolar, Vera, and Rubenstain, Reva: "Developing the Science Component in a PRIMEX Program," *Nurs. Outlook, 21*:325, (May) 1973.

Chapter 6

Plans of Care

Importance of a Unified Plan

The importance of having a plan of care (including nursing care) for the patient in a hospital or nursing home is now recognized by the Joint Commission on Accreditation of Hospitals and the Social Security Administration of the United States government.[1,2] Both of these organizations require that institutions include a written care plan as part of the complete patient record for purposes of accreditation and certification for public funding. However, it would be misleading to imply that written plans of patient care, as interpreted by the authors, with stated goals for therapy and rehabilitation can be found in all or even the majority of health agencies. Rudy L. Ciuca,[3] in 1972, reported that a survey of 235 randomly chosen nursing care plans from six hospitals on the West Coast showed that almost 75 percent of the notations were concerned with functional duties such as medications given, treatments completed, the monitoring of vital signs, intake and output (how much fluid the patient takes in and eliminates), and diagnostic studies. Only 1.7 percent of the notations on the nursing care plans related to rehabilitation or planning for discharge.

One of the many reasons why nursing care plans have been inadequately used is that they are of necessity complex, and a single, universally acceptable form has not yet been developed. *It is hard to imagine anything requiring more insight, knowledge, skill, and cooperative effort on the part of the sick person, the family, and health workers than making a plan of care as interpreted here.*

When several workers are responsible for planning and giving care to a patient, it goes without saying that some means must be devised to coordinate their efforts and direct them toward a common goal. In some institutions and health agencies, regular time is set aside for discussing the care and progress of patients. These meetings, called *"case,"* or *patient conferences,* may be attended by doctors, nurses, dietitians, social workers, and others. In some of them, patients and their families are invited into the conference so that they can contribute to it and learn from the discussion how to take care of themselves when they go home. If patients and families participate, health workers can learn far more about how they can help patients change their patterns of living to meet their health needs than they can otherwise. Mental health agencies are perhaps most likely to ask patients and families to participate in conferences and encourage patients to set their own goals so the most constructive use may be made of the agency and its personnel. *Nursing rounds* that include all nursing personnel with perhaps a nurse specialist, a head nurse, or a team leader are used in some hospitals as a way of identifying patients' problems, discussing nursing plans, and coordinating nursing care of patients. The "rounds" are conducted at the bedside.[4,5] For people who have roommates it is desirable to take them to a conference room since patients rarely like to discuss their problems within the hearing of other patients. Some method for exchange of information and planning of care should be used; otherwise, many of the patient's needs may not be considered and therapy for these may go unplanned.

Although many nurses believe that gathering necessary information about a patient and writing a plan for comprehensive care require too much time from a schedule that is already full; others, who have used various tools for these purposes, have found that time is simply put to a better use when they make a plan. L. Mae McPhetridge[6] found that most "nursing history" interviews required about 30 minutes to complete, and while the information gathered might also have been acquired over a period of several days, having it early in the patient's hospital stay was considered a great advantage. Philothea R. Sweet and Irmagene Stark[7] say that when a Nursing Information Record was developed for obstetric patients and used on initial contact and accompanied them throughout their prenatal parturient, and postnatal periods (with all nurses using the information and adding to it) there was less duplication of information and therefore less duplication of effort by various health workers in planning for and caring for these women. Also, patients were better informed, seemed less apprehensive about their pregnancies, and were better prepared for motherhood. Continuity of care was assured.

Effective nursing has always involved problem-solving, planning, and evaluation. There has been a concerted effort in recent decades to establish a definition of nursing, a theory (or theories) of nursing, and a science of nursing. Some persons find it helpful to use the term "the nursing process." In 1961, Ida Jean Orlando presented *The Dynamic Nurse–Patient Relationship: Function, Process and Principles*. She says, "A nursing situation is comprised of three basic elements: (1) the behavior of the patient, (2) the reaction of the nurse, and (3) the nursing actions which are designed for the patient's benefit. *The interaction of these elements with each other is nursing process.*"[a] Obviously she looks upon the term as explaining the essential momentary, hourly, and daily activity of anyone who nurses analytically. Her most helpful contribution to the development of nursing is, in our opinion, the insistence that nurses tell the patient what their reactions are and how they interpret the patient's behavior. This gives the patient a chance to correct the nurses' interpretation before it is acted upon.

In 1973 the Nursing Development Conference Group presented *Concept Formalization in Nursing: Process and Product*,[7a] in which are discussed and diagrammed "dominant themes" in concepts of nursing from Florence Nightingale to contemporary concepts. Looking at the index of this book under "Nursing Process" one finds "*See* Practice of Nursing." So, "nursing" is an adequate term for some, "nursing process" more helpful for others, and "nursing practice" may be synonymous with both.

Other nurses[8,9] have described steps or phases within the process of planning patient care: (1) taking a history; (2) identifying health problems; (3) setting goals with and for the client, or patient; (4) describing nursing action (or intervention); and (5) evaluating the client's, or patient's, progress (by use of selected criteria) both concurrently and when care is terminated.

One way to see how these steps in the process of planning patient care are employed jointly by all members of a health care team is to study patient care plans. In some institutions where the problem-oriented medical record (POMR) is used, nurses help to build the data base. The nursing history may be separate from or combined with the medical and psychosocial history. In the POMR system, progress notes for the client, or patient, include, in chronologic order, the reports and observations of all professional personnel involved in caring for the patient.[10-14] Whether this particular method helps the nurse evaluate or audit nursing care as separate from medical care has not been determined.

Health Problems and Determining the Patient's Need for Nursing

A *health problem* has been defined as an interruption in the individual's ability to meet a need, and a *nursing need* has been defined as whatever the person requires in knowledge, will, or strength to perform his or her daily activities and to carry out treatments prescribed for him or her, or as a "requirement of the patient which, if supplied, relieves or diminishes his [or her] . . distress or improves his [or her] . . . sense of adequacy or well-being."[b]

When identifying an individual's health problems and needs, nurses must analyze the information they got through observations and interviewing, and call upon all their knowledge about people's behavior that can inhibit or improve their functioning. A number of models for the organization of problems and needs have been proposed and may be helpful.[15-20e]

Setting Goals

The establishment of goals or objectives as part of the patient's plan of care not only gives the nurse and patient a specific point to be reached but also provides a basis for evaluating the patient's progress and the care given by nurses, physicians, and other health workers. Some goals for patient care are formulated by nurses based on their areas of expertise and interest and some are complex goals requiring that a team of health workers confer on the appropriate statement of the goal and the means to reach it. Berniece M. Wagner[21] urges that goals be stated as patient behavior (not as nursing action); they are to be stated in specific terms and should deal with the patient's future as well as the present. She thinks nurses should not hesitate to state them in physiologic or pathologic terms. Marlene G. Mayers[22] makes the point that too often the established goals, particularly those that are short-term, are not assigned a time deadline. She believes that saying when the goal should be reached is one way of determining the patient's progress. If the goal is not being reached, a revision of nursing action may be necessary.

Dolores E. Little and Doris L. Carnevali[23] caution that in some cases a too specific or narrow goal focuses attention on only a small part of the problem when a somewhat more general goal might help the patient more and permit a greater diversity of nursing action. For instance, the nursing objective for a 4-year-old boy hospitalized with pneumonia and there without his mother was "To decrease crying by using operant conditioning."[c] A more general objective, but one that focused on the basic problem, might have been "To relieve fears of abandonment and punishment."

Whatever objectives or goals (with their related problems) are established, the order in which they will be met should also be considered by the patient, family, and nurse. Fay L. Bower[25] says that problems that threaten the life and integrity of an individual, family, or community should have the highest priority; problems that threaten a destructive change in the individual, family, or community the next priority; and problems that affect normal growth of the individual, family, or community the next priority.

As goals or objectives are met in a priority order, short-term and long-term goals become apparent. New goals may develop as more is learned about the person, or, as immediate goals are reached, those with a lower priority in the initial plan may advance to a higher priority. Nurses also should consider that more than one goal can be reached in a single situation. For instance, when giving a preschool child an oral medication the goal of helping the child grow in self-mastery and carry out distasteful tasks can be met at the same time.

Long-term illness, or one that is chronic, threatening to life, or threatening to the body image, often increases *dependency*. The nurse should therefore help the person develop specific objectives early in the nursing care plan that will foster independence.

Types of Plans and Forms Used

The plan of care for patients includes an immediate and a long-term program designed with reference to each patient's problems and needs and the conditions under which he or she lives. In some cases, the latter type is all that is needed. The program or plan is made by the physician in collaboration with the patient and his or her family or possibly a friend, the nurse, the dietitian, the social worker, special therapists, and other health workers associated in care of the patient: in some cases, the clergyman may play a significant role. The person for whom the plan is made, if he or she is not too sick and has reached the age of reason, participates in making and executing the plan, since the patient's acceptance of the plan is essential to its success. It is important that all concerned with the program of care should know the central therapeutic aim and related goals. It is equally important that there should be a schedule of care for the patient, known to all those who are responsible for its execution, in order to prevent omissions and overlapping.

There are differing opinions about the amount of detail that should be in a written plan.[26-28] Some experienced nurses believe that with a patient objective such as "Increase oral fluid intake to 1500 ml daily," details about the kinds of drinks enjoyed by the patient, whether he needs or wants help with drinking, whether he abhors paper cups or cannot use a cup of any kind, or whether he needs constant, consistent reminding about taking fluids should be in the written plan. Others believe this kind of information should be found in the health history or obtained in nursing conferences and believe writing this information consumes unnecessary time and creates an inflexible plan. But the inclusion of details increases the continuity of care and gives patients assurance that the nursing staff considers them as individuals since they are not repeatedly questioned about likes and dislikes or abilities and disabilities. Usually the nurse, or other health worker, has less than complete information about patients and their situations, but to wait until the information is complete drastically limits necessary care. Nurses, with the patient and any others involved, therefore should make a decision for action weighing the probability of risk against the probability of benefit. An excellent description of the decision-making process can be found in Bower's *The Process of Planning Nursing Care*.[29]

Cooperation among workers and consistency in treatment and care are fostered by patient conferences and by the use of written plans of care kept with the patient's record. Written plans of care seem to provide the surest means of making the schedule known to all concerned. Planning treatment and care on an individual basis means that those who plan it must acquire a certain amount of information about the patient in order that they may analyze his or her problems and needs. Such data make up the *patient studies* in medicine, nursing, and social work. All professional workers in attendance on the patient share the responsibility for continuously assessing the patient's needs; therefore a record system that makes the findings or observations of each available to all should be used. All categories of health workers should have a clear understanding of their functions in relation to planning and executing the care of the patient. If they are not defined, there are apt to be overlapping and omissions.

Collecting all pertinent information about a patient is known as a *patient study*. William Osler and great doctors in all ages have stressed the present practice of teaching medicine through the study of individual cases. It seems self-evident that nurses cannot make effective plans for care of the patient without preparing such studies. The study need not necessarily take written form. If nurses are to discuss the patient's care in a conference, however, they may find it valuable to make notes on the salient facts and the way in which they affect nursing care; or, if they are preparing a study of a patient to be published or read by others, they may give this information in a narrative form.

Notes

---

[a]Orlando, Ida Jean: *The Dynamic Nurse–Patient Relationship: Function, Process, and Principles.* G. P. Putnam's Sons, New York, 1961, p. 36.

[b]Orlando, Ida Jean: *op. cit.*, p. 5.

[c]Operant conditioning also called reinforcement therapy, and sometimes behavior modification, is based on B. F. Skinner's work in the psychology of learning. Briefly, the basic tenets are that behavior is learned; learning is the result of reinforcement; behavior that is rewarded becomes pleasurable and is repeated; and behavior that is ignored or not rewarded gradually fades and finally stops.[24]

References

---

1. Joint Commission on Accreditation of Hospitals; *Standards for Accreditation of Hospitals.* The Joint Commission, Chicago, 1969, p. 22.

2. US Social Security Administration: *Conditions of Participation for Hospitals: Federal Health Insurance for the Aged.* (Code of Federal Regulations, Title 20, Chapter 3, Part 405, Section 1024–g.) U.S. Government Printing Office, Washington, D.C., June 1967.

3. Ciuca, Rudy L.: "Over the Years with the Nursing Care Plan," *Nurs. Outlook, 20*:706, (Nov.) 1972.

4. Alman, Beatrice: "Patients Participate in Nursing Care Conferences,"*Am. J. Nurs., 67*:2331, (Nov.) 1967.

5. Unangst, Carol: "The Clinician's Use of Nursing Rounds," *Am. J. Nurs., 71*:1566, (Aug.) 1971.

6. McPhetridge, L. Mae: "Nursing History: One Means to Personalize Care," *Am. J. Nurs., 68*:68, (Jan.) 1968.

7. Sweet, Philothea R. and Stark, Irmagene: "The Circle Care Nursing Plan," *Am. J. Nurs., 70*:1300 (June)1970.

7a. Nursing Development Conference Group: *Concept Formalization in Nursing. Process and Product.* Little, Brown & Co., Boston, 1973.

8. Mauksch, Ingeborg G., and David, Miriam L.: "Prescription for Survival," *Am. J. Nurs., 72*:2189, (Dec.) 1972.

9. Carrieri, Virginia K., and Sitzman, Judith: "Components of the Nursing Process," *Nurs. Clin. North Am., 6*:115, (Mar.) 1971.

10. Hurst, J. Willis, and Walker, H. Kenneth (eds.): *The Problem-Oriented System*. Medcom, Inc,. New York, 1972.

11. Bloom, Judith T., et al.: "Problem-Oriented Charting," *Am. J. Nurs., 71*:2144, (Nov.) 1971.

12. Schell, Pamela L., and Campbell, Alla T.: "POMR—Not Just Another Way to Chart," *Nurs. Outlook, 20*:510, (Aug.) 1972.

13. Bonkowsky, Marilyn L.: "Adapting the POMR to Community Child Health Care,"*Nurs. Outlook, 20*:515, (Aug.) 1972.

14. Field, Frances W.: "Communication Between Community, Nurse, and Physician," *Nurs. Outlook, 19*:722, (Nov.) 1971.

15. Aiken, Linda H.: "Patient Problems Are Problems in Learning," *Am. J. Nurs., 70*:1916, (Sept.) 1970.

16. Pierce, Lillian M.: "A Patient-Care Model," *Am. J. Nurs., 69*:1700, (Aug.) 1969.

17. Nadler, Gerald, and Sahney, Vinod: "A Descriptive Model of Nursing Care," *Am. J. Nurs., 69*:336, (Feb.) 1969.

18. Tayrien, Dorothy, and Lipchak, Amelia: "The Single-Problem Approach," *Am. J. Nurs., 67*:2523, (Dec.) 1967.

19. Kraegel, Janet M., et al.: "A System of Patient Care Based on Patient Needs," *Nurs. Outlook, 20*:257, (Apr.) 1972.

20a. Smith, Dorothy M.: "Writing Objectives as a Nursing Practice Skill," *Am. J. Nurs., 71*:319, (Feb.) 1971.

20b Vitale, Barbara, et al.: *A Problem Solving Approach to Nursing Care Plans*. C. V. Mosby Co., St. Louis, 1974.

20c. Hefferin, Elizabeth A. and Hunter, Ruth E.: "Nursing Assessment and Care Plan Statements," *Nurs. Res., 24*:360, (Sept.–Oct.) 1975.

20d. Schaefer, Jeanette: "The Interrelatedness of Decision Making and the Nursing Process," *Am. J. Nurs., 74*:1852, (Oct.) 1974.

20e. Gebbie, Kristine, and Lavin, Mary Ann (eds.): *Classification of Nursing Diagnoses. Proceedings of First National Conference*, Oct. 1–5, 1973. C. V. Mosby, Co., St. Louis, 1975.

21. Wagner, Berniece M.: "Care Plans—Right, Reasonable and Reachable," *Am. J. Nurs., 69*:986, (May) 1969.

22. Mayers, Marlene G.: *A Systematic Approach to the Nursing Care Plan*. Appleton-Century-Crofts, New York, 1972.

23. Little, Dolores E. and Carnevali, Doris L.: *Nursing Care Planning.* J. B. Lippincott Co., Philadelphia, 1969, p. 164.

24. Baumeister, Alfred A. (ed.): *Mental Retardation.* Aldine Publishing Co., Chicago, 1967, p. 196.

25. Bower, Fay L.: *The Process of Planning Nursing Care.* C. V. Mosby Co., St. Louis, 1972. p. 14.

26. White, Marguerite B.: "Importance of Selected Nursing Activities," *Nurs. Res., 21*:4, (Jan.–Feb.) 1972.

27. Kaufmann, Margaret A.: "Autonomic Responses as Related to Nursing Comfort Measures," *Nurs. Res., 13*:45, (Winter) 1964.

28. Hallstrom, Betty J.: "Contact Comfort: Its Application to Immunization Injections," *Nurs. Res., 17*:130, (Mar.–Apr.) 1968.

29. Bower, Fay L.: *op. cit.*

Chapter 7

Preserving the Essence of Nursing in a Technological Age[1]

T he impersonal character of health service is the commonest criticism of it in our Western culture, but we imply that the essence of nursing lies in its personal, individualized and human character. I hope our inference is substantiated in fact; that those who value the "essence of nursing" do, indeed, give holistic rather than disease-centered care.

In 1976 I spoke at the Commonwealth University of Richmond, Virginia, on the essence of nursing. I said then what I believe I must, in all honesty, say here.

> Because rapid transit has made this a small world and because I believe human welfare depends upon international cooperation rather than competition I am drawn to a global, rather than a national consideration of nursing or health care. And because I believe that we cannot possibly understand nursing in any age unless we see it as an aspect of the social scene I must wonder whether the essence of nursing can be stated except in relation to the society in which it exists. I also believe that no one category of health workers should stake out a claim to their share of the burden—say they will do this but not that—without reference to the shares claimed by other workers and the effect on human welfare if some essential tasks involved in health care are disclaimed, or shunned, by all. (Henderson, 1977)

[1]"The Nursing Lecture 1979", sponsored by the Royal College of Nursing of the United Kingdom and delivered in Birmingham, England on 7 November 1979.

So you can see that I have no ready answer to the question, "What is the essence of nursing?"

I went on to ask whether nursing is a distinct entity, different from other health services; to what extent it overlaps medicine, social science, health education and other disciplines. I concluded then, as I do now, that there is overlapping of nursing with many other fields but that, perhaps, because it is the only 24-hour, 7-day-week service, nurses do have a unique function.

While I will necessarily repeat some of the things I said in 1977 it seems almost necessary to set forth what I believe to be the unique function of the nurse, or the essence of nursing, to help persons, sick or well, from birth to death, with those activities of daily living that they would perform unaided if they had the strength, the will and the knowledge. At the same time, and throughout this relationship, nurses help people to gain or regain their independence and when independence is impossible, to cope with handicaps and irreversible disease, and finally, to die with dignity when death is inevitable. This unique function of the nurse is a helping art, it is also a science. This concept is by no means new. Dr. R. P. Howard who was one of Dr. Osler's teachers advocated a liberal education for nurses similar to that of physicians followed by a 3-year professional education. He said nursing should be a scientific art (MacDermot, 1950). Nurses are rehabilitators par excellence and might have coined the phrase and described the process had they been more thoroughly educated, more analytical, and more aware of their potential role in society.

Florence Nightingale said that what nurses do is to put people in the best condition for nature to cure them and she added that nature alone cures—that neither doctors nor nurses cure (Nightingale, 1969 edn.). I see no conflict between Miss Nightingale's statement and my own attempt to describe what we are calling today "the essence of nursing." But along with this "essence" or unique function of nursing (of which nurses are masters—whose method of implementation they design and prescribe) nurses also help people carry out treatment prescribed by physicians. And, just as in the absence of physicians, all peoples treat themselves or may be treated by persons other than physicians, so in the absence of physicians, nurses perform functions ordinarily considered medical. Just as many a doctor in the absence of nurses performs the nurse's function or just as, in the absence of social workers, nurses and doctors help people with social problems. In Great Britain, Canada and the United States, there are many more nurses than doctors; in India the reverse is true. Could we expect nurses and doctors in India to function as they do in the industrialized Western countries?

(Some people disagree with me in this analysis of the nurse's function. They say, for example, that the nurse is the patient's advocate, the nurse is the promoter of health—concerned with care rather than cure, and so on. However, I maintain that the concept offered here is so open-ended that it can include all of these more limited definitions of nursing and many more that have been proposed.)

The role of the nurse-midwife most clearly demonstrates the overlapping function of nurse and physician. The so-called extended role of nurses in the care of children, the care of the aged and the chronically ill and, in fact, the care of all those without access to physicians, is coming to be as fully accepted as the role of the nurse-midwife. She is the established prototype of the nurse specialist.

Today we cannot prolong this discussion of the function of the nurse. For practical purposes I must assume that we are talking about the same thing when we say "the essence of nursing."

The question raised in this paper is, how can we make it possible for nurses to "get inside the skin" of patients, or clients, and discover what help they need and can use; what sort of health regimen or plan of care can then be developed with them and their families that will foster independence, optimum coping behaviour, or a peaceful death, and how can nurses then preserve this basic function while, at the same time, they meet the increasing demand for technical skill. Evelyn R. Anderson's (1973) study of the role of the nurse in England showed that nurses and patients stressed emotional support from the nurse while doctors stressed technical competence. It would be unfortunate if nurses seemed indifferent to the latter, however. Technical skills increase in number and complexity; they include physical and psychosocial evaluations and diagnostic tests, assisting with pre- and post-surgical care that involves the operation of sensitive and dangerous machines; also the administration of drugs whose numbers proliferate hourly and whose possible threats to human welfare should haunt those who give and those who take them.

To illustrate the conflict between the humane and the technical aspects of nursing, I will describe a single incident that will be familiar to most of you: on a summer afternoon I went to a hospital hoping to spend a few hours with a very ill friend in an intensive care unit. After waiting some time in a small waiting room filled with anxious relatives, I was told that I could see my friend for 5 minutes. He was one of a dozen men and women in a large, cold, almost windowless room furnished with beds, straight chairs, and forbidding monitoring and other equipment. Vigorous young nurses wearing stethoscopes around their necks seemed normally busy and, by contrast with the patients, outrageously cheerful—and more or less unconcerned. At no point did a nurse approach me to find out whether I might be able to give any support to this elderly widower who had no close relatives to visit him. My friend looked frightened and was very cold when I touched him. He said he had been "freezing all day." When I asked him whether he had told the nurses, he said, "Oh no; the nurses are so busy!" After less than 12 hours in this anxiety-laden, machine-dominated atmosphere even the patients were discounting the importance of simple human fear and physical discomfort as factors in recovery! The patient's doctor, a notably humanistic practitioner, came to see him while I was there. We went out together and the doctor said, sadly, "There is something very wrong here but I don't know what to do about it."

Humane service from all health workers is, in the last analysis, dependent on what societies value. Nurses are part of these societies and do, of course, influence those values. If nurses themselves think it as important to meet the fundamental, universal needs of all mankind as to meet the demands of a small fragment of society for treatment that requires a high degree of technical proficiency, they will influence the public to support a health service that supplies humanistic care as generously, or more generously, than it supplies technologically sound treatment.

The nurses of Great Britain have a long history of being politically aware and effective (Abel-Smith, 1960; Schröck, 1977; White, 1978). The laws affecting health and social welfare in a country such as yours, which is committed to the concept of health care as a human right, determine the numbers and kinds of health workers and their functions, and how the money will be spent in the services they give. It therefore goes without saying that being a good citizen and helping to create effective legislation should have priority for all health workers, including nurses.

The Royal College of Nursing has published many documents that show the statesmanship of its officers, staff and working parties or commissions. I am especially impressed with the document Evidence to the Royal Commission on the National Health Service (Royal College of Nursing, 1977). I have not, therefore, in this paper, ventured into the realm of politics. I mention it here because it is naive to ignore its importance (National League for Nursing, 1978). Instead, I will point to some characteristics in administering nursing services, in educating nurses, in conducting research and, most importantly, in practicing nursing that I believe will help preserve the essence of nursing in a technological age.

As far as possible, I will refer to persons who are advocating these characteristics and places where they have proved effective, or places in which experiments are in progress.

What Kind of Administration Will Help Preserve the Essence of Nursing in a Technological Age?

Some of the characteristics of administration that might encourage "holistic," or humanistic, nursing care are, I suggest, the following:

1. A democratic pattern that encourages group decisions and individual initiative in both health care providers and consumers, and group decisions rather than autocratic decisions by administrators.
2. Decentralization of authority with the creation of clinical units small enough to allow those caring for patients, or clients, to know them and get interested in them, their families and friends.
3. The assignment of patients or clients to nurses rather than the assignment of tasks, functions, duties or activities.
4. An organizational structure that gives nurses the same professional responsibility and accountability for patient care that is given other health care providers, as for example, doctors, dentists, social workers, speech therapists or physical therapists.
5. A system of joint appointments that enables those who give nursing service, if they wish, to also teach or conduct research.

The preceding list could, of course, be expanded until it would be impossible to discuss any one of the characteristics mentioned. The list probably illustrates my bias and it might be challenged by almost anyone who has made a study of administration.

I have put democratic administration first because I believe so strongly in Jeffersonian principles. Thomas Jefferson's idea that a university faculty might elect from its members a chairman-president for a 5-year term is an example, and one that suggests the extent to which administration might encourage the potential development of individuals.

Hospital administration, especially administration of nursing services, has been repressive and its nature could be explained historically if there were time. Student nurses for many decades gave most of the nursing care. These students were in various stages of learning and were, in many cases minors.

Administrative practices were designed to protect the hospital, the patients and the students themselves rather than to foster creative nursing by well prepared adult professional practitioners. It may be many more years before we are able to discard the repressive elements that are inappropriate for this age when student labor is not the problem it once was.

Throughout this century, critics have urged nurses to revolt against patriarchal and matriarchal dominance. This is, of course, no news to the reader, but it is hard for younger nurses to understand why change has come slowly. In the forties, a doctor in Australia and one in England said that nurses were "exploited and scantily recognized" and suggested that the "first thing to discard is obsolete ideas"; nurses were advised to take an active role in planning and not to accept the role of "handmaiden to the gods" (Walker, 1944; Smith, 1942).

While progress has undoubtedly been made, the picture has not changed entirely. Joycelyn Evans, a patient's wife, writing about a London hospital in 1971, commented on a "sister" who ruled her underlings with a rod of iron, treating them like schoolgirls or domestic servants and yet taking for granted a professional dedication that would be highly prized in any other calling (Evans, 1971). Writing in 1974, Joan Ashley, an American nurse, clearly says that the hospital is still paternalistic (Ashley, 1976).

The administration of nursing services in community health agencies has been far more democratic than in hospitals, clinics and nursing homes but, since hospitals are training grounds for all health personnel, practices within them leave their mark on doctors, nurses, social workers and practically all health care providers except dentists who, generally speaking, escape the system. But the system is changing. Now we hear "participatory administration" extolled on every hand. Administrators are called "facilitators" and their worth is measured in terms of their ability to promote the potential ability of workers. The concept of administration that develops the potential ability of patients or clients for self-care and the potential ability of families for helping sick or disabled members is rare, however. Some psychiatric hospitals are exceptions and, probably, our best models of participatory administration by patients. Bruno Bettelheim's (1974) *A Home for the Heart* describes a Chicago hospital where patients are first-class citizens; Elisebeth Barnes edited a report of studies in the Cassell Hospital in London where patients help make the policy (Barnes, 1968). Many practices in these psychiatric institutions could be adapted to other types of hospitals, hospices, and nursing homes.

Decentralization of authority with the creation of autonomous, relatively small, clinical units is not new. Hospitals within the Kaiser-Permanente System in the Western part of the United States established this pattern in the 1950s where the patient unit was reduced to eight beds and supervisory nursing personnel eliminated. Relatively new hospitals in Canada and the United States that I have visited recently, present comparable, perhaps less radical, patterns of decentralization. Martha Haber discusses the merits of decentralization in a description of the nursing service at the University of California Hospital in San Francisco (Haber, 1979). In 1978, 81% of the nursing staff there were registered nurses and more than half of them degree holders. At this center an earnest effort is made to personalize patient care and to give the staff nurse responsibility for assessing, planning, implementing plans and evaluating nursing care. The principle of putting decision-making on patient care within the clinical unit is, I believe, gaining ground rapidly. It is widely recognized that decisions that should be based on a knowledge of patients and their families cannot often be made in a central office.

Patient assignment rather than task assignment, would do more to preserve the essence of nursing in a technological age than any other administrative characteristic, in my opinion. Marie Manthey calls this "primary nursing" and describes it as a "return to 'my patient,' 'my nurse'" (Manthey, 1970). Functional nursing, or job assignment, is a product of an industrial age and has been promoted as an efficiency measure. (I think it is unfortunate that the term "primary nursing" has been adopted for a system of patient assignment since it can so easily be confused with primary (health) care, which means the initial visit of the patient to a physician or nurse who follows-up this care and either provides the needed service or refers the patient to appropriate health workers.) Health care providers have not yet fully realized the danger of uncritically applying industrial management methods to health care systems. (The fact that we refer to "the health care industry" is itself disturbing to me.)

The centers in the United States that are reintroducing or adopting the patient assignment system are too numerous to mention. However, because the nursing staff has recently made a film showing its happy effect on patient and nursing satisfaction, I would like to call attention to the programme at the Beth-Israel Hospital in Boston, Massachusetts. In this acute care, general hospital, used by the Harvard Medical School for the most advanced technological medical practice, the care of patients is personal and humane. The nursing is provided largely by degree-holding graduate nurses. I have never seen higher morale among staff nurses. Joyce Clifford, the Director of Nursing Services, has, with Marie Manthey, gone as far afield as Germany to discuss the advantages of primary nursing.

Another centre that shall be mentioned in discussing the patient assignment system is that connected with Rush University in Chicago, Illinois. The School of Nursing there, under the deanship of Luther Christman, has received a large grant from the Kellogg Foundation to establish a "centre of excellence." The 4.5 million grant is from the John L. and Helen Kellogg Foundation. The Center of Excellence is committed to superior clinical care, a "complete school of nursing, continuing education, clinical research, demonstration programmes, multidisciplinary projects, and international programmes. The primary nursing philosophy was introduced there in 1972 and has been adopted in varying degrees in all units. The school is committed to the development of a self-governing, competent nursing staff composed of degree-holding graduate nurses and to the continuous monitoring of nursing care (Christman, 1978; Pryma, 1978; Hegyvary, 1978). (Sue Hegyvary, Associate Dean at Rush, tells a nice story about a patient who, after admission to a unit that did not use the primary care system, asked to see a nurse who had been "his nurse" on another unit where they did have primary nursing. When he found her he said, "You know I'm on that specialty floor now. There's a special person to take my temperature, somebody else gives me a bath, somebody else takes my blood pressure, another specialist gives me my medicine, but there's nobody to tie my shoes.")

At all of these centres, where a graduate nurse is taking responsibility for planning and giving much of the nursing care of each patient, nurses are enjoying a professional status comparable to that enjoyed by doctors, special therapists, and social workers. The superstructure of management has been reduced to a minimum and nursing competence is diverted from management to patient care. It is no wonder that such places report no difficulty in recruiting nurses who like to nurse.

Under an organizational pattern that encourages the development of clinical judgement and skill acquired through experience, and increased knowledge acquired through continuing education, staff nurses can, if interested in teaching, be valuable members of nursing faculties. If staff nurses are academically prepared, part-time faculty appointments on nursing faculties might be as open to them as they are to medical clinicians on medical faculties. It seems equally appropriate to free the clinical nurse interested in research to conduct investigations of clinical problems. A common criticism of nursing research in the past has been that even if applied it would have little effect on practice, for the problems studied have so seldom been those encountered in the care of patients. If nurse practitioners were free to conduct research it is unlikely that this criticism would be levelled at their work.

In summary, then, administrators can help to preserve the essence of nursing in a technological age by providing practicing nurses with settings in which they can practice both the art and the science of nursing.

What Kind of Education Will Help Preserve the Essence of Nursing in a Technological Age?

1. Admission requirements for nursing students that provide a balanced educational background. Nursing education that includes some of the following: language, history, religions, philosophy, government and economics, as well as the physical, biological, and psycho-social and nursing and medical arts and sciences.
2. Emphasis in the beginning of the generic nursing programme on the fundamental needs of man; on the assessment of patients' total health needs rather than those related only to the disease diagnosis.
3. Focus on representative theories of health and disease; especially the interdependence of spiritual, emotional, and physical health and some different approaches to health care world-wide.
4. Emphasis in the generic programme on the habits and skills of inquiry; on the problem approach, and on the value of scientific investigation, while at the same time recognizing the momentary necessity of instinctive, or intuitive, behaviour and the value of authority as a basis for action.
5. An opportunity to observe clinically expert role models in giving patient care; to help these experts give care and finally to assume sufficient responsibility for assessing nursing needs, planning, implementing plans and evaluating care to experience the satisfaction of giving effective care and to recognize care that is ineffective.
6. Opportunity for continuing education (of the patient-centered variety) throughout the working years of the nurse.

Again, I admit that my bias is showing in this very incomplete list of the characteristics of nursing education which might preserve the essence of nursing in a technological age. Some of the same points are made by medi-

cal educators who want humanistic values preserved by medical practitioners. Among present-day medical philosophers in the United States whose
writings are worth particular attention are: René Dubos, Edmund Pellegrino
and Lewis Thomas. All of them are urging medical schools, as I would urge
nursing schools, to select candidates who bring a humanistic educational
background to the study of health care (Dubos, 1959; Pellegrino, 1979;
Thomas, 1979).

A friend of mine, a nurse, who is now in her last year of medical school
wrote this tome on a Christmas card: "I am learning a lot about medicine
but the human aspect of man is sadly lacking. I find myself reminding myself to concentrate on that instead of the disease state. It is so easy to forget
the person!"

When I see a student nurse, as I did recently, ask a patient who is enjoying her lunch to put it aside while she, the student, checked her blood pressure, I wonder whether nursing education isn't tarred with the same stick.

In *The Nature of Nursing* and in the 6th edition of *Principles and Practice of Nursing* there is a suggested generic, or basic, nursing curriculum
outline that puts equal emphasis on the art and science of nursing (Henderson, 1966; Henderson & Nite, 1978). Strong components of the physical, biological, and psycho-social sciences are proposed, but a humanistic approach to the study of the clinical nursing aspect of the nursing curriculum
is given in some detail. It is urged that students concentrate first on studying the universal needs of all patients rather than on studying specific needs
due to a disease or a disability. It is suggested that students first learn how to
help individuals with their daily activities: with breathing; eating and drinking; with elimination; with maintenance of posture, moving and exercising;
with sleep and rest; with dressing and undressing; with maintaining body
temperatures in a normal range; with keeping clean and well groomed; with
avoiding dangers in the environment; with communication—expressing
emotions, needs, fears, questions and ideas; with forms of worship; with
work or productive activity; with play or recreation, and with learning, discovering and developing—especially as this relates to health.

After the period of study devoted to helping patients and their families
with meeting these fundamental needs, students might next study the problems that arise as a result of aberrations of function: abnormal respiration,
elimination, movement, communication, and so forth. Even in this stage of
the clinical curriculum the emphasis is not on the disease diagnosis, but on
the universal functions or activities of daily living. If, for every person assigned to them, the students made a study along these lines, and if this

study became a habit it would be almost impossible for them to give anything but individualized care. Not until the third phase of the clinical curriculum would the emphasis be placed on the modification of care necessitated by a specific disease entity—as for example, measles, diabetes, or muscular dystrophy. Ruth Hubbard discussing an understanding of health in nursing quotes Sir William Osler as saying, "Have no teaching without a patient for a text, and the best teaching is that taught by the patient himself." She added no patient is concerned about his diagnosis as such, but what his illness means to him and his work (Hubbard, 1943).

The Yale School of Nursing was started as an experiment to see whether students in a basic programme could be prepared for public health nursing. When asked how she was trying to accomplish this, Annie W. Goodrich, the first dean of the school, said it was accomplished by having students make a thorough study of each patient assigned to them (Goodrich, 1973). Yale graduates, at that time, left a selection of these patient studies in their folders in the school's office. Reviewing these studies, it is clear that the students were free to make home visits and to give imaginative creative care in the hospital and the home. While medical care at the University Hospital was not highly technical by today's standards, it was highly technical for that era. Malcolm T. MacEachern, then Director of the American College of Surgeons, was impressed by the programme at the Yale School of Nursing. Discussing hospitals with and without a future, he said the hospital with a future must be "human." He added that the Yale school had largely "solved this problem by having each student make a social study of the patient assigned to her" (MacEachern, 1926).

Western schools of medicine and nursing have tended to teach only the dominant Western theories of disease and therapy. The West is often said to be physically and materially rich, but spiritually weak, unwilling to admit the existence of forces it cannot comprehend or explain. In any event, until recently, treatment of a metaphysical nature has been scoffed at in the West. Today even the most "scientific" of therapists are, at least, withholding judgment. Western doctors are working with "medicine men." They are recognizing hypnosis, acupuncture, and transcendental meditation as accepted therapies. Norman Cousins, a layman, who is sometimes said to have "laughed himself well" is a senior lecturer in the School of Medicine at the University of California, and a consulting editor to *Man and Medicine*, published by the College of Physicians and Surgeons at Columbia University, New York City (Cousins, 1979). All students of health care might profit by studying the different approaches to health service reported by, for example, the World Health Organization (Djukanovic & Mach, 1975). WHO has largely abandoned its earlier efforts to transplant Western technology in soil that is foreign to it.

In case you believe I am belittling the importance of scientific inquiry, let me assure you that I think far too little is expected of nursing students and graduates along these lines. While acknowledging the necessity of acting intuitively most of the time and recognizing the value of expert opinion as a basis for action some of the time, I believe it difficult to survive in a technological age without making decisions based on research findings. I think our profession has put too little emphasis on knowing how to find and apply relevant data and has too much reverence for irrelevant studies made by nurses simply to qualify themselves as scientists or researchers. The habitual practice of identifying the basis on which an action is taken or recommended, is priceless, in my opinion, and should be expected of nursing students (undergraduate and graduate), of nurse educators and practitioners.

No experience offered by educators to students is as important as seeing expert nurses practice; then participating in this practice, and finally having an opportunity to practice as effectively as they can themselves, with help from the expert. The commonest, and I think most valid, criticism of nursing education at present, is that teachers are not role models and that students are not given sufficient time with their assigned patients to feel any satisfaction in accomplishment, to sense continuity of care or even to be reasonably skillful in giving basic nursing care.

Nursing schools offering faculty members joint appointments in service are able to provide students with role models that are clinically expert. University Hospitals of Cleveland associated with the Case Western Reserve University School of Nursing, announced a merger of education and service in 1966 that has contributed largely to its excellent reputation. A nurse director of each clinical nursing department is responsible for programmes of nursing education, nursing care and research (University Hospitals of Cleveland, 1966). This school has put its basic programme on a doctoral level, the emphasis being the art of nursing and the science of health.

In summary, nurse educators can help preserve the essence of nursing in a technological age by focusing on the humanistic and psycho-social aspects of care as well as the technical skills. Most particularly, they can demonstrate these aspects of care as role models and can help students to individualize the care they give.

What Kind of Research Will Help Preserve the Essence of Nursing in a Technological Age?

1. Research on basic human needs as related to health.
2. Research on problems involved in basic nursing care, or helping people meet their basic health needs.
3. Research which if applied would influence the effectiveness of basic nursing.
4. Research on nursing problems that recognizes the value of related studies and builds on them no matter what the discipline, be it psychology, sociology, physiology, pharmacology, physics, chemistry, economics or other.

Nurse researchers and those who believe that nursing should be a "research-based profession" can preserve the essence of nursing by finding or producing data on the non-technical, as well as the technical aspects of administration, teaching, and practice or by demonstrating that the problems nurses face in helping people meet their universal health needs are as susceptible to study in depth as the technological aspects of treatment. Researchers can help demonstrate the complexity of basic nursing care and the value of humanistic nursing.

Studies that demonstrate the dangers of bedrest, compare natural with drug-induced sleep, identify the causes of bed sores and effective preventive measures, the studies on biofeedback and hundreds of other clinical investigations, relate to problems nurses face in giving basic nursing care. The problems nurses face in helping people with breathing, eating, sleeping, exercising, communicating, and so on are as susceptible to study in depth as are the problems physicians face in disease diagnosis and treatment.

Most texts from which student nurses have learned the fundamentals of nursing have not presented practice problematically with a choice of method; nor have the suggested methods been based on research findings. While medical students might, for instance, be expected to know several theories on blood clotting and how to prevent or induce it, student nurses are rarely expected to know theories on sleep and how to delay or induce it, or theories on pain and how to control or relieve it. Many nursing texts have been little more than manuals or cookbooks dealing sketchily with the "why" and dogmatically with the "how." Generally speaking, nurses have not been prepared to present data as a basis for recommending change, in spite of the fact that the founder of modern nursing, Florence Nightingale, was past master at this. She was elected to fellowship in the Royal Statistical Society in 1858 and to honorary membership in the American Statistical Association in 1874 (Grier & Grier, 1978). Through statistical studies she was able to show that with basic nursing care she and her associates could reduce the mortality in the Crimean hospitals dramatically. Through persuasive statistical studies she brought about changes in the living conditions for soldiers in Army hospitals and in the Indian service. Miss Nightingale accomplished all this because she had not only reformed basic hygienic care, but used sound research methods to demonstrate its effectiveness. In her day she was a master of the science of health, although she said almost nothing was known about it.

In our *Survey and Assessment of Nursing Research*, Leo Simmons and I called attention to the rarity of studies dealing with clinical problems between 1900 and 1960 (Simmons & Henderson, 1964). More recent surveys suggest that there is now a tendency on the part of funding agencies to give preference to clinical investigations, and with post-basic programmes clinically focused, more students elect to do clinical research (Gortner & Nahm, 1977). In the *Abstracts of Papers* presented at the Royal College of Nursing Research Society Conference in 1978 I counted sixteen papers that dealt with practice, nine with research methods, six with education, five with management and one I couldn't fit into any of those categories (RCNR, 1979).

We need imaginative and bold nurse researchers who can, through demonstrations and sound evaluative research, bring about radical changes in the basic health care of the chronically ill, the mentally retarded, the prison population and the institutionalized aged—but to mention a few categories of society that are conspicuously neglected and whose fate might be radically altered by expert humanistic nursing. Such studies might persuade nurses themselves, as well as the public, that basic nursing is, indeed, as important as the technological advances in medical care.

Dorothy Johnson discussing the state of the art of theory development in nursing says, "There is as yet no circumscribed body of knowledge that is widely recognized and accepted as nursing science" (Johnson, 1978). Others believe, as I do, that all health disciplines are applied sciences and that medicine, nursing, nutrition, physical therapy, and so on, must of necessity, draw on the more basic sciences of physics, chemistry, physiology, microbiology, and psychology.

In summary, nurses might more drastically affect the quality of basic nursing if nurses developed the habits and skills of inquiry, if they applied existing research findings and if they thought of "theory" underlying nursing as having no circumscribed limits.

What Kind of Practice Will Help Preserve the Essence of Nursing in a Technological Age?

1. Helping patients and their families with health problems as well as focusing on the cure or control of disease, emphasizing self-help, family and community help rather than fostering dependency and institutionalization.
2. Basing nursing care on a continuous process of evaluating, planning (with patients and families), implementing plans, and evaluating and modifying care for each person so that it is effective and consistent with goals that are mutually acceptable to those who receive and those who give care.
3. Providing for continuity of care from one setting to another—from one institution and agency to another.
4. Assuming responsibility for decision-making and effective action within the legal definition of nursing but coordinating nursing care with other aspects of health care.

Practitioners of nursing are those who, in the last analysis, must preserve the essence of nursing. It is they who must value it and demonstrate its value.

There is, in nursing circles, a good deal of talk about how to improve the public image of the nurse. Only the practicing nurse can do this, I believe. The public's concept of nursing will always be what the average nurse does or the majority of nurses do. If this is true and if it is important to preserve the essence of nursing, it must be made possible for the average nurse or the majority of nurses to practice humanistic nursing. The reward for this practice must be commensurate with the reward for administering, teaching or researching nursing so that practitioners will remain practitioners, and through experience and continued study be increasingly proficient in the art and science of nursing.

It is likely that people who choose nursing as an occupation do so because they want to help others. They see people whole—mind and body "animated by that divine spark we call spirit" (as Miss Goodrich used to say) rather than as broken backs, cardiac failures, or cases of pernicious anemia. Young students tend to approach patients as personalities, individually and humanely. I am aware that this statement can be challenged; that some people think medical and nursing students choose these occupations because they offer a chance to dominate others, even a chance for the physician or nurse to work through their hostile feelings.

I can prove neither of these theories but would stress that the educational programme and conditions in health care settings should foster a humane approach and discourage the impersonal, indifferent or negative approach.

Using the term "practitioners" in its generic sense, it is essential that those who practice nursing be allowed to spend enough time with patients and their families and friends to understand them as individuals and know something about how they live. The fact that nursing is the only 24-hour, 7-day-a-week service makes it easier for nurses than for any other health workers to really know patients. (It is possible that this fact is what gives nursing its unique function, as I suggested earlier.)

While no one nurse can give a person constant care there can be *a* nurse who takes the dominant role in the care of each patient—in assessing strengths, weaknesses and needs; in planning and in implementing plans and evaluating care. This type of patient assignment (rather than task assignment) has been discussed under other headings. The advantages for patients and their families and for the caregivers are generally recognized. It has been pointed out that more and more centers are adopting this "my nurse," "my patient," system (now usually called "primary nursing"). The successful practitioner or primary nurse is rewarded by a patient's recovery, by his or her increased ability to cope with a handicap or a peaceful death; the unsuccessful practitioners will at least have the opportunity to identify their failures and to get the help they need to improve their practice (American Academy of Nursing, 1977).

Practitioners who see role models functioning effectively in one-to-one relationships with their patients and who have the opportunity to practice creatively within this system are not likely to function mechanically or to see the human aspect of nursing as less important than the technical aspects.

Primary nurses who know that their patients must be self-reliant on discharge will concentrate on self-help measures. Primary nurses who know that family members, friends, or neighbors will help patients on discharge will concentrate on teaching such persons how to give the necessary help. The New York University Hospital in New York City has a floor to which relatives or friends are admitted with patients and are taught how to nurse them. In some institutions staff nurses can make home visits and serve as consultants to families and home health workers after patients leave the hospital.

Few subjects are currently receiving more attention than self-help. Ivan Illich's book on "the expropriation of health" (by health workers) is much discussed (Illich, 1975; Thomas, 1979). His idea, with which Lewis Thomas seems to concur, is that we needlessly make people "patients" from the cradle to the grave—that we foster hypochondria. Health service, including that of the nurse, must take into account not only the emotional value of self-reliance, but the economic necessity of eliminating unnecessary services (Maxwell, 1974; Levin, 1976). Many developing countries are making startling advances in the health of their citizens by emphasizing self-care, care by relatives, friends, and neighbors and by organizing communities to deal with health problems. One such approach is to have the deaf help the blind, the emotionally disturbed help the physical handicapped, and so on. In some cases, the most effective nurses may be those who can help others preserve the essence of nursing.

Continuity of care is a problem nurse practitioners must help to solve by making it possible to move from one health care setting to another or by establishing better communication between nurses and others in and outside health institutions and agencies. Nurses are supporting the right of patients to own copies of their health and medical records and the rights of patients to give or withhold consent for treatment (Kelly, 1976). It seems likely that this will help preserve basic nursing care as much, or more than, the technological aspects since it will be necessary to make care and treatment understandable to patients and their families.

As the role of the nurse expands and includes more and more of the activities formerly considered medical, clarification of the respective authority, responsibility and accountability of nurses, physicians and others is necessary. This is so complex a question that it is impossible to discuss it in this paper. In the United States the National Joint Practice Commission (medicine and nursing) issued a report on a survey of statutory regulations of the scope of nursing practice. This report included the startling recommendation that medical practice acts exclude nurses from the prohibition to practice medicine (Hall, 1975)! Certainly nurses are "practicing medicine" in any community lacking physicians and have been throughout this century.

As the ratio of nurses and physicians to populations rises and falls from one country to another and one decade to another their functions will inevitably change. Unless the public is to suffer, nurses and doctors (and other health workers) must establish committees, councils or commissions in every agency, every community, every state, county, province or country to continuously assess the role or functions of each category of worker.

Conclusion

It has been suggested by Edmund Pellegrino (1979) and others that there are too many types of health workers, that we might do better if they were reduced to, say, six. If we were able to objectively assess health care and our role within it, we might see that both society and ourselves would profit by a redefinition of the nurse's function. Whatever the role of future nurses, however, I cannot believe that the essence of nursing, or basic nursing care, will ever be seen as anything less than essential to the welfare of the human race. Not until human beings are born, live, and die in an independent state—and not until the special knowledge and skill of the nurse becomes common knowledge and skill, can we abandon what we think of as basic nursing care.

References

Abel-Smith, B. (1960). *A History of the Nursing Profession*. Heinemann, London.

American Academy of Nursing (1977). *Primary care by nurses: Sphere of responsibility and accountability.* Papers presented at the Annual Meeting, September 1976. American Nurses Association, Kansas City.

Anderson, E. R. (1973). *The role of the nurse.* The Study of Nursing Care Research Project. Royal College of Nursing and National Council of Nurses of the United Kingdom, London.

Ashley, J. (1976). *Hospitals, paternalism and the role of the nurse.* Teachers College Press, Columbia University, New York.

Barnes, E. (Ed.) (1968). *Psychosocial nursing: Studies from the Cassell Hospital*. Tavistock Publications, London.

Bettelheim, B. (1974). *A home for the heart*. Alfred A. Knopf, New York.

Christman, L. (1976). The autonomous nursing staff in the hospital. *Nursing Administration Quarterly 1*, 37–44.

Christman, L. (1978). *An organizational perspective for nursing practice.*

Paper presented at workshop colleagues in patient care: The Rush model for nursing. Chicago, Illinois.

Cousins, N. (1979). *Anatomy of an illness as perceived by the patient.* W.W. Norton & Co., New York.

Djukanovic, V., & Mach, E. P. (Eds.) (1975). *Alternative approaches to meeting basic health needs in developing countries. A Joint UNICEF/WHO study.* World Health Organization, Geneva.

Dubos, R. (1959). *Mirage of health.* Doubleday and Co., Garden City, New York.

Evans, J. (1971). *Living with a man who is dying.* Taplinger Publishing Company, New York.

Goodrich, A. W. (1973). *The social and ethical significance of nursing.* The Yale University School of Nursing, New Haven, CT.

Gortner, S., & Nahm, H. (1977). An overview of nursing research in the United States. *Nursing Research, 26*(10), 3.

Grier, B., & Grier, M. (1978). Contributions of a passionate statistician. *Research in Nursing and Health 1,* 103.

Haber, M. E. (1979). Structuring a nursing service in an urban hospital. *Nursing service in a specialty, a rural and an urban hospital.* National League for Nursing, New York.

Hall, V. (1975). *Statutory regulation of the scope of nursing practice—A critical survey.* National Joint Practice Commission, Chicago.

Hegyvary, S. (1978). Primary nursing. Rush–Presbyterian: St Luke's Medical Center. *The Magazine, 2.*

Henderson, V. (1966). *The nature of nursing.* Macmillan Publishing Co., New York.

Henderson, V. (1977). The Essence of Nursing. *Virginia Nurse,* 78.

Henderson, V., & Nite, G. (1978). *Principles and practice of nursing.* Macmillan Publishing Co., New York.

Hubbard, R. W. (1943). An understanding of health in nursing. *Public Health Nurse, 35.*

Illich, I. (1975). *Medical nemesis—The expropriation of health.* McClelland & Stewart, London.

Johnson, D. E. (1978). State of the art of theory development in nursing. In *Theory development—What, why, how?* National League for Nursing, New York.

Kelly, L. Y. (1976). The patient's right to know. *Nursing Outlook,* 24.

Levin, L. (1976). *Self care: Lay initiatives in health.* Prodist, New York.

MacDermot, H. E. (1950). Nursing in Osler's student days. *Canadian Nurse* 46, 222.

MacEachern, M. T. (1926). The hospital with and without a future. *Hospital Progress, 6.*

Manthey, M. (1970). Primary nursing: A return to the concept of "my nurse" and "my patient." *Nursing Forum 9,* 65–83.

Maxwell, R. (1974). *Health care: The proving dilemma: Needs* versus *resources in Western Europe, the U.S. and U.S.S.R.* McKinsey & Co., New York.

National League for Nursing (1978). *Political, social and educational forces on nursing: Impact of political forces.* New York: The League.

Nightingale, F. (1969 edn). *Notes on nursing.* Dover Publications, New York.

Pellegrino, E. D. (1979). Collected papers. University of Tennessee Press, Memphis.

Pryma, R. (1978). Primary nursing—A working philosophy—An organizational style. Rush Presbyterian, St. Luke's Medical Center. *The Magazine 2,* Spring 1978.

Royal College of Nursing Research Society Conference (1979). Abstracts of papers. RCN, London.

Royal College of Nursing of the United Kingdom (1977). *Evidence to the Royal Commission, the National Health Service.* RCN, London.

Schröck, R. A. (1977). On political consciousness in nurses. *Journal of Advanced Nursing 2,* 41–5.

Simmons, L. W., & Henderson, V. (1964). *Nursing research, a survey and assessment.* Appleton-Century-Crofts, New York.

Smith, S. M. (1942). Nurses in a cooperative health service. *The Australia Nurses' Journal,* July 1, 195.

Thomas, L. (1979). *The medusa and the snail.* The Viking Press, New York.

University Hospitals of Cleveland (1966). *News release* (March 21). Cleveland, Ohio.

Walker, G. F. (1944). A medical superintendent gives his suggestions for reforms in hospital organization. *Nursing Mirror, 78,* 15 January.

White, R. (1978). *Social change and development of the nursing profession: A study of the poor I, nursing service 1848–1948.* Henry Kimpton, London.

Chapter 8

Care of the Dying Person

The Effect of the Setting on the Kind of Care that is Possible

If most people want to die at home, care anywhere else may be less than ideal.[a] In the United States, more people die in hospitals than anywhere else, and the number that die in nursing homes is increasing.

As has been noted, patients who die in the general hospital are likely to be in the emergency room or in the intensive care unit, both organized and equipped for heroic life-saving measures. Some patients are brought to the emergency room for the physician to confirm or "pronounce" their death; others arrive mortally sick or injured, and for these persons measures designed to arrive at an immediate diagnosis and vigorous resuscitation are mobilized. When a patient is managed as an acute emergency, physicians and nurses don't have time to note that these may be the last moments of the patient's life, that family and friends who are there should be instantly summoned, and that they should be given professional support. Many hospitals have an individual, such as an ombudsman, or staff member in a department of religious ministry available who can help the emergency personnel meet the needs of the patient and the family. Some hospitals have social workers or psychiatrists especially prepared to help families and friends of patients.

While many clients of the emergency room will have been well up until the moment of a heart attack or an accident that brought them to the hospital, other patients will arrive just as ill, yet quite aware and prepared for death. A patient may have been at home or in another institution, such as a nursing home, and have to come to the emergency room either because help was needed for symptoms, such as air hunger, weakness, or hemorrhage, or because the family or those caring for needed physical or psychologic support through the very last phases of life. Thus the emergency room staff is confronted with patients who are dead or dying, but whose ways of coming to terms with death are completely unknown to the staff. Emergency room workers must decide quickly, with little information, whether to resuscitate the patient or to give supportive care only.

In sharp contrast with the emergency room of the acute hospital are the small specialized units where extended, personalized care helps patients and their families come to terms with an illness until it no longer responds to curative treatment. From the moment the patient is greeted at the door by the nurse who will be giving care, the approach is human being to human being. There are in England between 20 and 30 facilities of this sort; some are called hospices. One of the most widely known is St. Christopher's Hospice in London. There the treatment of choice is palliative, that is, skillful management of the symptoms of disease. By minimizing such symptoms as pain, weakness, anxiety, and nausea, patients facing death are kept comfortable, alert, and able to sustain activity and social relationships. In a setting such as this, nurses can attend to the particular needs of the dying with little conflict and confusion, and the patient and the family can be helped to live fully until the end. The majority of these institutions offer home care as well as an inpatient service and so provide both alternatives.

Death may occur in either of these contrasting institutional settings. Wherever it occurs, the family and friends of the dying patient, if they are present, require help. As will be discussed later, involvement of family is important. Most persons are comforted by the presence of those they love, so, for the patients' benefit as well as for their sake, family and friends should be part of the dying scene. Nurses and physicians may have to focus on the patient but they should not forget that relatives and friends of the dying are suffering and when left behind will need physical and psychologic help. In fact, such help should be available before as well as after the patient's death.

Even if patients come to terms with death and are ready to relinquish life, those around them may not reach that point at the same time. Family members or the patient's helpers (nurses, physicians, and others) may be ready to "let go" before or after the patient is ready. If nurses understand this, they can sense, mitigate, or relieve the tension emanating from a conflict created by differing expectations between themselves and others. Clues to such conflicts are varied. For example, a child said her mother would not have died "If only she had put up a better fight!" Another 6-year-old referred to his father with childish disappointment in saying, "Mean Daddy, he died on me." Both of these children expressed natural feelings of disappointment and loss of a very significant person in their lives.

The feeling of being left behind or abandoned is often a cause of suffering and a reason for the relative's or friend's need to cling to the patient. Equally understandable is the family's desire to see the end of a life that has come to be meaningless. For example, a 40-year-old husband whose wife had been comatose for a month following cardiac arrest on the operating table and who realized hope for her recovery was not realistic, did not want her death delayed. To him and to his teenage daughters, the wife and mother was already dead, but to the staff of the nursing home where every other patient was over 65 this young and beautiful woman was very much alive. The staff's well-meant efforts to prolong the patient's life with tube feedings were painful for the family to watch or to accept as useful, but the nursing home staff thought she deserved their concentrated attention, more perhaps than the old persons there, even though the young woman was unresponsive and their older patients were responsive.

Differences in the expectations and attitudes of those concerned with the dying person create tensions that charge the atmosphere with emotion. Decisions are difficult and differences between right and wrong are not obvious. Whether in the hospital or at home, nurses must be capable of providing suggestions about who should be called, what help professionals, friends, and family can give, and what help all involved need, including the staff. Nurses and doctors often overlook the impact of the loss of a patient on themselves, or feel that, as professionals, they should not show their emotions. In studies by Glaser and Strauss and by Quint and others, this observation was made repeatedly, partially accounting for what is interpreted as the withdrawal of the staff from the patient and the family. In homes or in homelike institutional settings such as hospices, it is possible for everyone to behave more naturally, more individually, more personally than in large hospitals. Saunders, talking about a setting in which a person (in this case, a child) can feel secure says: "Gossiping is very important and I suppose playing and reading with a child are its equivalents. I am sure I do not have to emphasize the importance of delight, of beauty and fantasy, and of parties."[b]

T. S. West, deputy medical director of St. Christopher's Hospice, makes the following observation on individualizing care:

> Death has become a fashionable subject to talk about and to write about. It is clothed with such words as "dignity" and many who approach the subject hope that "the specialists in death" will have some formula that can be handed round to make the "dignity" a reality.
> There is no such formula.
> Members of an institution whose main concern is to care for people whose terminal disease is causing them suffering know only too well that no formula can be applied to more than one patient. At St. Christopher's we have begun to learn that just as each patient will approach death in his own particular way, so each member of staff must find his own and special way to approach each patient. We know that patients and staff have to learn to deal not only with each other, but also with themselves.[c]

Wherever care is given the dying patient, the *environment* is important. In private homes it may be desirable for the patient to be in a room on the ground floor so that he or she can walk or be wheeled outdoors and eat meals with the family as long as possible. Nearby bathroom facilities are important, and the cheerfulness and comfort of the furnishings of the patient's room. Familiar and beloved objects in the room to which they are accustomed, may, however, make persons prefer not to move to another seemingly more suitable room.

In general hospitals or nursing homes, every effort should be made to provide privacy when it is desirable for patients and their families. If death is imminent, a private room is often preferred. However, if patients are expected to live for weeks or possibly months, they may be happier in a multiple-bed unit where they will not feel isolated between visits from family or friends. Multiple-bed units are especially desirable for solitary persons who have no visitors.

Henry Wald, who has studied the architectural designs of hospices and special units for the terminally ill, thinks that the preference in acute care hospital design for private rooms for most, if not all, patients does not apply to hospices. In his 1971 master's thesis for the Columbia University School of Architecture, he supports the following US Department of Health, Education, and Welfare recommendation for four-bed units:

The terminal phase of life is an area that has just begun to be investigated in an objective way, and the results raise some surprising psychological issues. Reactions to imminent death vary as much as reactions to familiar life circumstances. But research has shown that during the last few months of life the individual has an increased feeling that his body is inadequate. The dying person experiences a growing feeling of helplessness because of loss of influence over his environment but he has an increased interest in other people. A study comparing interviews (1) with persons who died within a year and (2) with those who survived, showed that the individuals closest to the time of their death, showed a much greater interest in their immediate environment. Information such as this suggests that perhaps the greatest disservice that can be done to the dying person is to isolate him.

To deny the dying person access to others and to the information of his normal environment, therefore, would seem to reduce the likelihood that he will resolve his own departure with dignity. Isolation of the dying is, perhaps, a reflection of the attitudes of younger professionals who are disquieted by their own unresolved conflicts. The social and psychological, as well as the physiological, concomitants of dying should be considered carefully in design services for the terminally ill persons.[d]

Craven and Wald, describing the design of the hospice in Branford, Connecticut, say that

The four single rooms will be used as alternatives for those who are not helped by the multibed arrangement—a teenager who may need lots of loud companions, a writer trying to get work done, a couple who face the end of life simultaneously.[e]

They point out that the scale of the hospice "is human" and designed to help patients continue "life as usual"; to feel a part of on-going life. Patients have easy access to the outdoors, as well as to other parts of the hospice, including the chapel. They see children going to and from the nursery school within the hospice for children of personnel, and volunteers of all ages going about their various activities—gardening, folding linen, serving tea and coffee, etc.

In general hospitals it is common practice to hide the sight and sound of death. Saunders, in discussing the program at St. Christopher's Hospice, London, England, describes the acceptance of death on the ward as one of its advantages. One or more members of the staff, as well as family members, are present, and a prayer is usually said at the end. Other patients, who may never have witnessed death, see that it comes easily and that they will not be alone when they die. Patients can sometimes help each other and frequently want to do so. Just the presence of someone else is support for the dying, and in turn, those who see this as a more distant but inevitable event are reassured to know that dying patients are appropriately treated.

In the last days of life, though the pace is slower, patients' appreciation of peace, quiet, and beauty are frequently heightened. A flower or a beloved object put at close range, where it is seen by the dying, gives pleasure. Ample and comfortable seating should be available to make the patient's visitors feel they are wanted and seats arranged so that the patient can easily see and hear them. In any setting, every effort should be made to prevent disagreeable odors in the room. If anything is used to mask unavoidable odors, it should probably have an aromatic smell, like that of ammonia or camphor, rather than either an acrid or sweet smell. For the sake of patients and their families, whatever makes for beauty in the environment should be kept until the end. It is possible that music might help many who are dying. They should be surrounded with what they most like at the last.

Care of the Dying Person—Principles and Goals

Principles and Goals of Terminal Care in Any Setting

The principles and goals of terminal care are emerging from those who are providing and evaluating care in hospices, hospitals, at home, and in nursing homes. They are applicable to any setting.

An interdisciplinary group called the International Work Group on Death. Dying and Bereavement has prepared a working document on standards of care and will develop outcome measures, using these standards as working hypotheses.[f] The standards in this working document touch upon the need for palliative treatment of highest quality; the need for spiritual support, care and respect for the family; open communication, shared decision-making and support for the patient's family who are searching for meaning. The document also emphasizes need for an interdisciplinary team and an atmosphere of concern and support.

Saunders, writing about the management of fatal illness in childhood, and the unusual strains it put on the staff, says: "We are all concerned . . . in trying to come to terms . . . with our own feelings of guilt and fear in the presence of death. It is easier when we know we are not alone. We . . . need frequent, informal meetings. *I would give for the first principle of terminal care co-operation or, perhaps better, community."* [Italics ours][8]

Edward Henderson, a physician, discussing the approach to patients with incurable diseases, makes the following points:

> In summary, those caring for the patient with an incurable illness should (a) provide him with knowledge as to the reasonable expectations and limitations imposed by his disease: (b) help him thoroughly and thoughtfully to obtain the greatest possible rewards from his truncated existence; (c) maintain as much as possible an emotional and social environment consistent with his pre-diagnosis status: and (d) preserve his self-esteem and self-recognition for as long as his illness permits, both by allowing and requiring of him a role and voice in the decisions of his life.[h]

In the following pages an effort is made to describe some ways in which these goals can be met.

Influence of Age on the Care of the Dying Person

It is easy to say that it is the quality rather than the length of a life that is important but almost everyone sees the death of a much wanted *infant* or the death of a beloved *child* as particularly sad. Some students of medicine and nursing who planned to specialize in child care have given up the idea because they couldn't cope with their own suffering and feeling of helplessness when faced with the fatally ill and dying child. Health workers share with parents the fear that more might have been done, a cure found, or the life prolonged until a cure was discovered. It is hard to help parents to accept the inevitability of death and to know when and how to face it with the child. Ida Martinson[i] has been giving nursing care and psychologic support to dying children and their parents. Most of her patients have had leukemia. Many of them with her help, have been able to stay at home longer and even die at home. Many children might die more happily at home if parents weren't clinging to the hope that a medical miracle would save them. But hospital life for sick children is becoming more bearable as institutions encourage parents to participate in the child's care, even making provision for parents to stay overnight.

There seems to be general agreement that children after the age of 5 know what death means. Before this, they may not think of death as a permanent separation. Children, like adults, sense the imminence of death and ask questions which, if not answered adequately and truthfully, isolate them with their fears of death. Wessel says, "The basic need for a grieving child is to have open and honest relationships with trusted adults."[j] Their fears may be so much worse than the reality of death that protecting children from the sight of dying and death may be a great disservice. Saunders reports the following conversation between a nurse and a dying child:

> A boy with sarcomatosis died with us not very long ago. Towards the end of his four months' stay with us Sister suddenly knew that the time had come to speak directly while she was doing something practical for him. She just said quietly: "Are you afraid about dying, David?" "Yes," he said. "You've seen other people here. . . . You know we won't let you down. It will be all right." He said: "Yes, it *is* all right" and never needed to say anything else.[k]

This conversation suggests the importance of allowing the child to see others die—easily and supported by those they love. Maria H. Nagy,[1] Delphie J. Fredlund,[2] and Erna Furman,[3] among others, have studied the meaning of death to children.[l] Readers will find their reports helpful. Special chapters in texts on child care describe the care of the dying child and helping parents in more detail than can be included here.

While the death of those who haven't had a chance to live fully is particularly sad, the death of *young adults*, and especially young parents, is also hard to accept. They weigh heavily in the scale of social worth emphasized by Glaser and Strauss. Like fatally ill children, they are likely to get the best physical care available in a general hospital. Heroic life-saving measures may be used long after the staff realizes these measures are useless.

The difficulty of facing death with the parent and with the children may result in complete avoidance of the subject. This isolates the fatally ill patients with their instinctive knowledge that death is imminent. W. E. Wynant, as a clergyman, describes the help he was able to give a husband in facing death with his dying wife and the support he gave her in seeing her children who had withdrawn from their mother, feeling themselves unloved and forsaken by her.

Death in *middle* and *old age* rarely has the poignancy that death in youth has. However, age is not a matter of years alone. In some cultures, men and women are old at 45 or 50; in others, they retain their zest for living far beyond the Biblical threescore years and ten. In every culture, there are individuals whose death at 80, or even older, is a social loss. For example, there are statesmen and scientists whose life work is nearing fruition, artists who are producing masterpieces in their maturity, and men and women who are, for one reason or another, holding families together. In 1945, Leo W. Simmons published a study of the aged in primitive society[5] and in 1970, with Dorothea Jaeger, he reported a study of the care of the aged in the United States.[6] Such works should be consulted for data on this subject, but the generalization may be justifiable that isolation and withdrawal in the care of the dying apply particularly to the elderly. On the other hand, the aged may not be subjected to prolonged dying through the use of respiratory aids and artificial feeding. Kastenbaum, under the title "While the Old Man Dies: Our Conflicting Attitudes Toward the Elderly," describes the thoughts of the son who has witnessed the death of a father when they could not communicate with each other:

> The core problem is the one to concentrate upon: many of us have misgivings about the prospects of our own aging and death, and we have mixed feelings about people in our own lives who are aged. We are quick to project our own attitudes and expectations upon elderly men and women. This projection can exert powerful influence over the lives and deaths of the elderly as we are generally in a position of greater socioeconomic leverage. If we are convinced it is right or necessary for an old person to die, then we may be making it extraordinarily difficult for him to live. We may fail to bolster his chances of remaining in good health, we may fail to recognize when, in fact, his preterminal process has begun, and we may remain so closeted in our own assumptions that we do not bother to find out what it is that he really needs in his last hours.
>
> And then, one of these days, there is somebody over us with all the ignorant benevolence we have taught him . . .[m]

Such experiences represent not only an unsatisfactory end to a life but a lasting source of unhappiness to the witness.

If the staff can give the kind of care to the elderly that relieves them of pain and discomfort and that makes them feel wanted, and if the institution encourages the presence of relatives (adults and children, and Saunders says, "even the dog"), it is unlikely that the death of an elderly parent will leave this traumatic memory. In the same way, families caring for the elderly at home can be helped by the clergy, by doctors, and by nurses on a home care staff to give the elderly a chance to die in peace and dignity. The family that observes its older members face death with equanimity can see the ultimate achievement and so experience strength and pride, and the person who has so died may be an inspiration to those who go on.

Roles of Caregivers

Helping the Patient with "Getting the House in Order"[n]

A peaceful death is difficult as long as the persons who are dying are struggling to complete unfinished tasks; as long as they feel there are persons they have injured to whom they have never made amends; as long as relatives or friends who have depended on them are not provided for. Giving the dying person an opportunity to complete the tasks of life, as nearly as this is possible, is one of the principal arguments for giving them the best professional assessment of the time they have left. Saunders titles an article on the care of the dying person "The Moment of Truth" and she gives the following explanation:

> The title . . . includes far more than the question "Who should tell—or should you tell—a patient that his death is near?" I think that the title includes many more of the realities and challenges of the situation. It is a situation that concerns all of us, whether we are doctors, nurses, psychiatrists, psychologists, social workers, or theologians. (I have deliberately made the list alphabetical, because all are of equal importance.) Perhaps most of all the situation concerns us when a member of our family or a friend is dying. This is or should be, a "moment of truth". . . it is the patient who is, or who should be, in the center. The question is *his* because it is his situation and he is the person who matters.[o]

One of the practical aspects of "getting the house in order" is making or changing a will, as the patient often wants to do. State laws require wills to be signed in the presence of two or three witnesses. The nurse may be asked to witness a signature on a will and to get one or more persons to act in this capacity. It is unwise for medical personnel to witness signatures unless there is no alternative. There may be subsequent litigation that will require their presence in court and that will interrupt the work for which they are best fitted. In addition to the patient's attorney, the hospital nurse can turn to its ombudsman, the hospital's attorney, social worker, or administrator; outside the hospital, nurses can guide the patient or family to the Legal Aid Society or its equivalent if they don't have their own attorney.

Putting the house in order, arriving at the point where death can be faced calmly—and even gratefully for some—may require the help of family, friends, and professionals. The roles of the various workers who may be involved in the care of the dying are discussed briefly in the following paragraphs. Their roles are overlapping and they may have to substitute for each other according to who is available when help is needed. The importance of working together, of coordinating the various competencies represented in a community and reaching decisions in harmony, cannot be overstressed. Coordination is most likely when, as Saunders says, everyone sees the dying as "the person that matters."

Role of the Family and Friends

There is no substitute for the presence of the family at the bedside of dying persons when they want them there. Those closest to patients can communicate with them effortlessly; a word, a question, a glance can speak volumes. Expressions of family love and loyalty can make persons who are not particularly proud of their accomplishments realize that their life has not been wasted and that they will live on in the memory of their kin. The presence of intimate friends can be equally important. Those who are experienced in the care of dying patients say that the patient and family should be treated as a unit. Craven and Wald make the following observations:

> A family group can be compared to a mobile made up of infinite numbers and kinds of members suspended from a single strand. Each member can move and change independently to some degree, but every shift cannot help but precipitate movement of every other member and the whole. Terminal illness has immediate and long-range effects on this equilibrium.[P]

When a person dies at home, the family may give some part, even most, of the physical care. The role of professional health workers is to share their skills with the family and help them learn how to relieve pain and discomfort: also to identify the tension and conflicts that illness creates and to help the family solve or cope with their problems. When people die in hospitals, nursing homes, and hospices, the staff can encourage the family and friends to participate in the care of the patient. Every effort should be made to sense when they would like to be left alone with each other and when the presence of another person enables them to do or say something that they want to have done or said.

Patients and families have taken the initiative themselves in forming mutual aid and support. In the United States Orville Kelly and his family have built a nationwide network of patients and their families who are facing death. In addition to providing mutual support, its members (particularly Orville Kelly and his wife Wanda) have lectured to community groups and health workers. This organization is called "Make Today Count."

The founders of The Foundation of Thanatology, Austin and Lillian Kutscher, developed that institution because of the experiences both had in the loss of a spouse.

One of the characteristics of present-day hospices that help account for the contentment expressed by patients is the welcome they offer the family and friends; the opportunity to share the life of the dying patient. Rooms are available where family members can stay overnight. As Saunders put it, a family "moved in" to the room of a youth who was dying, bringing games and pets— anything that would make his last days as normal and content as possible.

The treatment of the bereaved begins while the patient is living, for bereavement is least traumatic for those who can believe that they have done everything that was possible for the one who has died.

Books such as John Gunther's *Death Be Not Proud*,[7] Jocelyn Evans' *Living With A Man Who Is Dying*,[8] and C. S. Lewis' *A Grief Observed*[9] describe the satisfaction there is in sharing the pain of separation but living each day as fully as possible until the end.

Role of the Clergy

The role of the clergy is important. Death strikes at the roots of people's lives; it sometimes shakes but also strengthens their faith, and, if they have time to think, impending death makes them question their ethical values. A religion may or may not include belief in an afterlife. In a sample of 30,000 Americans, E. S. Shneidman[10] reported in 1971 that 43 per cent were convinced there was life after death or tended to believe in it. Only 11 percent preferred not to believe in an afterlife. Ninian Smart,[11] writing in *Man's Concern with Death*, edited by Arnold Toynbee and his associates, estimated that about half the people in Great Britain believed in life after death. Alan L. Berman,[12] reviewing other studies and his own data, concluded that "religiously active Catholics and Protestants" are more likely to believe in an afterlife than inactive members of these faiths. Fewer Jews, whether they are active or inactive, believe in an afterlife. Lifton and Olson contrast the teachings of Freud and Jung in the following excerpt from their chapter on symbolic immortality:

> Jung described the psychic vitality of "primitive" peoples who live in tune with archetypal truth. And he observed the positive effects of belief in myths for persons nearing death. He said that when man's conscious thinking is in harmony with the deep truths of the unconscious revealed in mythology, then fear of death is no longer overwhelming. Life can then be lived to the fullest until the end. Therefore, Jung, in contrast to Freud, encouraged belief in religious teachings because he thought such belief was, in his words, "hygienic—necessary for healthy living." He wrote: "When I live in a house that I know will fall about my head within the next two weeks, all my vital functions will be impaired by this thought, but if, on the contrary, I feel myself to be safe, I can dwell there in a normal comfortable way."[q]

There are certain observances and religious practices that help persons of each faith. Ministers of all denominations are expected to give the services of their church to the dying, and will administer them at the patient's request whether they are at home or in an institution. Some religions have no sacraments; others have sacraments of vital significance. This is, however, not the only, or chief, reason why sick people may want to see their ministers. When a relationship exists between the sick and their religious representative, a patient's faith can be strengthened. The clergyman can be a friend and confidant who will discuss with the dying their hopes and fears, their plans for their families, the fact that they are dying, and the consequences of their death. The ability of the clergy to help patients and families in crisis varies widely and is affected by religious and social issues. Many members of a congregation may be at odds with their clergyman over changes in forms of worship or the church's involvement with current events. An example of the first case is the modernization of Roman Catholic or Protestant liturgies; an example of the second, the church's position on women's rights or on wars such as those in Israel, Vietnam, Ireland, Lebanon, or Angola. Some clergymen have had so little experience with seriously ill and dying persons that they have not learned how to give adequate help. It is easier for the priest, minister, rabbi, swami, or other religious representative to help patients if they have been seeing them throughout their illness. If there are resident chaplains in the hospitals, their visits are made routinely; if not, the family, the doctor, or the nurse should help find an appropriate person, whether clergy or lay person, who will give the patient spiritual comfort.

Patients should know that a minister is coming to see them. If nurses have any reason to believe that patients do not realize the seriousness of their condition and might assume that a visit from a clergyman means they are thought to be dying, nurses may assure them that patients are often visited by clergymen on a hospital service. The Catholic Church adopted the term "sacraments of the sick" in 1968 to replace the "sacraments of the Viaticum" (last rites) in order to avoid the finality of "last rites."

Communities where ministries reach out to help people in need regardless of religious creed provide patient, family, and health workers with support that spans all creeds and acknowledge the patient's need to be cared for with or without ritual. It is worth repeating that the clergy, the patient, the family, and other health workers should have as long a time to know one another as possible.

On the clergyman's first visit to the patient, nurses can help by telling them what they think will he helpful about the patient's physical condition, problems, and needs, and, in turn, ask the clergyman what relevant information he has. The minister, priest, rabbi, swami, or other religious representative may prefer to go to the patient unaccompanied, but nurses should offer to take them to patients and make the introduction. It is desirable for this visit to be so timed that the patients are as alert and rational as possible. Among Christians, the Catholics—Roman, Western Non-Roman, and Eastern Orthodox—attach the greatest importance to the sacraments. The Episcopalian, Lutheran, and Moravian are spoken of as "bridge faiths" between Catholicism and Protestantism and have some sacraments and rituals in common. If patients belong to any of these groups, it is desirable to have ready a few simple things the clergyman will need for the administration of the sacraments—usually a table covered with a white cloth and on it a glass, a small bowl of water, a spoon, and a linen napkin or a towel. A glass, a tube, and fresh drinking water should be on the bedside table. Most ministers bring what is needed; if not, they may ask the nurse for certain articles. In denominational hospitals, sacred objects, such as holy oil and crucifixes, are kept in a special place ready for use. If nurses of the same faith are available, they may be of special help to the patient, the family, and the clergyman.

Those involved should be asked whether they prefer privacy or sharing the ritual with others. It can be a rewarding and moving experience for the staff and other patients to see or participate in the ritual, even though they are not of the same faith. The religious observance can be a bridge for others on the periphery to share the suffering of patient and family and the offered help. When privacy is preferred, this should be provided with screens or curtains in an open space, or by putting signs on doors of private rooms.

The Roman Catholics especially believe that the sacraments are essential to a "state of grace" and admission to heaven. The sacraments administered to the dying are Baptism (if the person has not been baptized), Penance (Confession), Holy Eucharist (Communion), and Extreme Unction, formerly called Viaticum when received by a dying person. If the dying person is a Roman Catholic and has not been baptized (as in the case of an infant), nurses should make every effort to get a priest to baptize the person. If this is not possible, a Roman Catholic member of the staff should be asked to administer the sacrament. In the last resort, a non-Catholic can do so.

It is not possible to describe the ministrations of the spiritual adviser to the various Protestant, Catholic, Jewish, Hindu, Mohammedan, and other faiths, but nurses should know something about all the great religions. Many people have a belief in faith healing and laying on of hands. Nurses serve dying patients best by seeing that the proper representatives of their churches are present and then by providing the clergymen as nearly as they can with the conditions they indicate are essential to, or helpful to, their ministry. Visits of clergymen should be recorded. The name of the person administering the sacraments, and the time at which they were received, should be included in the record.

Dicks[13] so long ago warned those who attend dying persons against trying to make them conform to their theological beliefs, and contemporary writers are emphatic on this score.[14–16]

Role of Doctors

The role of doctors has been touched on throughout this chapter. Traditionally they bear the professional responsibility for deciding when it is inappropriate to continue using so-called heroic measures to prolong life. Many opinions have been cited on this subject and the reader is referred to Hinton's volume *Dying*[17] that includes a review of the literature up to 1972. The volume, *The Dying Patient*,[18] edited by Orville Brim, Jr. and his associates includes discussions of the physician's role by Osler Peterson and by Anselm Strauss and Barney G. Glaser. Avery D. Weisman, a physician who has devoted years to the study of the psychosocial aspects of dying, makes the following observation:

> What the Doctor can do about death has two sides, professional and personal. As a professional, he tries to diagnose and treat. If he cannot, then he relieves anguish. But if this, too, fails, he continues to give of himself. Then, when death approaches, he stands by, guiding, assisting, ameliorating. This is his "professional" responsibility, which can be assigned to

others, but cannot be routinely relegated. Like most ethical ideals, it can rarely be fulfilled. Lacking time as well as training, he may perform the essentials of his skill, and allow competent paraprofessionals to take over. However, the Doctor may not realize that he cannot fulfill his own ethical expectations. His traditional role at the pinnacle of the professional pyramid may create an illusion that everything is under his control, because he has not assigned his job to anyone else. What has happened is that having other obligations prevents the doctor from following his obligations to the dying. He does not delegate; he has already forfeited.[r]

Edmund Pellegrino, who has spoken and written widely on the importance of a humane and authentic relationship between patients and health workers, especially physicians, includes the following in a 1975 lecture:

> For most of its history, the relationship of physician and patient has been dominated by the physician's point of view. Ethical codes have been established more on the basis of the obligation physicians feel than those patients may impose. The image of physicians which dominates the profession and society is still based in the Hippocratic ideal. . . . Hippocratic physicians assume responsibility as set forth in the Oath—not to harm patients, not to induce abortion, not to practice euthanasia, to preserve confidentiality, and to take a paternal interest in their students as the future members of a select group. . . . *The Law, Decorum, The Physician,* and *Precepts.* . . . enjoin physicians to attend carefully to their comportment, to be dignified, and reserved, to use common sense, to be moderate, and to reveal nothing of their secrets to those outside of the brotherhood, or even to their patients.
>
> We no longer have consensus as a nation about what we expect from physicians and from medicine. Our attitudes about the authority, privileges and superiority of professional groups have changed drastically. In a democratic society, we expect everyone to participate in decisions which will affect them.
>
> In a democratic society . . . the crucial issues [are] how to enable people to participate as free individuals in the choices which affect them.
>
> There are particular features of illness which diminish and obstruct patients' capacity to live a specifically human existence to its fullest. These features create a relationship of inherent inequality between two human beings—one a physician, the other a patient.
>
> By virtue of the event of illness, these patients lose their freedom to act; they lack the knowledge upon which to make rational choices or to regain their freedom to act; they must place themselves in the power of another human, as petitioners, to regain their humanity, their integrity—i.e., self-image. . . . The sick person lacks knowledge of almost all the essential in-

formation needed to make rational choices and decisions of the utmost importance to his life. He does not know what is wrong; he is not sure of how he became ill, or why; he does not know how serious his problem may be, whether he can recover, what treatments are available, whether they are effective, and with what risk, cost, pain or loss of dignity.

[And so,] in making his competence available to the patient, the physician must also attend to the other deficiencies created by illness. His technical decisions must be congruent with the patient's needs to participate in the choices as freely and rationally as education, time and the circumstances permit. Disclosure of the facts of the illness, the degree of its gravity, the alternatives open, their relative effectiveness, costs and dangers, the physician's own experience and skill in comparison with others, and the likelihood of success or failure must all be explicated. Only with the closing of the information gap can patients approach truly valid consent, one which permits participation as a human and enables the patient to incorporate the decision into his own value system.[s]

Krant, a medical educator, in the following statement makes a plea for the preparation of physicians who can and will share the responsibility for decision-making with others:

Care of the dying patient and of his family obviously involves extensive professional performance, and frequently the best caregivers may be nurses, aides, psychologists, social workers, and others who come to know the patient and family. Yet it is the physician who is the ultimate power in any unit, and he can effectively block an open program of care. The physician may view himself as the lonely, solitary figure in decision-making and care-giving. In a way, the educational process he is put through fosters such an exclusiveness.[t]

While it is part of the physician's traditional role to discuss the imminence of death with the patient's family and to notify the family when death occurs, systems in which the physician bears sole responsibility for telling the patient have severe critics. Hinton[19] called attention to studies showing that the majority of doctors (80 to 90 percent) say they rarely tell their patients the illness is terminal even though studies have also shown that 80 percent of the patients interviewed want to be told.

Some health care practitioners argue that patients will crumble if the truth is disclosed. Other practitioners express opposing views and present practical difficulties that result from withholding the truth; for instance, patients die without getting their affairs in order. There are also ethical and moral issues and the legal right of the patient to be informed and participate in decisions affecting him or her is transgressed. Those who can continue to talk to the end can add an important dimension to their lives and help those around them to understand what it is like to be dying.

Saunders puts the principle in practical and clear terms: "Every patient needs an explanation of his illness that will be understandable and convincing to him if he is to cooperate in his treatment or be relieved of the burden of unknown fears. This is true whether it is a question of giving a diagnosis in a hopeful situation or of confirming a poor prognosis."[u]

Physicians are changing their views on informing patients. For example, Oliver Cope[20], professor emeritus of surgery at Harvard University, has recommended that when cancer of the breast is suspected, patients should be included in decisions, beginning with diagnostic procedures. He recommends that the diagnostic process have sequential steps, which begin with telling the patient that no therapy will be prescribed until a biopsy is made and until the pathology report can be reviewed by a team of physician–surgeon, oncologist, radiologist, and pathologist. The nature and extent of the pathology will be discussed by the team and the following questions answered: Is there blood vessel invasion? What is the chance of the disease spreading by way of the lymphatics? What are the relative merits of available types of treatment (modalities)? After consideration of these issues, the conferring physicians and pathologists agree on what treatment is best and why. At this point, the primary physician discusses the findings with the patient and they reach a decision, and so the patient can give an "informed consent" to treatment.

Alfred S. Ketchan, writing on a surgeon's approach to advanced cancer, expressed the following opinion:

> The doctor who takes it upon himself to be less than honest with the mentally alert cancer-bearing patient, who has family or financial responsibilities, is treading deeply in the realm of the Supreme Being. Although there is nothing sweeter to the ears of the physician than the words, "Thank you Doctor, for curing me," or "Here I am Doc, it's been five years since you told my wife I was going to die," it can be almost as satisfying and heart-warming to hear the sincere and heartfelt expression of the patient, "Thank you, Doctor, for being honest and frank with me in telling me what I need to know, if I am to properly prepare for what lies ahead of me."[v]

These changing views are amply supported in *A Patient's Bill of Rights*,[21] published by the American Hospital Association, which include the patient's right to know about treatment, the risks involved, and the right to refuse the treatment recommended.

Richard Lamerton, a physician of the Home Care Service of St. Joseph's Hospice, Hackney, England, puts the responsibility for deciding when to "abandon cure" (but not *care*) on the doctor, who "must decide who is dying." He says the next question is "who shall be told, and when." Lamerton says that patients tend to ask first-year nurses and medical students rather than the medical consultant and he makes the following observation:

> If the doctors will not be realistic . . . the nurses can find themselves required to deceive patients who are not fooled, and having to ask nurses from the previous shift which lie they are supposed to be supporting.
>
> Ward sisters should have a completely free hand to confirm or reassure as they see fit, and junior nurses should have had the opportunity to discuss in advance what their response should be. Patients . . . sooner or later . . . will lose faith in any one who deceives them.
>
> This kind of approach demands good communication between the nurses and doctors, and also with any other member of the caring team whom the patient may choose as his confidante.

Lamerton thinks that the caring team, including the chaplain and the social worker, should have access to all the information there is on diagnosis and prognosis and that regular conferences are essential. He says that "Only in this way can we really function as a team, learning to trust one another, and to serve the patient properly."[w]

In addition to making a diagnosis and a prognosis on the length of life and telling the patient and the family, it is traditional for the doctor to prescribe the medical management of symptoms and to pronounce death. While the physicians prescribe drugs for pain, nausea, dyspnea, and other symptoms, it is the nurses who give them and have the best opportunity to see their effects. As in the psychosocial aspects of care there is much to be gained by pooling judgment, by conferring frequently, and by inviting the opinion of the most experienced caregivers regardless of their appointed roles.

Pronouncement of death is by law the function of the physician. Robert H. Moser, discussing the doctor's role, notes what he calls "the new ethics." He makes the following observation on defining the border between life and death and contemporary problems:

> But there is now a new dimension. Our engineers and technologists have provided us with machines that have prodded and crowded Death onto a strange, unfamiliar terrain. The delicate yet definable border between life and

death that existed in the past now has new, ill-defined interfaces with philosophy and ethics. We are denied a simple physiological endpoint for death. What morality applies in choosing live donors for organ transplantation? When is the donor of an unpaired organ dead? Must we designate some arbitrary waiting period before removing critical organs that are becoming ischemic? Is it a violation of Hippocratic ethic to dialyze or infuse mannitol into the patient dying from a head injury just to preserve his kidneys for graft purposes? Dare we remove vital organs from a patient who is not judged, by all criteria, to be totally and irrevocably dead? Who will make the decision? Just what is our obligation to potential donors and potential recipients, for example, the mother of three who just happens to be the most compatible donor for a fourth child with end-stage kidney disease?

In this same article Moser says:

> The shifting, perhaps slightly tattered image of the physician in the public eye continues to evoke much thought and comment. When the tumult subsides, one thing will not have changed since the first aboriginal mother took her dying child to the village shaman: the status of the physician as life and death decisionmaker. Of his many roles, this role has always been the most difficult for the physician.[x]

Saunders, also discussing the inescapable distress for physicians in the care of the dying, says it is more difficult than the nurse's role because the latter can do something for the patient with their hands. This giving by touching is mutually comforting, it makes nurses feel useful to patients, while the doctors, with all their authority, feel frustrated and helpless. Perhaps the answer lies in shared decisions, always remembering that "informed patients" and their families should have the last word.

Among physicians, no specialists seem to have shown more interest in research on death than *psychiatrists*. They may be on the staff of institutions and home care services for the purpose of studying the meaning of death, the psychosocial needs of the dying, the reaction of others to the dying person, or the effect of bereavement. Psychiatrists may also have staff appointments so that they can be accessible to patients and their families or as consultants to the other physicians, to nurses, or to anyone involved in patient care. Psychiatrists in psychiatric hospitals are, of course, responsible for the total medical care of terminally ill patients. The staff also needs support so psychiatrists indirectly help the patient when they help the caregiver.

Role of Pharmacists

Pharmacists have a special role in institutions and agencies providing terminal care since the medical management of symptoms is in many cases dependent on knowledge of drugs, their actions and interactions.[21a] This is particularly true in the case of cancer. This era is characterized by proliferation of drugs. It is hard for physicians to keep up with the development of pharmacology. Doctors and nurses are more than ever inclined to consult pharmacists and use their special competence in the preparation of drugs and in assessing their interaction. In other eras nurses may have been expected to operate the pharmacy in the afternoon and at night after the pharmacist left for the day; in this age the danger of having any but experts prepare and dispense drugs (which was always present) is so generally recognized that pharmacists are available on a full-time basis. They may often participate in patient conferences. Many medical centers have a research pharmacist who can gather relevant data quickly and, using a computer, can make comprehensive up-to-date information available. The pharmacist increasingly helps the physician and nurse relieve the symptoms so that patients can lead a more active and comfortable life.

Role of the Nurse

The nurse's role in the care of dying patients depends upon whether the patients are at home or in an institution and on the amount of care family or friends want and are able to give. How nurses function depends also on how others expect or permit them to function, the environment created by administrative officers of an institution, the limiting, or inhibiting, rules and regulations, and time available to nurses for meeting the needs of dying patients.

Either directly or by teaching others, it is the function of the nurse to give patients the help they need with the activities of daily living, to help them maintain their independence as long as possible, and to make it possible for patients to have what they consider a good death.[y] It is also the function of the nurse to minimize any pain or discomfort associated with the dying process by helping patients and families use effectively the measures prescribed by physicians. In situations where physicians are unavailable, as in most emergencies, nurses may have to assume responsibility for using a relief measure that has not been prescribed. Physicians' directions ("orders") may stipulate a discretionary role of the nurse in relation to certain treatments.

In institutions and in some home care services, nurses are with the patient more than other trained health workers so it is they who have the best opportunity to sense patients' needs and wishes, their symptoms and responses to treatment, their fears and anxieties, their hopes and the way they want to die. Saunders repeatedly refers to the tendency of patients to "confide in the nurse." Ronald Gibson,[22] a British physician, says few nurses appreciate what they mean to patients and their families. Nurses are accessible and the physical care they give patients evokes a confidential relationship.

So many articles on nursing care of the dying have appeared recently in the *American Journal of Nursing* that Mary H. Browning and Edith P. Lewis compiled them in a volume—*The Dying Patient: A Nursing Perspective*.[23] Reports given at ANA Clinical Conferences have focused on care of the dying.[24,25] Reference has been made to Jeanne C. Quint's (Benoliel) study[26] and to the course she is teaching at the University of Washington School of Nursing, to a program at the University of Florida School of Nursing, described by Ramona Powell Davidson,[27] and to the experience of the investigation of terminal nursing care.[28] Counterparts of the American articles appear in nursing journals around the world.[29-35] Saunders' writings, dating from the 1950s, stress the importance of the nurse's (the "Sister's") role and she pays special tribute to the nurses in the Irish Order of the Sisters of Charity, who, at St. Joseph's Hospice in London, demonstrated their skilled and sensitive care of the dying— care on which she, as its founder, has based the program at St. Christopher's Hospice in London.

Barbara J. McNulty, nursing officer of the Domiciliary Service at St. Christopher's, hopes it will be part of every nurse's skill to give [effective] terminal care. She stresses the importance of nurses realizing that they are members of "a team" which means that the nurse may be the most important person to some patients, but "the back-up" for other workers in other cases. McNulty thinks it essential that nurses understand their attitudes toward death; that they individualize their care of patients and help to relatives; and that they learn to "feel without being overwhelmed, to care without being overcome, to participate without being identified."[z] Earlier, for an American audience, McNulty described St. Christopher's and its home care program.[36] And there is an illustrated description of Christmas there which shows how nurses join with other members of the staff in creating a "joyous" atmosphere.[36a]

D. H. Summers, another member of St. Christopher's nursing staff, discussing the role of the nurse in 1974, quotes Florence Nightingale as saying that the most dangerous maxim for a nurse is "What can't be cured must be endured." Summers says:

Let us refute this statement [that nothing more can be done] and accept
the challenge that at this point everything can and must be done, not to
prolong life, but to improve the quality of [life in] the time that remains.[aa]

Summers thinks nurses can be effective in their role if they become involved, if they function as one of a concerned group. She discusses the way
the nurse "shares" with the patient, the family, other nurses, doctors, the
clergy, social workers, nutritionists, occupational and physical therapists—
the various health workers serving the patient.

No rules can be laid down for the nurse's behavior with the dying and their
families or what they do for them since no two situations are alike. And so much
depends on the age of the patient; whether the death comes suddenly or after a
long illness, on the setting in which the death occurs; and on the availability of
other health workers. Even though nurses have had no previous experience with
death, they need not fear self-consciousness or embarrassment if they turn their
entire attention to their helping task. A great deal depends upon their sensitiveness to people, their judgment, and taste; or, in other words, the nurse's personality. People cannot give something they do not themselves possess. Nursing skills
can be learned that relieve or lessen the patient's physical discomfort and therefore the family's distress, but everyone concerned is supported by the nurse's
willingness to go with them through an experience with death. This willingness
is an attitude which is expressed in thoughtful actions even more than words. If
present, it helps the patient and family make use of the nurse's professional sus-
taining competence. Carol Ren Kneisl, a nurse, discussing thoughtful care for the
dying, stresses the importance of simply being with the patient. She thinks that
dying people suffer most from a sense of isolation and abandonment. She notes
that "the ancient Greeks believed the most fearful event was not dying but dying
alone."[bb] Ilse S. Wolfe, a psychiatric nurse, years ago, illustrated with clinical incidents this willingness to walk beside the patient. She called this "The Magnificence of Understanding."[37] Listening is, of course, essential to understanding.
The most experienced persons in the care of the dying keep saying that directly
or obliquely most patients will let caregivers know their needs if they will sit quietly and listen.

When death is imminent, nothing is more reassuring to patients and their families than the promise that someone will be there when the patient needs a comforting presence. And it goes without saying that such promises must be realistic
so that they can be kept. Reports of solitary hospital deaths and the literature
abounds in criticism of doctors who are not present, even in hospitals.[cc] Nurses
have the greatest opportunity and therefore should have the responsibility for

noting signs of approaching death and the authority to call the physician, and in his absence, or with his approval, the family and the clergy or a spiritual adviser of the patient's choice. While nurses cannot legally pronounce death, in the physician's absence and in the normal course of open communication with the family they should share their opinion that life is over. Nurses prepare the body to go to the undertaking establishment; this is discussed in a later section, as is their role in helping the bereaved.

Role of Social Workers

Social workers, Ruth D. Abrams says, are the most available counselors in many medical settings. They collaborate with chaplains, doctors, nurses, and others in helping patients and their relatives with a variety of problems. In some countries and in certain eras, the preparation and work of the public health nurse and the social worker are combined; in the United States, visiting nurse associations often have social workers on their staffs.

Abrams thinks there are common misconceptions about the role of the social worker whose function she sees as follows:

> Many people think of the social worker as a person who gives advice on how to manage the financial aspect of the illness. If they do not need such help, their first reaction is to reject the suggestion that such a person can be useful. I believe that changing the term "social worker" to "family counselor" would be a giant step toward ensuring acceptance by health workers and by the family. Her help should include practical matters, to be sure, but it goes well beyond that.[dd]

Abrams,[38,39] through excerpts from case studies, shows the problems and describes the kinds of help social workers at the Massachusetts General Hospital give patients with cancer and the families of these patients. Social workers may help them cope with financial problems or with the changes in the way the family lives when either parent dies. Knowing the resources in the community, social workers may be the best prepared persons to help patients and families make use of them. As, through regular visits and participation in patient conferences, they come to know the patients, their relatives, and friends, they may be in an admirable position to help patients' families to live as normally as possible during a terminal illness and to return to normal community life after the period of acute grief.

Notes

[a]Reed Nelson, formerly research coordinator at Hospice, Inc., New Haven, Conn., interviewed 100 close relatives of persons who died of cancer in New Haven between 1968 and 1971. Of these, 42 died in the hospital but only 21 had wanted to go there. Another 20 died in a nursing home while only 7 had wanted to go there. Only 38 died at home, although 65 had said they would like to stay at home with their families. Of the 100 persons interviewed, 72 were unable to keep the sick family member at home although 61 of them said they would have liked to do so had adequate support been available. (*Hospice* [Newsletter], Oct. 1974. p. 3.)

[b]Saunders, Cicely: "The Management of Fatal Illness in Childhood," *Proc. R. Soc. Med.,* 62:550, (June) 1969.

[c]West, T. S.: "Symposium on Care of the Dying. Approach to Death," *Nurs. Mirror,* 139:56, (Oct. 10) 1974.

[d]U.S. Department of Health, Education, and Welfare: *Working With Older People, Vol. II.* U.S. Government Printing OlElce, Washington, D.C., Apr. 1970 (PHS Pub. No. 1459), p. 7.

[e]Craven, Joan, and Wald, Florence: "Hospice Care for Dying Patients," *Am. J. Nurs.,* 75:1816, (Oct.) 1975.

[f]Working Document, International Work Group on Death, Dying and Bereavement, Yale University, 1976 Conference. Not available for publication in 1976.

[g]Saunders, Cicely: "The Management of Fatal Illness in Childhood," *Proc. R. Soc. Med.,* 62:550, (June) 1969.

[h]Henderson, Edward: "The Approach to the Patient with an Incurable Disease," in Schoenberg, Bernard, et al. (eds.): *Psychosocial Aspects of Terminal Care.* Columbia University Press, New York, 1972, p. 61.

[i]Martinson, Ida Marie (ed.): *Home Care for the Dying Child, Professional and Family Perspectives.* Appleton-Century-Crofts, New York, 1976.

[j]Wessel, Morris A.: "A Death in the Family. The Impact on Children," *J.A.M.A.,* 234:865 (Nov. 24) 1975.

[k]Saunders, Cicely: "The Management of Fatal Illness in Childhood," *Proc. R. Soc. Med.,* 63:550 (June) 1969.

[l]David Maddison and Beverley Raphael say that "Before the age of five years, death is equated with sleep and is not considered final. Through the years from five to nine, death is often personified and may be thought of as an event

contingent upon the aggressive fantasies or actions of others. It is only after the age of nine that death is seen as a process dependent upon natural laws and characterized by the permanent cessation of vital bodily functions. Fear of death in children is variously seen as a fear of the aggressive retaliation of others, together with a fear of emotional deprivation possibly related to separation anxiety. (Maddison, David, and Raphael, Beverley: "The Family of the Dying Patient," in Schoenberg, Bernard, et al. [eds.]: *Psychosocial Aspects of Terminal Care.* Columbia University Press, New York, 1972, p. 187.)

mKastenbaum, Robert: "While the Old Man Dies: Our Conflicting Attitudes Toward the Elderly. Concluding Note," in Schoenberg, Bernard, et al. (eds.): *Psychosocial Aspects of Terminal Care.* Columbia University Press, New York, 1972, p. 124.

nThis is a term which patients in my study frequently used. [Florence Wald]

oSaunders, Cicely: "The Moment of Truth: Care of the Dying Person," in Pearson, L. (ed.): *Death and Dying: Current Issues in the Treatment of the Dying Person.* Press of Case-Western Reserve University, Cleveland, 1969, p. 49.

pCraven, Joan, and Wald, Florence S.: "Hospice Care for Dying Patients," *Am. J. Nurs., 75*:1816 (Oct.) 1975.

qLifton, Robert Jay, and Olson, Eric: *Living and Dying.* Praeger Publishers, New York, p. 73.

rWeisman, Avery D.: *On Dying and Denying; a Psychiatric Study of Terminality.* Behavioral Publications, New York, 1972, p. 201.

sPellegrino, Edmund D.: *The Humanistic Base of Professional Ethics in Medicine.* Jubilee Lecture, Memorial University of Newfoundland, Canada, May 13, 1975.

tKrant, Melvin: "In the Context of Dying," in Schoenberg, Bernard, et al. (eds.): *Psychosocial aspects of Terminal Care.* Columbia University Press, New York, 1972, p. 203.

uSaunders, Cicely: "Telling Patients," *Dist. Nurs., 8*:149, (Sept.) 1965.

vKetchan, Alfred S.: "A Surgeon's Approach to the Patient with Advanced Cancer. Who Should Know," in Schoenberg, Bernard, et al. (eds.): *Psychosocial Aspects of Terminal Care.* Columbia University Press, New York, 1972, p. 97.

wLamerton, Richard: "Symposium on Care of the Dying. Ethical Questions in the Care of the Dying," *Nurs. Mirror, 139*:61, (Oct. 10) 1974.

xMoser, Robert H.: "The New Ethics," in Schoenberg, Bernard, et al. (eds.): *Psychosocial Aspects of Terminal Care.* Columbia University Press, New York, 1972, p. 43.

[y]It is interesting that Jocelyn Evans, a wife who took care of her dying husband, says that this role of the nurse, which she read in the *ICN Basic Principles of Nursing Care*, "reflects my attitude absolutely. 'The unique function of the nurse,' it says, 'is to assist the individual, sick or well, in the performance of those activities contributing to health or its recovery (or to peaceful death) that he would perform unaided if he had the necessary strength, will or knowledge.' The nurse assists her patient, it explains, by contributing to 'what is—*to him*—a good death.' " (Evans, Jocelyn: *Living with a Man Who Is Dying*. Taplinger Publishing Co., New York, 1971, p. 109.)

[z]McNulty, Barbara J.: "Symposium on Care of the Dying. The Nurse's Contribution in Terminal Care," *Nurs. Mirror, 139,*:59, (Oct. 10) 1974.

[aa]Summers, D. H.: "The Role of the Nurse," presented at Thanatology Nursing Symposium, New York City, Nov. 1–2, 1974.

[bb]Kneisl, Carol Ren: "Thoughtful Care for the Dying," *Am. J. Nurs., 68*:550, (Mar.) 1968.

[cc]Dorothy P. Geis, a nurse who interviewed 26 mothers who had lost a child, found that the doctor was present in 13 instances, the nurse in 8, the father and mother in 5, the mother alone in 4, the father in 1, others in 6 cases, and in 4 cases the mother did not know. The mothers thought physicians most helpful (11), the clergy next, and the nurse third. In 5 cases, no one was "most helpful." The sample is too small to have much significance but data of this sort are badly needed as a substitute for unfounded inferences on the needs of patients and families and who can and will meet them. (Geis, Dorothy P.: "Mothers' Perceptions of Care Given Their Dying Children," *Am. J. Nurs., 65*:105, [Feb.] 1965.)

[dd]Abrams, Ruth D.: *Not Alone With Cancer*. Charles C Thomas, Publisher, Springfield, Ill., 1974, p. 14.

References

---

1. Nagy, Maria H.: "The Child's View of Death," in Feifel, Herman (ed.): *The Meaning of Death*. McGraw-Hill Book Co., New York, 1959.

2. Fredlund, Delphia J.: "A Nurse Looks at Children's Questions About Death," in *ANA Clinical Conferences*, 1970. Appleton-Century-Crofts, New York, 1970.

3. Furman, Erna: *A Child's Parent Dies. Studies in Childhood Bereavement.* Yale University Press, New Haven, 1974.

4. Wynant, W. E.: "Dying But Not Alone," *Am. J. Nurs., 67*:574, (Mar.) 1967.

5. Simmons, Leo W.: *The Role of the Aged in Primitive society.* Yale University Press, New Haven, Conn., 1945.

6. Jaeger, Dorothea, and Simmons, Leo W.: *The Aged Ill; Coping with Problems in Geriatric Care.* Appleton-Century-Crofts, New York, 1970.

7. Gunther, John: *Death Be Not Proud.* Harper & Brothers, New York, 1949, pp. 250, 251.

8. Evans, Jocelyn: *op. cit.*

9. Lewis, C. S.: *A Grief Observed.* Sebury Press, New York, 1961.

10. Shneidman, E. S.: "You and Death," *Psychology Today, 5*:43, (June) 1971.

11. Smart, Ninian: "Death and the Decline of Religion in Western society," in Toynbee, Arnold, et al. (eds.) *Man's concern With Death.* McGraw-Hill Book Co., New York, 1968.

12. Berman, Alan L.: "Believe in Afterlife, Religion Religiosity, and Life-Threatening Experiences," *Omega, 5*:127, (Summer) 1974.

13. Dicks, Russell L.: *Who Is My Patient?* Macmillan Publishing Co., Inc., New York, 1941.

14. Feifel, Herman (ed.): *The Meaning of Death.* McGraw-Hill Book Co., New York, 1959.

15. Hinton, John: *Dying,* 2nd ed. Penguin Books, Harmondsworth, Eng., 1972

16. Schoenberg, Bernard, et al. (eds.): *Psychosocial Aspects of Terminal Care.* Columbia University Press, New York, 1972.

17. Hinton, John: *op cit.*

18. Brim, Orville G., Jr., et al. (eds.) *op. cit.*

19. Hinton, John: *op. cit.*

20. Cope, Oliver: "Has the Time Come for a Less Mutilating Treatment" *Radcliffe Q. Rev.,* June 1970.

21. American Hospital Association: *op. cit.*

21a. Lipman, Arthur C.: "Drug Therapy in the Care of Terminally Ill Patients," *Am. J. Hosp. Pharm., 32*:270, (Mar.) 1975.

22. Gibson, Ronald: "Symposium on Care of the Dying, Caring for the Bereaved," *Nurs. Mirrors, 139*:65, (Oct. 10) 1974.

23. Browning, Mary H., and Lewis, Edith P. (comps.) *The Dying Patient: A*

Nursing Perspective. American Journal of Nursing Co., New York, 1972 (Contemporary Nursing Series).

24. Aguilera, Donna Conant: "Crisis: Death and Dying," in *ANA Clinical Sessions, 1968.* Appleton-Century-Crofts, New York, 1968.

25. Wald, Florence S.: "Development of an Interdisciplinary Team to Care for Dying Patients and Their Families," in *ANA Clinical Conferences, 1969.* Appleton-Century-Crofts, New York, 1970.

26. Crofts, New York, 1970.

27. Davidson, Ramona Powell: "To Give Care in Terminal Illness," *Am. J. Nurs., 66*:74, (Jan.) 1966.

28. Wald, Florence S.: *A Nurse's Study of Care for Dying Patients.* U.S-.P.H.S. Nursing Resources Grant NU 00352–01, 02, Sept. 1, 1969–Aug. 30, 1971 (report in preparation).

29. Henderson, I., and Henderson, J. E.: "Psychological Care of Patients with Catastrophic Illness," *Can. Nurse, 61*:899, (Nov.) 1965.

30. Craig, Y.: "The Care of a Dying Child. The Needs of the Nurses, the Patient, and Parents," *Nurs. Mirror, 137*:14, (Sept. 28) 1973.

31. Cramond, W. A.: "The Psychological Care of Patients with Terminal Illness," N.Z. *Nurs. J., 66*:27, (Sept.) 1973.

32. Bennett, M. B.: "Care of the Dying," *S. Afr. Med. J., 47*:1558, (Sept. 1) 1973.

33. Goldfogel, L.: "Working with the Parents of a Dying Child," *Nurs. J. India, 62*:8, (Jan.) 1971.

34. Kono, H.: ["Death and Nursing"], *Jap. J. Nurs., 37*:98, (Jan.); 1046, (Aug.) 1973.

35. Cramond, W. A.: "The Psychological Care of Patients with Terminal Illness," *N.Z. Nurs. J., 66*:23, (Oct.) 1973.

36. McNulty, Barbara J.: "St. Christopher's Outpatients," *Am. J. Nurs., 71*:2328, (Dec.) 1971.

36a. _____: "Christmas at St. Christopher's," *Am. J. Nurs., 71*:2325, (Dec.) 1971.

37. Wolfe, Ilse S.: "The Magnificence of Understanding," in Standard, Samuel, and Nathan, Helmut (eds.): *Should the Patient Know the Truth.* Springer Publishing Co., New York, 1955.

38. Abrams, Ruth D.: "The Responsibility of Social Work in Terminal Cancer," in Schloenberg, Bernard, et al. (eds.): *Psychosocial Aspects of Terminal Care.* Columbia University Press, New York, 1972.

39. _____: *Not Alone with Cancer.* Charles C. Thomas, Publisher, Springfield, Ill., 1974.

PART II

Nursing Education

Introduction

U ntil Miss Henderson was 50 years of age and a well-established teacher in the nursing education program at Teacher's College, Columbia University, she frequently returned to the hospital or public health agency to practice nursing. Her associates hint that the reason she left her teaching position was because she was deprived of the opportunity to teach in the clinical section of graduate nursing courses. Her papers at the Mugar Library, Boston University, contain many of the clinical case reports her students at Teacher's College wrote. Miss Henderson believes that nursing is best taught by persons who practice.

Derek Bok (1991) says that the task of a faculty is to decide who teaches and what is taught. Miss Henderson answers these questions in the *Nature of Nursing* (1991). In it there is a curriculum plan that rationalizes the progress of a student through a professional nursing educational program. She advocates the expansion of nursing education to include the teaching of primary care and therapy.

The fact that clinical teaching is the most expensive part of nursing education—and its expense is given as rationale for separating the theory and practice components—has always alarmed her. She is supportive of those educational institutions that cultivated strong affiliations with hospitals that allowed practice privileges for faculty; Yale, Case-Western Reserve, Rush, and Rochester being a few outstanding examples. The separation of the professional functions of education from practice is a relatively new development and began with the wholesale replacement of hospital nursing schools with community college programs. The difference in the per graduate cost of these programs (diploma schools had small enrollments, large faculties and buildings; community colleges have small faculties, many matriculants, and few buildings) is ample testimony to the negative economic effects of the change from hospital to community college. That such changes occurred in a largely women's field, while Law, Medical, and Business schools flourished, may reflect the continued emphasis on societal investments in mens' education.

Miss Henderson has never criticized nurses for availing themselves of education in community college nursing programs but rather has advocated for a solid educational foundation and a strong professional education for all nurses. Perhaps we should consider the amalgamation of our state university nursing schools with our teaching hospitals to more closely couple education and practice. I have long been a convert of former dean Rozella Schlodtfelt, who successfully combined nursing education at the Frances Payne Bolton School of Nursing and service at University Hospitals of Cleveland so the activities were mutually supportive and efficient. Perhaps leaders in the profession can also begin to see Master's preparation in Nursing as the rule rather than the exception (only 5% of the 2.3 million American nurses have MSNs). This can be achieved by bypassing the Bachelor's degree where nurses have not been given the opportunity to obtain one. Our patients are better served by nurses who have strong educational backgrounds in clinical nursing, of the type now provided in university professional schools at the Master's level.

It is incumbent upon today's nurses to value their nursing education enough to seek it for all professional nurses, not just limiting it to a few privileged nurses. To the degree nurses believe that nursing education is for the well-being of persons who use nurses' services, and that professional schools serve patients through the nurses they educate, then targeting most nurses for advanced professional education will empower nurses to accomplish reform in health care more than any other activity. Nurses can participate more actively in primary care and other activities, thereby leading the population toward health services that encourage their independence, provided that their education is consistent with their responsibilities.

References

1. Bok, D. (1991). *Higher learning*. New York: Basic Books.
2. Henderson, V. (1991). *The Nature of Nursing: Reflections after 25 years*. New York: National League for Nursing Press.

Chapter 9

Preparation for General Nursing

Some Initial, or Basic, Professional Programs

The following pages are devoted mainly to the preparation in North America of the registered "professional" nurse as defined by the International Council of Nurses. The registered "professional" nurse is the worker referred to as "the nurse" throughout this book. There is no intention of disregarding or underestimating the contribution to health care of licensed practical nurses, nurse's assistants, nurse's aides, orderlies, and nursing personnel with other titles. The current trend toward identifying information and skills all health workers should acquire is, we believe, constructive. Making it possible for students to move from one educational program to another is also thought desirable by the writer. Nursing, as discussed here, will, we hope, interest all those who practice it regardless of their titles.

In 1975, Dorothy Ozimek[1] of the National League for Nursing, reviewing current studies, summarized recent changes and predicted the future of nursing education, noting major social trends that affect its future. Nothing characterizes nursing in this era more than experimentation in nursing education and rapid changes in curricula. Many institutions and agencies in the United States and elsewhere are trying to individualize student programs and to encourage independent study that allows a student to progress at his or her own pace.[2] Admission requirements have been liberalized so that young men and women with dissimilar social and ethnic backgrounds have equal opportunity to enter the nursing occupations, though minorities do not presently have proportional representation.[a] The "open curriculum" and the "ladder concept" in nursing education are widely discussed and encouraged by grants that make demonstration projects possible. Even a doctoral degree may be acquired from "the University without walls."[3,4]

The idea that continuing education will be available to all health workers makes the concept of watertight, dead-end programs obsolete. In the USSR and the People's Republic of China, radically new and productive systems of health care have been developed in surprisingly short time periods. These countries use health workers with relatively brief training programs. Since, however, these workers come from, live beside, and understand the needs of the people, and since in both countries continuing education and the ladder concept are part of the system, health workers with a limited initial training can make good use of what they know and can go as far as their innate ability allows them since they return again and again for additional study and experience in health centers. Health education programs for the public encourage self-help and effective use of all types of health workers and facilities.

Certain countries, for example, Canada, have discouraged the proliferation of health workers, even rejecting the idea of "intermediate" health workers as exemplified by the feldshers of the USSR or the physician's assistants of the United States. Claude Castonguay expressed the prevalent view when he said, with reference to proposed legislation, "Nurses . . . will as a group remain what is justly called the 'backbone' of the health establishment." He rejected the physician's assistant (feldsher type) because he thought no category of health worker should be an assistant "forever."[b]

Some students of health care systems in the United States and elsewhere believe that proliferation of health workers makes for fragmentation of care and they would like to see fewer varieties, each prepared to give a wider range of services or more effective service. To modify the present hierarchical system of health care in the United States, it has been suggested that new terms or titles be used that would do away with the present public and self-image of doctors, nurses, and others, for current images may be barriers to good working relationships and hence barriers to effective health care.

Suggestions for a single health profession, or for fewer or new kinds of health workers in the United States imply such radical changes in educational programs that no attempt can be made to identify them here. However, the practice in some North American universities of offering interdisciplinary courses for medical and nursing students and students in other health fields is a step in this direction, as is the requirement of continuing education for all health workers. Many students in one health occupation now take, as electives, courses designed primarily for those in a different occupation; nursing faculties include nonnurses such as physicians, social workers, and clinical psychologists, while medical faculties include many nonphysicians—sometimes nurses. The overlapping functions and responsibilities of physicians, nurses, social workers, health educators, and others is increasingly recognized and is modifying their preparation for practice.

Because rapid change characterizes this era, defining types of nursing personnel and their preparation must be tentative. Statements from the World Health Organization and the ICN may soon be of historical interest only. Both indicate, however, that registered nurses should be so prepared that they can offer a professional service.

In most countries, nursing personnel whose preparation is most like that of the registered nurse are prepared in a 1-year to 2-year planned program under educational or hospital auspices. In the United States, this category of worker is called a "licensed practical nurse" and in Canada a "qualified nursing assistant," although a 1976 Canadian publication refers to practical nursing schools.

The second category of nursing personnel with less preparation than that of the registered nurse was described as follows by the WHO:

> Nursing personnel able to perform specified tasks related to patient care that require considerably less use of judgment. They should be able to relate well to patients and to carry out dependably, under supervision, the tasks for which they have been trained.[c]

While in many countries, such workers are given in-service training which ranges considerably in length and thoroughness, the American Nurses' Association recommends short, intensive courses in vocational service institutions rather than on-the-job training.

In the United States, the ANA calls both categories just discussed "allied nursing personnel," saying that the licensed practical nurse is a distinct occupational group and that nurse's aides, orderlies, and home health aides constitute another group. In Canada, nursing personnel with less preparation than the registered nurse are called "auxiliary nursing personnel."

In the United States, the estimated numbers of employed allied nursing personnel (including practical nurses) in 1972 totalled 1,327,000, a considerably larger number than the 780,000 employed registered nurses and even more than the 1,127,657 registered nurses. In Canada, the licensed auxiliary nursing personnel totalled 45,945 in 1972, considerably less than the total 114,349 employed registered nurses in that country. However, since some auxiliary nursing personnel are not licensed, this comparison may be misleading.[5,6]

Allied or auxiliary nursing personnel are obviously giving a great deal of the nursing care in these (and other) countries, so it is of the utmost importance that their preparation be upgraded. While this question is not discussed here, it is recognized as part of the over-all aspect of nursing education.

Historical Background

Nursing education today is, like practice, changing rapidly, and these changes can be understood best by those who know its history. It has been the subject of more published volumes, more doctoral dissertations, and more journal articles than has any other nursing topic. National surveys of nursing schools and critical analyses of the system of nursing education in the United States date from Adelaide M. Nutting's study in 1912 to that of the current National Commission for the Study of Nursing and Nursing Education. At least five other major studies were reported in the intervening years. All of these reports have recommended that nursing schools be put under educational auspices rather than under hospitals, which are primarily service institutions, and that the preparation of nurses be comparable to that of other professionals, for example, teachers, doctors, and lawyers. In the United States, this means putting nursing schools in colleges and universities. Some individuals saw the desirability of this even in the nineteenth century. For example, Abby H. Woolsey,[7] the Civil War self-taught nurse, in 1876 recommended the equivalent of a normal school education for nurses. (Normal schools of that day were in some respects like community colleges of today. They prepared most teachers in the United States at that time.) Isabel A. Hampton made ardent appeals for a liberalized education for nurses, but she did not, according to Mary Roberts,[8] see the necessity of getting them out from under hospital control. In 1901, Mrs. Bedford Fenwick[9] of England gave four reasons behind her "plea for the higher education of trained nurses." Some physicians supported these nursing leaders. Among them was Richard C. Cabot,[10] who, in 1906, reported a local study showing the exploitation of nursing students by hospitals. One hospital earned

$12,845.36 from payment to the hospital for services of student nurses to patients in their homes.[d] In 1910, Richard Olding Beard,[11] a physician, described the creation of a nursing school under university auspices at the University of Minnesota.

In 1912, Annie W. Goodrich,[12] in an article, "The Complete Nurse," discussed the complexity of nursing and the importance of social experience and a thorough education for the nurse. Hers was a life-long struggle to get schools of nursing into the universities. In 1921, Ethel Johns,[13] a Canadian nurse, presented the logic of placing nursing schools in universities and she described one degree program offered nurses in four of the Canadian universities.

In 1931, Dean E. P. Lyon[14] of the University of Minnesota Medical School read a paper at several state nurses' association meetings entitled "Taking the Profit Out of Nursing Education." He reported that at the University Hospital connected with the Schools of Medicine and Nursing, pupil nurses saved the hospital "around $20,000" a year. He called on nursing to follow the example of the medical profession, which, after the Flexner Report and through the AMA Council on Medical Education, no longer countenanced a medical school "connected with a profit-making college." Lyon's article was duplicated in nonmedical journals which showed some public interest in the question. Martha Dreiblatt,[15] for example, asked, "Shall We Have Cheap Labor or Good Nurses?"

In 1937, a British physician, Harold Balme,[16] recommended the closing of non-approved schools and the inauguration of a "model college of nursing." In effect, he approved the position of nursing leaders in England and in North America, but college education for nurses in Great Britain has made comparatively little progress. In 1976 Roslyn Emblin and Michael J. Hill compiled descriptions of 14 degree courses in England, Scotland, and Wales. They made the following introductory statement: "Degree courses in nursing have evolved over a period of 15 years in this country and are therefore comparative newcomers to the scene of British nurse education."[e]

Isabel M. Stewart traced the evolution of collegiate nursing education in her monograph, *The Education of Nurses*.[17] Charles L. Russell, in 1958, reported a careful study of "liberal education and nursing,"[18] showing the overwhelming support the ideas of such persons as have been mentioned received throughout their lives; he also showed the forces that held back the movement.

In 1965, the American Nurses' Association published its first "Position on Education for Nursing." It included the following statements:

> The education for all those who are licensed to practice nursing should take place in institutions of higher education; minimum preparation for beginning professional nursing practice at the present time should be baccalaureate degree education in nursing; minimum preparation for beginning technical nursing practice at the present time should be associate degree education in nursing, education for assistants in the health service occupations should be short, intensive preservice programs in vocational education institutions rather than on-the-job training programs.[f]

While the U.S. President's Commission on Higher Education had made similar recommendations in 1947 and national studies of nursing education had repeatedly made some of these recommendations, the fact that the ANA's House of Delegates supported this position paper carried great weight.[g] In 1975, the ANA's Commission on Nursing Education issued *Standards for Nursing Education* covering graduate, basic (programs leading to baccalaureate and to associate degrees and to diplomas), and continuing education. The Commission claims "the responsibility for developing standards and devising methods for gaining acceptance and implementation through appropriate channels."[h] The ANA's increasing concern for the education of nurses and for quality assurance is indirectly affecting all programs.

Length and General Nature of the Curricula in Basic, or Initial, Programs

All registered nurses in the United States must currently complete a basic course of study that measures up to standards set by a state board of nurse examiners. Comparable boards or bodies have this regulating function in the provinces of Canada, in Great Britain, and in other countries.

The following description of initial nursing programs or curricula is based on a study of selected current bulletins or catalogues from 17 schools offering initial (Registered Nurse) baccalaureate programs in the North, South, East, and West of the United States.[i] Bulletins of diploma and associate degree programs were also studied, but less data on them is given here.

Diploma programs under hospital auspices are usually 3 years in length, associate degree programs in junior colleges 2 years in length, and baccalaureate programs 4 years in length, although nursing content may be concentrated in the last 2 years. Some initial nursing programs in universities may require a bachelor's degree from an academic program as an admission requirement. In such cases the program is usually 2 years in length and in several schools the student is awarded a master's degree in nursing.

Of 1372 initial (R.N.) programs in the United Slates in 1974, 461 were diploma, 598 were associate degree, and 313 were baccalaureate. However, of the total students admitted to these programs in the fall of 1974, 26,943 were admitted to diploma programs, 48,596 to associate degree programs, and 32,672 to baccalaureate programs.[19] Study of available data shows the number of graduations from diploma programs decreasing and the numbers of associate degree and baccalaureate programs increasing and graduations from them increasing. The highest growth rate in graduations is from the baccalaureate programs.

Purpose of Initial Programs

Most nursing school bulletins of this decade that were consulted gave the school's philosophy, and the goals or purposes growing out of the philosophy, which usually contains a definition of nursing. The following statement is from the Faculty of Nursing of Syracuse University:

> Professional nursing is a deliberative process of human interaction designed to promote, maintain, and restore the health of individuals, families, and communities. This is achieved through the provision of care and comfort while assisting in the channeling of energies for maximum use of extrinsic and intrinsic resources to cope with stress in order to move toward a state of effective adaptation, including a peaceful and dignified death.[j]

The University of Texas System School of Nursing (with branches in six cities) defined nursing in the following terms:

> Professional nursing practice involves assessing health needs, and planning, providing, directing, and evaluating nursing care for individuals and groups in a variety of settings. It is a scientifically based process devoted to helping individuals, families, and groups make maximum use of their resources in meeting their respective health needs. It further incorporates the individualities of nurse and patient/client and is most effective when the thoughts, feelings, and values of both are recognized; therefore, a high

degree of communication skill and sensitivity in interpersonal situations is required. The obligation to improve nursing practice encompasses the use of knowledge and skills as well as the systematic study of the effects of this practice on human health.[k]

This university system listed seven "beliefs and knowledge" which the graduate of the baccalaureate program would have, sixteen "skills" they would have in assessment, planning, implementation, and practice, and four characteristics of their practice. The purpose of the programs was to help students acquire these skills and characteristics.

The faculty of the School of Nursing at the University of Rochester, in describing its basic program, said:

> The faculty believe that nursing is a useful occupation, a service rendered by one human being for another, or for a group, in which knowledge is drawn from the health sciences and applied to the maintenance and restoration of physical and mental well-being of persons and in that the nurse acts in the interests of the person or persons being served.[1]

The University of Oregon School of Nursing defined nursing as "a process of interaction with the following characteristics":

(a) Nursing contributes to and makes use of the physical and behavioral sciences.
(b) An understanding of normal growth and development is basic to nursing.
(c) Nursing is an interpersonal process.
(d) Assessment, planning, intervention, and evaluation are components of nursing.
(e) Nurses, as members of the health team, work toward achieving optimum wellness for individuals, families and society.[m]

The University of Maryland School of Nursing said the baccalaureate program "is committed to the total well-being of an individual and demonstrates a respect for the dignity, worth, autonomy and uniqueness of people. In a variety of settings, the graduate will assist the individual and selected small groups at any point on the health continuum to attain and/or maintain their maximum level of health." [n]

The Faculty of the Frances Payne Bolton School of Nursing of Case Western Reserve University stated its "concept of professional nursing practice" as a collaborative process:

> Professional nursing shares with other health professionals responsibility for meeting the health needs of society. Nursing, as an integral part of the health care delivery system, shares responsibility for working collaboratively toward attaining optimal health for all members of society.[o]

In a lengthy statement the following paragraphs showed the emphasis placed on health as opposed to disease:

> Professional nursing is responsible for the promotion, restoration and maintenance of an optimal state of health for individuals, families, groups and the community. Professional nursing practice includes nursing actions which assist persons to cope with physiological, psychological, and sociocultural threats to health.
>
> Professional nursing is responsible for formulating a nursing diagnosis based upon systematic collection of data about the health status of the individual. The plan of care and subsequent nursing actions are goal directed, derived from the nursing diagnosis and based upon knowledge of social, behavioral, biological, physical, medical and nursing sciences. Nursing actions which are performed humanely and competently, are also based upon the creation of interpersonal relationships and an environment conducive to optimal functioning. These actions and plan of care are evaluated continually and systematically in terms of the stated goals and the person's responses.[p]

Later in the bulletin, under "Philosophy of Undergraduate Education," the purpose of the basic nursing education was briefly and clearly expressed:

> Baccalaureate education in nursing at Case Western Reserve University constitutes the essential minimal preparation for the beginning professional nurse practitioner, who is a generalist. The educational program prepares nurse practitioners to engage in primary, acute and long-term care of people of all ages and in a variety of settings.[q]

The preceding statements taken from six recent university nursing school bulletins from the North, South, West, East, and Middle of the United States suggest diversity rather than unanimity of thinking about basic programs, although the diversity may be more a matter of style than substance. At least the statements show that these initial baccalaureate nursing programs were designed to prepare graduates to give nursing care to people of all ages and in all settings.

"Nursing" was obviously believed to include promotion of health and prevention of disease as well as care of the sick. Some faculties saw the basic program as preparing "nurse generalists" and "nurse practitioners" to give "primary, acute, and long-term care."

Statements on philosophy and purpose in the bulletins of hospital diploma programs tended to be less elaborate than those of baccalaureate programs, and those consulted did not claim to prepare "nurse practitioners" for giving primary, acute, and long-term care.[r] All types of initial programs were said to prepare graduates for further study, either continuing education, admission to baccalaureate programs for diploma graduates, or admission to graduate (master's) programs.

Main Divisions of the Initial (Basic) Nursing Programs

According to their current bulletins the curricula of 17 initial baccalaureate nursing programs listed courses that might be classified into (1) *the humanities,* (2) *biological and physical sciences,* (3) *social sciences,* and (4) *medical and nursing arts and sciences.*

Programs leading to a baccalaureate degree in nursing were usually 4 years in length. Nursing courses might be concentrated in the last 2 years or might be distributed. Nursing courses were based on the assumption that the student had some knowledge of the humanities and sciences.

Of the 17 schools whose bulletins were analyzed, about half used the blanket term *humanities*, but all specified courses in English literature and composition (or "speech communication" or "nature of language"); a few specified ethics, philosophy, logic, religion, history, and music appreciation.

Physical and biological sciences were universally required, either as an element in the nursing curriculum or as prerequisites. These courses were listed under 20 different titles. All programs included human anatomy and physiology, either as separate or combined courses. Pathology might be combined with physiology and called pathophysiology. All programs examined included chemistry; two, biochemistry; one, nutritional biochemistry; one, biophysics and biochemistry; one, chemistry and physics of life; one program recommended but did not require physics; several listed zoology and biology; one offered a course entitled "Science, Elegance, and Discovery." All programs included microbiology, or bacteriology (the more common term); one listed advanced microbiology and immunology. Only ten programs listed nutrition—normal and therapeutic; one, food and nutrition; one, nutrition and dietetics. Physical education was listed as a requirement in five programs. While the above titles vary, there seems to be far more uniformity in thinking about the biologic and physical sciences than any other aspects of initial nursing curricula.

Required or recommended *social sciences* were listed under 43 different titles, some so vague or ambiguous, even in the course description, as to defy classification under any traditional terms. All programs included straight sociology, although the following titles might belong under this heading: Social Change, American Society, Social Systems Analysis, and Marriage and Family. Psychology was included in all 17 programs, and the following courses, either required or recommended, might fall under psychology: Human Life Cycle, Growth Development, Human Development, Deviations in Growth and Development, Abnormal Psychology, Group Dynamics, Psychological Adaptation in Health and Illness, Behavioral Science, Human Behavior, Behavioral Social Science, Child Psychology, and Adolescent and Adult Psychology.

Anthropology was required in eight programs, and some courses mentioned above, for instance, American Society, might fall under this heading rather than sociology.

There was little indication that schools of nursing were trying to help their graduates understand political forces underlying health care systems, or how to effect changes in them. However, one program included Principles of Management, one included Health and Illness in American Society, another Social Systems Analysis, and another Health Care Systems. Statistics, required in four programs, and Man and the Computer required in one, might be mentioned in this connection, although these courses are probably more related to the conduct of research in health and disease, health sciences, or medical and nursing arts and sciences than to the politics of health care.

Courses here classified as *nursing or medical arts and sciences* were listed under 140 titles in 17 bulletins analyzed and it is hard to group them under such traditional terms as hygiene, epidemiology, public health, pathology, therapeutics, maternal and child care (obstetrical and pediatric nursing), geriatric nursing, mental health, or neurologic and psychiatric nursing. Nor can they be classified under nursing in various settings such as hospitals, clinics, schools, homes, or industries. Some designers of nursing programs were obviously trying to get away from emphasis on the hospital setting and were stressing health promotion rather than care of the ill. Medical terminology seems to be rejected in part but not totally.

Studying current bulletins, it is hard to find how much experience students have in any setting, although most state board requirements are still relatively specific about the clinical experience students must have, so this information may be available in the school's records.

The following is an attempt to show the main subdivisions of the category which we, in this analysis, arbitrarily call *Medical and Nursing Arts and Sciences,* since, as courses are now titled, it is impossible to separate them. Nursing students were once introduced to health promotion and the prevention of disease in courses with titles such as hygiene, sanitation, epidemiology, and public health. Such terms seem to be in disuse, but the following titles may be related to them. Introduction to Public Health Science, Principles of Epidemiology and Research, Health and Society, Health Care Delivery, Health Promotion, Human Awareness in the Health Professions, Comprehensive Health Planning, and Public Health Fundamentals. Such courses are sometimes tied to the students' experience in so-called community (extra-hospital) nursing, which, in some form, is probably common to all baccalaureate programs.

Nursing students were formerly or traditionally introduced to pathology and therapeutics under courses so titled or, perhaps, called Introduction to Medical Sciences. Two schools listed a course entitled Pathology, but some other courses listed in the 17 bulletins analyzed that might relate to pathology and therapeutics included the following: Medical Science, Biomedical Science, Pathophysiology, Pathophysiological Basis of Nursing Practice (two programs), Basic Nursing Science, Clinical Nursing Science. Systemic Investigation, Introduction to Basic Concepts of Illness, and possibly an interdisciplinary course entitled Patient, Professional, and Society.

Nursing students were traditionally introduced to nursing practice or the science and art of nursing by giving aspects of care to selected patients on medical, surgical, and maternal and child care services of the hospital, with an accompanying course that emphasized the acquisition of basic nursing skills. An obvious effort is now made to offer students early experiences that are not hospital- or sickness-dominated and that may be creative rather than technical. The words "procedures," "skills," and "techniques" are used infrequently. Some schools build the nursing curriculum around such concepts as Man and Health, Man and Stress, Man and Adaptation, Health Issues Affecting Family and Community Life, Dynamics of Nursing, the Nursing Process, Nursing in Health Crises, Nursing Intervention in Health Crises, Crisis Theory. One school listed seven courses under the over-all title of Nursing Science; another listed four courses under Foundations of Nursing. One school offered a course that reviewed or studied current concepts or theories of nursing, and many listed courses in Nursing Process, although course descriptions suggested that this term meant different things to different faculties.

Some schools had titles for beginning nursing courses that were quite specific. For example five schools listed Introduction to Nursing, four listed Nursing Fundamentals, one listed Health Skills, another Principles of Nursing Care, another Basic Nursing Sciences and Clinical Nursing Science. It is not easy to find out where students participate in the care of either well clients or sick patients.

Obviously, all schools offered study of and experience in care of mothers and children, but even here terminology was far from uniform. The following are titles that specifically related to maternal and child care: Maternal–Child Nursing (six programs offered this course), Maternal and Newborn Nursing, Nursing of Children, Nursing in the Beginning of Life Cycle, Nursing in the Evolving Life Cycle, Nursing with Individual Families and Groups in Health and Illness. Other related titles included Family and Community Patterns in Health and Illness, Growth and Development, Obstetrical Nursing and Clinical Experience in Obstetrical Nursing (two programs), Maternity Nursing, Pediatric Nursing (two programs), and Clinical Experience in Pediatric Nursing, Nursing Care of Adults and Children, Family Centered Adult–Child Nursing, Health Issues Affecting Family and Community Life. Only one bulletin listed the course Human Sexuality.

Geriatric nursing was not listed as such and mentioned only once under Care of Adult Patients (Medical–Surgical Geriatrics), but might be included in many of the courses that were organized around the development of man from birth to death. Specific preparation in the care of the dying did not seem to have been considered by faculties of the baccalaureate programs sampled except to be mentioned as a topic in several course descriptions.

There is little doubt that all nursing students in these schools have experience in the units of a hospital where patients are treated medically and surgically. In graduate programs medical–surgical nursing courses were commonly listed but in the 17 bulletins that described baccalaureate programs, only four listed Medical and Surgical Nursing, or Medical–Surgical Nursing. However, six schools listed Pharmacology, one listed Introduction to the

Administration of Medications, one listed Operating Room–Continuous Care Experience, and one listed Care.of the Chronically Ill.

Psychiatric Nursing was listed in five bulletins, Psychiatric and Mental Health Nursing in two programs. Courses under the following titles are probably substitutes for or related to psychiatric nursing: Modern Concepts in Psychiatric Nursing, Reading in Psychiatric Nursing, Communication and Interviewing, Crises Theory, Dynamics of Interpersonal Relationships, Behavioral Concepts in Nursing, Dynamics of Nursing, Human Behavior, Human Relations, Psychopathology, Man and Stress, Man and Adaptation, Intervention in Crises Throughout Life, Therapeutic Strategies of Mental Health, Therapeutic Communication and Psychopathology, Psychosocial Dynamics in Nursing, Nursing Communications (two programs), and Dynamics of Human Relations.

In only three bulletins was Public Health Nursing listed; two bulletins listed Community Health Nursing. It is quite clear, however, that most schools offered nursing experience in and related study of health care outside the hospital. Some courses that suggested this include the following: Family and Community Patterns in Health and Illness, Nursing in the Social Order, Ecology of Nursing, Nursing with Individual Families, Group Concepts in Health and Illness, Comprehensive Health Planning, Public Health Fundamentals, Nursing in Society, Introduction to Public Health Science, Family and Community Nursing, Family Counseling, Rural County Nursing, and Nursing in Health Care Systems. The nature and scope of extra-hospital nursing experience offered students is hard to assess, but programs seem quite dissimilar in this respect.

Seven bulletins listed Independent Study and a number said that students might elect to concentrate on an "area"; one listed Senior Clinical Nursing, others Advanced Nursing, Individual Study in Nursing, Advanced Clinical Experience in Nursing, Advanced Nursing Process in Major Health Areas, and Senior Seminar (supporting independent study, specialized topics in nursing). Courses entitled Nursing Research were offered in four programs, but Explorations in Nursing, Directed Reading or Research, and Senior Honors Thesis were other titles suggesting that students were introduced to research. It is obvious that many baccalaureate programs were trying to prepare graduates for the (admittedly ill-defined but much-discussed) "expanded role." Two schools listed Nursing Assessment, one school listed Health Assessment, another Process of Clinical Judgment, another Concepts of Illness, another Clinical Health Skills, one Physical Examination, and another Systemic Investigation. Descriptions of clinical courses and independent study stress the intent of helping the student acquire independence in making clinical judgment. One bulletin listed courses, Introduction to Primary Health Care and Introduction to Secondary Health Care.

Initial or basic nursing programs traditionally included courses in nursing history, current trends, and problems and opportunities within the profession. Only one bulletin listed History of Nursing, but three listed Issues and Trends in Nursing and Health Care; two listed Legal Aspects of Health Care, one Nursing in the Social Order, three Nursing Leadership and Management in Nursing, one Principles of Administration and Leadership, one Nursing in the Changing Order, one Study of the Nursing Profession, one Nursing in Society, one Background for Nursing, one Patterns of Organization for Nursing Leadership, one Perspectives in Nursing, and one Principles of Management and Leadership.

Differences in Baccalaureate Programs

For those unfamiliar with nursing in the United States, the preceding pages must present a confused picture. It is an indication that the selected schools represented here are experimenting and trying to develop a new pattern of nursing education. Nursing is a new profession and nursing education in the United States *is* obviously floundering. Nurse educators Claire M. Fagin, Margaret McClure, and Rozella Schlotfeldt, in the January, 1976, issue of the *American Journal of Nursing,* try to answer the question "Can We Bring Order Out of the Chaos of Nursing Education?" They noted that three programs ranging from 2 to 4 years in length prepared graduates to write state board examinations enabling them to be registered nurses. Functions or competences of associate degree (2-year), diploma (3-year), and baccalaureate (4-year) graduates have never been satisfactorily differentiated, and Fagin thinks the public is unaware of the differences. (Actually, in the writer's opinion, the public finds difficulty in differentiating between the registered nurse and the practical nurse in the United States.)

Fagin and McClure concluded that registered "professional" nurses should be at least graduates of baccalaureate programs in universities and that practical nurse programs should be merged with associate degree programs in junior colleges to prepare a second category of nursing personnel. They pointed out that this conclusion was reached repeatedly in national studies of nursing education from 1948 on. They would retain the two nursing licenses since new ones would only add to public confusion. The baccalaureate program would prepare persons licensed as the professional nurse (RN) who is capable of "self-directed" work and the associate degree program would prepare the "technical" or practical nurse. Both writers admitted the drawbacks in these terms and they failed, in our opinion, to clearly state the difference between the role of the technical or practical nurse and that of the professional nurse.

Schlotfeldt took a different position. She said professional nurses should be as thoroughly prepared for their special function as are physicians for theirs, and she recommended a doctor of nursing (D.N.) as the initial degree. She thinks the promotion of health and the prevention of disease—the nurses' special contribution—as important and as difficult as treatment, which is the physician's special province, and she aligned her position on the nurse's role with that of Florence Nightingale's, the founder of "modern" nursing. She put her position in the following terms:

> Nursing's right to create a future in which nurses can provide people with the kind of care that promotes healthy, productive, rewarding, and happy lives inheres in its magnificent heritage.
>
> It was Florence Nightingale, the brilliant and visionary founder of modern nursing, who, over a century ago, explicated the nature of nursing in terms of its goals and outcomes. She clearly established nursing's practice focus to be that of assessing and promoting the health status, health assets, and health potential of human beings of all ages, all nationalities, all races, and all varieties of human circumstances.[5]

The New York State Nurses' Association has proposed legislation to make a baccalaureate base mandatory for professional nurse licensure. The American Association of Colleges of Nursing has developed a model licensure law that makes a B.S. a base for "nurse" licensure and the junior college degree a base for the "nursing associate." Even these proposals are meeting with opposition, so it would be difficult to implement the Schlotfeldt recommendations in the near future, even if nurses, physicians, and the public could accept the assumption that health promotion and prevention of disease is a function separate from the cure of disease. While it may be generally accepted that the nurse is more expert in care than is the physician and the physician more expert in cure than is the nurse, these two workers presently perform both functions. As long as there are situations in which nurses are the best prepared health workers available to the public, they are forced into the curing role, and, in rare cases, when there is no nurse available, physicians must assume the caring role or their patients will die.

Nursing education has for many years accepted medical education as its model. The care of patients has usually been organized, patients actually housed, around the physician's diagnosis and treatment plan. Patients of all ages with tuberculosis or with cancer were once segregated, for example, or patients to undergo surgery were often segregated according to the region of the body or the surgical specialist performing the operation, for example, the orthopedic surgeon or the neurosurgeon. Diseases have been classified under the *systems* affected and formal instruction organized this way. Nursing State Boards have required a certain number of weeks' experience in hospital divisions established to a large extent for the convenience of physicians and surgeons under the systems classification.

It has been, and still is, most convenient for urologists to have all their patients in one place, although they are of both sexes and all ages; some bedfast, others ambulatory. The same thing holds for the cardiologist, the ophthalmologist, or the dermatologist. In recent years, this system of segregating patients has been questioned and other schemes substituted. Some medical centers have, for example, segregated patients according to the amount of help they need from the institution's staff. People who come to the center for diagnosis and can take care of themselves may stay in a unit that is run very much like an inn or hotel; those who are ambulatory but need some help are housed in another unit and so on until those who need most help are in intensive care units. Some large state neuropsychiatric hospitals have been broken down into small autonomous units that house patients according to the county, city, or town of which they are residents. Infants and children may or may not be segregated.

This reassembling of patients is one reason why some faculties believe that medical–surgical nursing and pediatric nursing are no longer valid courses in the curriculum. Another reason that these courses are questioned is that they have been hospital-oriented and disease-oriented. Nurse educators are trying to give students experience as observers or participants in extra-hospital health services, for example, private homes, schools, industries, neighborhood health maintenance units, and even penal institutions, and are searching for terminology in describing courses that will convey the prevalent philosophy that health care is an inherent right of all people everywhere.

The multiplicity of nursing courses, or titles used to describe them, suggests that, while faculties are striving to break the hospital- and disease-oriented mold that has dominated both nursing and medical education, it is not easy to identify a new pattern for the current initial or basic program.

While the traditional pattern of nursing education seems to be under fire, all the 17 baccalaureate programs examined have not relinquished it. The Frances Payne Bolton School of Nursing at Case Western Reserve University gives the following courses in "a typical program plan": General Chemistry, Organic Chemistry, General Biology, Anatomy, Human Physiology, Microbiology, Sociology or Anthropology, Growth and Development, Introduction to Basic Concepts of Illness, Pharmacology, Nutrition, Statistics, Fundamentals of Nursing, Medical and Surgical Nursing, Maternal and Newborn Nursing, Nursing of Children, Nursing in the Social Order, Public Health Nursing, Psychiatric Nursing, and Senior Clinical Nursing.[f]

Because this section has presented such a confusing picture of current basic or initial curricula, the writer offers in the next sections some curricula suggestions. It is hoped that among other concepts they may encourage interdisciplinary study, emphasize helping people everywhere with health problems (rather than nursing the acutely ill in hospitals), and encourage the self-reliance of patients or clients (rather than fostering dependence).

Notes

---

[a]The US Department of Health, Education, and Welfare reports that of 700,000 employed nurses in 1970 3.6 per cent (25,000) were black and 0.06 per cent (450) were American Indians. (Bureau of Health Resources Development, Health Resources Administration, US Department of Health, Education, and Welfare: *Nursing Student Loan Programs.* The Bureau, Bethesda, Md., p. 1.)

[b]"ANPQ [Association of Nurses of the Province of Quebec] Hears Claude Castonguay on Proposed Legislation," *Can. Nurse,* 68:13, (Dec.) 1972.

[c]World Health Organization: *Fifth Report of the Expert Committee on Nursing.* The Organization, Geneva, Switzerland, 1966 (Tech. Report Series No. 347).

[d]In most educational systems, students can decide whether they will work to pay for their tuition; student nurses in the early schools had no choice; they all paid for their "training" by giving nursing service, or they worked their way through training.

[e]Emblin, Roslyn, and Hill, Michael J. (comps.): *Degree Courses in Nursing.* Nursing and Hospital Course Information Centre, London, and Association

of Integrated and Degree Courses in Nursing, Guildford (Surrey), England, 1976, p. 1.

[f]American Nurses' Association, Committee on Education: "American Nurses" Association First Position on Education for Nursing," *Am. J. Nurs.,* 65:106, (Dec.) 1965.

[g]The US President's Commission on Higher Education's *Higher Education for American Democracy* (US Government Printing Office, Washington, D.C., 1948, 6 pam.) included the discussion of educating practical nurses in junior colleges and of educating professional nurses in universities.

[h]American Nurses' Association, Commission on Nursing Education: *Standards for Nursing Education.* The Association, Kansas City, Mo., 1975, p. 33.

[i]The present dissimilarity in initial programs and the varied and often ambiguous titles of courses (especially nursing courses) may lead to another effort on the part of national nursing organizations and concerned citizens to clearly define the purpose and nature of the preparation for general nursing.

[j]Syracuse University: *Bulletin School of Nursing.* The University, Syracuse, N.Y., Dec. 1971, p. 6.

[k]University of Texas System School of Nursing: *1975–1976 Catalogue.* The University, Austin, El Paso, Fort Worth, etc., p. 52.

[l]University of Rochester: *Official Bulletin, University of Rochester, 1974–1975, Undergraduate Studies.* The University, Rochester, N.Y., p. 217.

[m]University of Oregon: *Bulletin, University of Oregon School of Nursing, Portland, 1974–1975.* The University, Portland, p. 12.

[n]University of Maryland: *School of Nursing, University of Maryland at Baltimore, 1974–1975.* The University, Baltimore, p. 27.

[o]Case Western Reserve University: *Frances Payne Bolton School of Nursing Bulletin: 1974–1975.* The University, Cleveland, p. 8.

[p]*Ibid.*

[q]*Ibid.,* p. 13.

[r]For definitions of these terms, see pages 347 and 348. Bulletins using these terms would do well to define them since they presently have different meanings.

⁵Schlotfeldt, Rozella: "Can We Bring Order Out of the Chaos of Nursing Education? Rozella Schlolfeldt says . . . ," *Am. J. Nurs., 76*:105, (Jan.) 1976.
ᵗCase Western Reserve University: *op. cit.*

References

1. Ozimek, Dorothy: *The Future of Nursing Education*. National League for Nursing, New York, 1975 (Pub. No. 15–1581).

2. Rufflin, Janice: "Issues for the Black Nurse Today. Competence and Commitment," in National League for Nursing, Council of Baccalaureate and Higher Degree Programs: *Current Issues in Nursing Education*. The League, New York, 1974.

3. Lenburg, Carrie, and Johnson, Walter: "Career Mobility Through Nursing Education," *Nurs. Outlook, 22*:266, (Apr.) 1974.

4. American Nurses' Association, Council of State Boards of Nursing: *Boards of Nursing—Open Curriculum. Proceedings of the ANA Conference for Members and Professional Employees of State Boards of Nursing, June 7, 1974.* The Association, Kansas City, Mo., 1975.

5. American Nurses' Association: *Facts About Nursing, 72–73.* The Association, Kansas City Mo., 1974, pp. 6, 167, 181.

6. Canadian Nurses' Association: *Countdown 1973.* The Association, Ottawa, 1974, p. 114.

7. Woolsey, Abby H.: "Hospitals and Training Schools," in *A Century of Nursing*. G. P. Putnam's Sons, New York, 1950, p. 133.

8. Roberts, Mary: *American Nursing: History and Interpretation*. Macmillan Publishing Co., Inc., New York, 1954, p. 22.

9. Fenwick, Ethel Gordon: "A Plea for the Higher Education of Trained Nurses," *Am. J. Nurs., 2*:4, (Oct.) 1901.

10. Cabot, Richard C.: "A Statistical Study of the Educational Opportunities Offered in the Massachusetts Training School for Nurses," *Am. J. Nurs., 6*:438, (Apr.) 1906.

11. Beard, Richard Olding: "The University Education of the Nurse," *Teach. Coll. Rec., 11*:28, (May) 1910.

12. Goodrich, Annie Warburton: "The Complete Nurse," *Am. J. Nurs., 12*:799, (July) 1912.

13. Johns, Ethel: "The University in Relation to Nursing," *Public Health J. Can., 12*:6, (Jan.) 1921.

14. Lyon, E. P.: "Taking the Profit Out of Nursing Education," *Mod. Hosp.* *37*:122, (Nov.) 1931.

15. Dreiblatt, Martha: "Shall We Have Cheap Labor or Good Nurses?" *Am. Mercury*, Apr. 1931.

16. Balme, Harold: *A Criticism of Nursing Education with Suggestions for Constructive Reform.* Oxford University Press, London, 1937.

17. Stewart, Isabel M.: *The Education of Nurses. Historical Foundations and Modern Trends.* Macmillan Publishing Co., Inc., New York, 1943.

18. Russell, Charles H.: "Liberal Education and Nursing," *Nurs. Res.,* 7:116, (Oct.) 1958.

19. National League for Nursing, Division of Research: "Educational Preparation for Nursing—1974," *Nurs. Outlook, 23*:578 (Sept.) 1975.

Chapter 10

Suggestions for Basic Nursing Curricula

Suggestions for Initial, or Basic Nursing Curricula

An Interdisciplinary Approach

The Division of Health Manpower Development in the World Health Organization seems to recognize the interrelation of education for health workers. Two of its publications are entitled, *Development of Educational Programmes for the Health Professions* (1973)[1] and *Educational Strategies for the Health Professions* (1974).[2] Various contributors to these publications discuss program planning, educational objectives, curricula design, preparation of faculty, and methods of teaching. Most of the studies reported were conducted at the Center for Educational Development, University of Illinois College of Medicine, which has been made a WHO Collaborating Institute; most focus on the education of medical students, but Tamás Fülöp, director of the Division of Health Manpower Development in WHO, stresses the organization's "comprehensive, coordinated long-term programs for teachers of medical and allied health sciences."[a] Lippard was quoted on page 61 as saying that the medical school faculty as an entity might cease to exist. Pellegrino,[3] in 1972, discussed the Carnegie Commission's recommendation that 126 area health education centers be established to "improve education in the health professions." As its Dean, Pellegrino described the health "consortium" at the New York State University Center at Stony Brook—the

Health Science Center-Medical School" which is an implementation of this concept. There students of "medicine, dentistry, nursing, allied health, basic health sciences and social work" can study together in many courses and use the same facilities. Since we believe this to be the prototype of future schools for health workers, a nursing curriculum is suggested in the following pages that seems to the writer to fit into a health-science center. The prerequisite courses could be taken with students in any other discipline, and the third phase of nursing, which is focused on adapting care to the needs of patients with particular disease or conditions, could be studied in part with medical students in "clinical clerkships." In studying certain aspects of care, students of social work, physical therapy, clinical psychology, and even dentistry, might participate. Since graduates of all these schools must collaborate as practitioners if patients are to be well served, it seems highly desirable that they study together.

Courses Prerequisite to or Supporting the Nursing Courses

Either as prerequisite to the study of nursing or included in the initial program there should be courses in the *humanities* that ensure students' ability to use language effectively, to consider the present in the light of history, and to have some understanding of logic and the dominant philosophies and religions of the world.[b] It is certainly desirable that nursing students have some art appreciation, including music appreciation, and have an opportunity to continue to cultivate any special artistic talents they may have. Among the *social sciences*, psychology is of outstanding importance—developmental psychology (human development from birth to death) especially. The study of sociology and anthropology provides a background that is almost essential to the understanding of society. It is desirable that students in the health professions know about governmental processes not only the governmental systems within their own country but those in other parts of the world, including international law. It is especially important that they understand the ways in which governments promote the welfare of citizens—their education and health care. This may involve an introduction to economics and political theory.

There is little question that nursing students profit by a strong background in the *biologic and physical sciences*. In the opinion of the writer, this cannot be too strong. Whether these courses are taught separately or combined, they should include chemistry, physics, anatomy, and physiology. Physiology is particularly important. Knowledge of cell structure and function has been so enhanced by use of the electron microscope and special photographic techniques that students now entering nursing schools may bring with them more advanced concepts of anatomy and physiology than were held by experts before recent techniques were developed. Certainly the physiology made available to nursing students should include cell physiology and some of the theories of electronic balance within the cell.

The physiology of nutrition is usually singled out for emphasis in a special course because good nutrition is so essential to health but it is possible that the same emphasis should be put on neuromotor physiology and other essential functions modifiable by daily living habits and by medical treatment. It is desirable that students in the health field understand man's relationship to other living organisms, and for this reason general courses in biology and zoology are recommended. The study of microorganisms should include the essential nature of microscopic life as well as its role in causing disease—epidemic and sporadic.

In the 1955 revision of the book, *Principles and Practice of Nursing* (5th ed.), an effort was made to suggest an *ordering of nursing education* around the needs of clients or patients. The ideas expressed there were elaborated on in *The Nature of Nursing* (Macmillan Publishing Co., Inc., New York, 1966). The following is, to some extent, a synthesis of the discussion in these two sources. It constitutes an effort to show the implications for initial or basic nursing education in the definition of nursing underlying nursing practice.

Adaptation of Treatment and Nursing Care to the Needs of the Patient as an Over-All Goal

Those who see the skill and confidence of successful physicians and nurses often marvel at their ability to adapt treatment and nursing care to the particular needs of their patients, no matter how ill they are, what disease they have, or what age they may be. Obviously, even those medical workers with the widest experience have not always seen similar conditions, and since each personality is unique, each client or patient presents a unique problem. The success of health workers must therefore lie in a knowledge of guiding principles and in their ability to study patients and provide the care and treatment that each demands.[c] The development of this ability should be the major aim of all nursing curricula. Nursing faculties are constantly trying to find satisfactory answers to the following question: How much and what kind of experience is necessary to enable the graduate to adapt nursing care to particular patients and situations?

Classification and Organization of Subject Matter and Its Influence on Medical and Nursing Thought

Courses in nursing and medicine in the past were most often based on anatomic classifications of disease. For example, units of clinical study might be entitled "Treatment and Nursing Care of Diseases of the Respiratory System," or of the genitourinary system or the nervous system. A great effort was formerly made to enable medical and nursing students to see as many operations, conditions, or diseases as they could and to take part in the care of these patients. It is no wonder that students of both professions, brought up under such an educational plan, tended to refer to "the cardiac in Bed 2," or "the hysterectomy in Room 15." With emphasis on the disease or the operation rather on the individual with certain symptoms and difficulties, it is not surprising that students of both medicine and nursing were likely to assume that all persons with the same disease should be treated in the same way.

There are today marked changes in medical as well as nursing education. There is, for example, the effort to stress health promotion and disease prevention, to develop awareness in the medical student of people's needs as they see them, and to individualize care. Developing the public's self-reliance is stressed. This is often expressed as "the self-help movement." The fact that physicians are required to get "informed consent" for treatment implies knowledge of disease and the rationale of treatment on the part of the public. Television programs are making everyone aware of the signs of cancer, drug addiction, venereal disease, depressive psychoses, and many other forms of pathology and means of preventing them.

In spite of this emphasis on health education and the prevention of disease, the medical curricula in most American universities are still focused on the physician's functions of diagnosis, prognosis, and therapy. Diagnosis is based on a physical examination of the anatomic systems of the body. It is often called a "systems' review." Diseases are classified under systems, and texts and courses are organized under systems. William R. Houston,[4] a physician of long experience writing in 1936, expressed the opinion that this was *not* the most effective way to teach therapy. In his *Art of Treatment*, he pointed out, for example, that grouping a deviated nasal septum or pharyngitis with lung cancer did not facilitate learning, even though all these conditions might be diseases or defects of the respiratory system. He suggested grouping diseases around the main lines of therapy, which he identified as administration of specifics, psychotherapy, limiting or modifying the living pattern, altering the physiology, supplying nursing, or giving supportive care (where there was no other effective therapy), and using an experimental or tentative approach.

Recently, some medical schools, trying to develop a health-centered, individualized approach to medicine, have assigned beginning medical students to families in their homes when a baby is to be born to the parents.[d] Students study psychologic and physiologic problems associated with pregnancy and seek help from appropriate resources within the medical school as they work with the families and the nurses and social workers who are also interested in the families. But whether or not the medical curriculum is didactic and planned or grows out of assigned experience, it is usually focused on the physician's principal functions. The nursing curriculum, whether planned or growing out of assigned experience, should, it seems to the writer, focus on the nurse's principal functions. Where the functions of doctors and nurses overlap, joint study seems appropriate. For example, medical and nursing students need the same knowledge of the health care system, the health resources of the country and the smaller community where they work; both medical and nursing students must be able to assess health or conduct health examinations effectively. While medical students need a broader knowledge of diagnostic procedures, nurses are now using or requesting the more common ones. Medical students study pathologic changes ("pathophysiology") in greater depth, but nursing students must have considerable knowledge of them and may elect to study them intensively. It is not possible for either medical or nursing students to study the hundreds of diseases affecting humans; it is possible to study disease processes, for example, the body's response to a bacterial invasion, prolonged emotional stress, vitamin or protein deficiency, blood loss, or oxygen want.

While therapy is the main focus of the medical curriculum, nursing curricula that prepare graduates to give primary care must also offer students an opportunity to study therapeutics. In order to help patients carry out therapy prescribed by physicians, nurses have always needed an understanding of therapeutics, but their present need is even greater. The extent to which the study of therapeutics should be interdisciplinary is debatable.

Obstetricians and nurse-midwives need common knowledge and skills, as do pediatricians and pediatric nurses, psychiatrists and psychiatric nurses. Physicians and nurses in medical services, especially those serving the elderly and the chronically ill, also have common needs. Only on surgical services is the preparation of a surgeon quite different from the preparation of a surgical nurse.

If and when medical and nursing students study diagnosis and therapy on an interdisciplinary basis, faculties should make an effort to classify or organize the content of such courses into units that have meaning for both, that emphasize causes and prevention as well as cure, that give guiding principles rather than rules, and that stress the treatment of the person rather than the condition or the disease.

It is suggested that the nursing courses in the initial curriculum be organized into the three following blocks representing three stages of learning: *Basic Nursing Care* (see Table 10.1); *Symptomatic Nursing, or Common Problems in Nursing* (see Table 10.2); *and Disease-Oriented Nursing* and *Mother, Infant, and Child Care* (see Table 10.3). All focus on the nurse's principal function of supplementing the patient's strength, will, or knowledge in performing his or her daily activities or carrying out prescribed therapy, with the ultimate goal of independence or rehabilitation for the client or patient when this is possible and an ability to cope with incurable chronic disease or achieve a "good death" (see Chapter 8) when neither a cure nor "coping" is possible.

The first block of experience (Nursing 1. Basic Nursing Care) and related instruction is organized around helping people with their daily activities or providing conditions that enable them to perform them without help. This experience is available in almost any health service or clinical unit of the hospital, in nursing homes, or in private homes. The needs of clients or patients are analyzed according to age, temperament, social or cultural status, and physical and intellectual capacity (see Table 10.1). In this first phase of the curriculum, there is no emphasis on the patient's diagnosis or the therapeutic plan, although students with inquiring minds will learn a good deal about both. During this stage of learning, students are participant observers or assistants to more experienced students or to graduates who are helping patients with daily activities and prescribed treatment. At the end of Nursing I. Basic Nursing Care, the student should have acquired many skills, as well as the ability to plan with patients for the 14 daily functions listed in Table 10.1 to help them with their activities as they need help, and to become independent of help as soon as possible.

TABLE 10.1 Nursing I. Basic Nursing Care. Contents of Course Organized Around the Fundamental Needs of Man, Around Planning Care, and the Nurse's Unique Function of Helping Patients with their Daily Activities

1. Breathe normally.
2. Eat and drink adequately.
3. Eliminate by all avenues of elimination.
4. Move and maintain desirable posture (walking, sitting, lying, and changing from one to the other).
5. Sleep and rest.
6. Select suitable clothing, dress and undress.
7. Maintain body temperature within normal range by adjusting clothing and modifying the environment.
8. Keep the body clean and well groomed and protect the integument.
9. Avoid dangers in the environment and avoid injuring others.
10. Communicate with others in expressing emotions, needs, fears, questions, and ideas.
11. Worship according to his faith.
12. Work at something that provides a sense of accomplishment.
13. Play, or participate in various forms of recreation.
14. Learn, discover, or satisfy the curiosity that leads to "normal" development and health.

This includes making a plan for such assistance, taking into consideration the following factors always present that affect the person's needs.

1. Age: newborn, child, youth, adult, middle-aged, aged, and dying.
2. Temperament, emotional state, or passing mood:
   a. "Normal" or
   b. Euphoric and hyperactive
   c. Anxious, fearful, agitated, or hysterical or
   d. Depressed and hypoactive
3. Social or cultural status:
   A member of a family unit with friends and status or a person relatively alone and/or maladjusted, destitute.
   a. Normal weight
   b. Underweight
   c. Overweight
   d. Normal mentality
   e. Subnormal mentality
   f. Gifted mentality
   g. Normal sense of hearing, sight, equilibrium, and touch
   h. Loss of special sense
   i. Normal motor power
   j. Loss of motor power

Note: From Henderson, Virginia: *The Nature of Nursing.* Macmillan Publishing Co., Inc., New York, 1966, p. 49. Used with permission.

TABLE 10.2 Nursing II. Symptomatic Nursing, or Common Problems in Nursing. Content Organized Around Symptoms, Syndromes, or States (Common to Many Diagnoses) Encountered by Nurses in Many Settings

1. Marked disturbance of intake and output of gases demanding medical intervention such as administration of oxygen.
2. Marked disturbance of nutrition, fluid and electrolyte balance, starvation, obesity, pernicious vomiting, diarrhea.
3. Marked disturbance of elimination with constipation, suppression or retention of urine, incontinence of urine or feces.
4. Motor disturbance limiting motion; also prescribed immobilization.
5. Hyperactivity, with or without convulsions or hysteria.
6. Fainting, dizziness (loss of equilibrium), transitory and prolonged coma, or unconsciousness, disorientation, delirium.
7. Insomnia, anxiety, depression.
8. Hyperthermia or hypothermia as a result of exposure to environmental temperatures or as prescribed treatment.
9. Local injury, or wound, with infection.
10. A systemic infection, a communicable condition transmitted by various channels, with or without febrile states.
11. Shock, or collapse, with or without hemorrhage.
12. Disorders of communication attributable to congenital defects of sight, hearing, or speech (including deafness and mutism), and such handicaps when imposed by illness or treatment.
13. Preoperative state.
14. Postoperative state.
15. Persistent, or intractable pain.
16. Dying state.

Note: From Henderson, Virginia: *The Nature of Nursing.* Macmillan Publishing Co., Inc., New York, 1966, p. 52. Used with permission.

The second phase of the suggested clinical, or nursing, curriculum is Nursing II. Symptomatic Nursing. Student experience is focused on helping patients meet their momentary, hourly, daily, or future needs when there are marked disturbances of one or more of the 14 functions listed in Table 10.1. These disturbances, regardless of the disease diagnosis, constitute problems for patients and those who nurse them, and they demand modifications in daily living that must be made by the patient or the nurse, or both, if the symptom is to be relieved or made tolerable. Table 10.2 lists 16 symptoms or disturbances of function that create problems for patients and nurses. They may occur in both sexes, in all ages, and in almost any setting, although in order to have experience with these common nursing problems, students may have to be assigned to a number of services, including the emergency, medical, surgical, psychiatric, and pediatric services. Patients are chosen for the specific symptoms or states they present; the stu-

TABLE 10.3 Nursing III. Disease-Oriented Nursing and Mother, Infant, and Child Care. Content Organized Around Prescribed Therapy and the Modification of Daily Activities Indicated by Disease or Physiologic Developmental States

ON MEDICAL SERVICES

Therapy related to general conditions such as:	Therapy related to specific diseases such as:
Long-term illness	Arthritis
Metabolic disorders	Osteomalacia
Endocrine disorders	Addison's disease
Functional disorders	Anemia
Neoplasms	Leukemia
Infections	Tuberculosis
Degenerative processes	Cardiovascular diseases

ON SURGICAL SERVICES

Therapy related to general conditions such as:	Therapy related to specific diseases such as:
Preoperative state, operative, and postoperative state in	Brain tumor removal
Head and neck	Thyroidectomy
Chest	Lobectomy (lung)
Areal surgery Abdomen	Colostomy
Pelvis	Nephrectomy
Extremities	Reduction and fixation of fracture of an extremity

ON MATERNAL AND CHILD CARE SERVICES

Therapy related to general states such as:	Therapy related to specific diseases such as:
Prenatal	Eclampsia
Natal	Cesarean birth
Postnatal	Mastitis
Newborn	Erythroblastosis fetalis
Infancy	Eczema
Preschool children	Cerebral palsy
Middle childhood	Poliomyelitis
Adolescence	Rheumatic fever

TABLE 10.3 Continued

ON NEUROPSYCHIATRIC SERVICES

Therapy related to general conditions such as:	Therapy related to specific diseases such as:
Mental deficiency	Hydrocephalus
Pathological personality development	Alcoholism and drug addiction
Anxiety states-psychoneuroses	Manic-depressive psychoses
Acute depression with suicidal tendencies	Schizophrenia
Maniacal states	
Paranoid states	

Note: From Henderson, Virginia: *The Nature of Nursing.* Macmillan Publishing Co., Inc., New York, 1966, p. 54. Used with permission.

dent studies the pathologic changes in patient physiology and the rationale of therapy prescribed to relieve symptoms or make them tolerable. Some of the common nursing problems, for instance, the care of those who have intractable pain or those who are dying, are extremely complex. Volumes are written on these subjects, and health workers are devoting their lives to the study of these states. Students in the initial or basic program cannot be expected to learn all there is to know about them, but society expects every registered nurse to be able to help people cope with them and so every basic program should offer an opportunity to do just this. Faculties may very well identify other or different aberrations of body functions, human states, or common nursing problems with which students should have experience. Faye G. Abdellah and her associates in *Patient-Centered Approaches to Nursing*[5] in 1961 listed 21 problems with which they thought students should have experience.[e]

It is obviously desirable for students to help people with these commonly encountered problems in settings outside as well as inside hospitals and clinics where all kinds of experts, equipment, and supplies are available. It is desirable that the skills patients and nurses (one or both) must learn in order to cope with these problems be identified and efforts made to help nursing students acquire these skills. It is a common criticism of present-day registered nurses that they lack certain skills that employers expect them to have.[f] It is even more disturbing that graduates of some basic programs lose their self-confidence, finding themselves lacking in the ability to give patients the kind of help they would like to be able to give them, including the ability to perform, or teach patients to perform, necessary procedures. For example, while it is essential that nurses understand the physiology of respiration and the common pathology involved in oxygen want, it is also essential that they be able to use the mechanical devices and teach patients or their families to use mechanical devices that increase the oxygen supply to the patient; knowledge of the causes of coma, the pathology involved, is certainly necessary for those who nurse the unconscious patient, but skill in cleaning their mouths, in moving and lifting them, and in preventing pressure sores is also essential. While this second phase of the nursing curriculum focuses on symptomatic treatment, it includes helping the patient with the 14 daily activities stressed in the first phase of the curriculum and all the skills, abilities, or competences essential to both the first and second phase. In this phase, nursing students might study with medical students but, most particularly, with students of physical, occupational, and speech therapy who also help patients with activities of daily living.

The third phase of the suggested clinical, or nursing, curriculum is Nursing III. Disease-Oriented Nursing and the Care of Mothers, Infants, and Children (see Table 10.3). Here, the focus is on the modification of care demanded, or on the particular problem patients face because of a specific disease or an operation that requires special preparation or postoperative care or because they are in a phase of reproduction or a growth cycle that makes them dependent.

There have been many attempts to identify the diseases, the conditions, and the operations with which nursing (and medical) students should have some experience. As noted earlier, it is obviously impossible for either to study the care of patients with all the diseases, conditions, and operations they may encounter as physicians or nurses. It is therefore suggested that educators stress the care and therapy associated with *types* of conditions, as shown in Table 10.2. On medical services, some types are long-term illness, metabolic, endocrine, and functional disorders, neoplasms, infections, and degenerative processes. Experience can be provided students in the care of some patients with conditions of each type. Patients should be selected so that students have experience in the care of males and females of all ages. Experience in maternal and child care should include the normal and abnormal. While previous phases of the clinical curriculum should have stressed developmental needs, special emphasis should be put on them in this phase of the curriculum. Some faculties may offer a special course in geriatrics, as they do in pediatrics. It seems even more important to take a developmental approach in all clinical courses, helping students to see that every patient has to make adjustments in care and treatment imposed by his or her age.

In this third phase of the clinical curriculum, "classes" (discussions, seminars, conferences) are around particular patients. Lippard,[6] with reference to medical teaching, says patient-centered clinical teaching is never "behind the times" since the student is learning about the diseases and treatments of the day. Christman,[7] describing the new nursing program at Rush University, Chicago, emphasizes the importance of the practitioner-teacher who teaches students around "his or her own set of patients."

On surgical services, experience can be provided in the care of patients with each category of regional surgery since there are, for example, commonalities in the care of all patients having abdominal surgery or operations on the extremities. In maternal, infant, and child nursing, experience can be offered in the care of patients with representative pathologic conditions in the prenatal, natal, and postnatal states, in infancy and childhood, and through adolescence. In neuropsychiatric services, students might have experience in the care of patients in all age groups, in mental deficiency, in abnormal personality development, in anxiety states or psychoneuroses, in depression or suicidal states, in maniacal and paranoid states. In the second column (Table 10.3), *examples* of diagnosis falling within these general categories are given, but they are examples only. It is not our intention to suggest either the most common or the most important examples. The experience available and the judgment of faculty and interests of students will determine in every school the assignment to patients in hospitals, clinics, nursing homes, home care programs, and other settings.

In this third phase of the student nurse's clinical program, he or she should have the opportunity to help patients with all aspects of care, including planning: in other words, an opportunity to practice nursing as students as they will be expected to practice as graduates. Presently, this includes conducting physical examinations, assessing health, determining the diagnostic procedures and referrals to other health workers that are indicated, and in some cases suggesting a plan of therapy.

Students should have an opportunity to give the best care of which they are capable, and to study thoroughly the prescribed therapy and the patient's responses to it. Experience should be planned so that students can follow at least some patients through all stages of treatment, for example, preoperative, operative, and postoperative care or prenatal, natal, and postnatal care. If students are to graduate with a concept of family-centered nursing, it is important that they visit patients before hospitalization, that they care for hospital patients when they go home, and that they make home visits with community, school, industrial, or prison nurses and hospital nurses assigned to home care programs.

In this third phase of the clinical nursing program, students should have an opportunity to give as nearly "ideal" nursing care as possible to both sexes and all ages; at the same time, they should learn the realities of health service as it exists today and should see some effective efforts made to maintain the better services or improve the inadequate ones. If students see only ideal conditions, they may be unfitted for work in existing agencies and institutions. Obviously, as long as students are students, the faculty is responsible for the judgments they make and the care they give. At any point where either is contrary to the patient's welfare, the faculty must so advise students and help them make appropriate changes, or themselves make the decision or give the care for which the student is unprepared.

Clinical nursing curricula—however they are organized, however they are taught—should foster an inquiring attitude toward practice. While students need the assurance that the care they learn to give is safe and effective in the light of present knowledge, they should accept the fact that the boundaries of knowledge are constantly expanding, that health workers, in fact, everyone, should be open to new ideas—ready to modify practice as new findings in the physical, biologic, and social sciences invalidate current practice.

Nursing students must be able to find pertinent research, read it, evaluate it, and apply it as they seek answers to clinical problems. Therefore, they need a course that introduces them to the scientific method of investigation if their prenursing education has not included research experience. It is desirable that the initial nursing program include some experience in conducting a clinical study, and possibly a course in statistics and the use of computers. However, students are not likely to think of nursing research as the basis on which changes are made in nursing practice unless they see this happening in the centers where they study nursing.

Finally, the initial nursing curriculum should prepare graduates to play a constructive role as members of a major health profession. They can understand the current opportunities, obligations, and problems of nursing only if they have some knowledge of the history of health care in general and of nursing in particular. Nursing students should have firsthand experience as active members, associate members, or observers in nursing and other health organizations, as well as the opportunity to see and discuss the work of those who are maintaining effective services or helping to bring about change in the health structure. Knowledge of medical and nursing ethics and jurisprudence is increasingly important. If students have an opportunity to see health legislation in the making or participate in efforts to enact legislation, they are more likely as graduates to help effect change in a variety of ways.[8] Health care is presently accepted all over the world as a human right. The United States occupies a unique position among the developed nations in its fee-for-service system. Nurses who believe that health opportunities should be equalized and wish to work toward that end must be knowledgeable in the governmental and legal processes inherent in a national health insurance system that covers all citizens. For nurses who believe the United States should remain unique in retaining its fee-for-service system, knowledge of governmental and legal processes will also serve their needs.

A basic curriculum, however designed, is only the beginning of a lifetime of study for the practicing nurse; the succeeding sections describe postbasic study, graduate programs, and continuing and staff education.

Baccalaureate Programs for Registered Nurses with Diplomas or Associate Degrees in Nursing

Need for Baccalaureate Programs for Registered Nurses with Diplomas or Associate Degrees

In discussing initial nursing programs, it was noted that there is a movement, which is gaining momentum in the United States and other countries, to make a baccalaureate degree essential to the licensure of the professional registered nurse. If this becomes fact, and if the requirement should be made retroactive (which is most unlikely), registered nurses who graduated from initial diploma and associate degree programs must go to institutions offering baccalaureate degrees to registered nurses.

Perhaps more important is the growing demand by employers for degree-holding nurses, or nurses prepared to work independently and creatively. An over-all shortage of nurses may be debatable, but few question the undersupply of well-prepared nurses. Some hospitals are closing in the United States and Canada because hospital occupancy is falling and there is a realization that there may be too many hospitals. This may result in unemployed nurses and create an impression of a surplus. In any economically depressed country, nurses, like all other workers, fear unemployment. A thorough preparation for work (if it is not accompanied by a demand for a disproportionate rise in salary) is the best guarantee against unemployment. It is economically desirable in North America for graduate nurses to hold a baccalaureate degree which makes them more effective in generalized nursing, makes possible subsequent preparation for specialized nursing in graduate programs, and promotes economic security.

The Purpose of Baccalaureate Programs for Registered Nurses

The goal of all baccalaureate programs for registered nurses is to give them the learning opportunities offered by initial baccalaureate programs that they have missed as students in diploma or associate degree programs. It is not easy to identify these opportunities, so baccalaureate programs for registered nurses in the United States vary considerably. Colleges and universities offering such programs expect their graduates to be at least as competent as graduates of initial or basic baccalaureate nursing programs. Depending largely on the nursing experience these registered nurses bring with them into the program, they may be more competent.

Nature of the Programs

Since diploma and associate degree programs cannot offer, and rarely demand as prerequisites, the humanities and sciences required for the initial baccalaureate programs, registered nurse students are offered and may be required to include some courses in both areas, depending on the student's former educational experience—the strengths and weaknesses in their backgrounds. It is generally believed that courses in the medical and nursing arts and sciences are taught differently in the associate and diploma programs from the way they are taught in the baccalaureate programs. Registered nurses are, therefore, not exempt from courses in maternal and child care, medical-surgical nursing, psychiatric nursing, or community nursing just because their initial programs included such courses.

In some universities, registered nurses have been put in nursing classes with initial baccalaureate students. Few educators believe this is justifiable. It means a great deal of repetition, which alienates the registered nurse student. Most schools have exemption examinations or self-pacing systems that enable students, with help from the faculty, to select the units or modules of learning they need or to use various types of media for self-teaching. Many schools offer special clinical courses designed especially for the registered nurse student. Because they are at home in the clinical setting and have usually learned the basic nursing skills, the clinical experience (sometimes called "the practicum") can be of a different nature from that of the student in the initial baccalaureate program. Experienced and able registered nurse students may be allowed more electives, may have more independent study assignments, or may be able to follow their special clinical interests to a greater extent than students in the initial or basic baccalaureate program. Courses of study should be individually planned so that students see them as opportunities for useful and interesting learning rather than the fulfillment of a stereotyped requirement.

Notes

[a]Miller, George E., and Fülöp, Tamás (eds.): *Educational Strategies for the Health Professions*. World Health Organization, Geneva, 1974, p. 89 (Public Health Paper No. 61).

[b]Nursing students will find it useful to know languages other than their own but this should probably not be a prerequisite or a requirement.

[c]Vernon W. Lippard, discussing medical education, said that "all thought of total coverage" has been abandoned. Basic concepts are stressed, "the mechanisms of disease; continuing self-education; the development of a scientific critique; the cultivation of skills; and the inculcation of ideals." (*A Half Century of American Medical Education: 1920–1970*. Josiah Macy, Jr. Foundation, New York, 1974, p. 17.)

[d]Vernon W. Lippard described the curriculum of the medical school of Case Western Reserve University as follows: "The four-year curriculum was divided into three phases: the first, lasting one year, was concerned with normal structure, function, growth and development; the second, lasting one-and-a-half years, was concerned with alterations of normal structure, function, and development and the study of disease; the third, also lasting one-and-a-half years, was devoted to clinical application of the knowledge previously acquired." (*Ibid.*, p. 18.)

[e]Olga Andruskiw and Betsy L. B. Battick in 1964 studied two of these problems (oxygen want and electrolyte imbalance) and identified diseases and

conditions in which they occur. ("Identification of Nursing Problems," *Nurs. Res.,* *13*:75, [Winter] 1964.)

[f]Eleanor Gill, dean of the School of Nursing at the University of Connecticut, told the writer in 1975 that the faculty of this school has "gone back" to the practice of having a checklist of skills, procedures, or techniques with which students must have experience.

[g]There is considerable evidence that nurses are helping to effect change. A survey conducted by the ANA in 1975 through the state nurses' associations showed 15 RNs in 13 state legislatures, nine of whom were serving on health or social service committees. ("15 Nurse Legislators Reported in 13 States," *Am. Nurse,* 7:5 (May) 1975.

References

---

1. World Health Organization: *Development of Educational Programmes for the Health Professions*. The Organization, Geneva, 1973 (Public Health Paper No. 52).

2. Miler, George E., and Fülöp, Tamás (eds.): *Educational Strategies for the Health Professions*. World Health Organization, Geneva, 1974 (Public Health Paper No. 61).

3. Pellegrino, Edmund D.: "The Regionalization of Academic Medicine: The Metamorphosis of a Concept," *J. Med. Educ., 48*:119, (Feb.) 1973.

4. Houston, William R.: *Art of Treatment*. Macmillan Publishing Co., Inc., New York, 1936.

5. Abdellah, Faye G., et al.: *Patient-Centered Approaches to Nursing*. Macmillan Publishing Co., Inc., New York, 1960.

6. Lippard, Vernon W.: *A Half-Century of American Medical Education 1920–1970*. Josiah Macy, Jr. Foundation, New York, 1974, p. 11.

7. Christman, Luther: "The Practitioner-Teacher: A Working Paper," unpublished, 1973. (Rush University, Chicago.)

Chapter 11

Preparation for Specialized Nursing Graduate Programs

Need for Nurse Specialists with Graduate Degrees

The major national nursing surveys in the United States have for decades stressed the need for nurses with preparation in specialized practice, for teaching, administration, and research. Initial baccalaureate programs are not designed to prepare specialists in maternal and child health, medical and surgical nursing or any of its subspecialties, or in psychiatric nursing, although many are preparing graduates for generalized primary nursing. Nor do baccalaureate programs offer more than an introduction to teaching, administration, or research, or to the special problems of nursing in public (or community) health agencies, schools and colleges, industries, penal institutions, and other settings.[a] There is a demand for well-qualified nurses in all settings and for nurses who have advanced study in the care of patients in every age group and clinical category. Most graduates of initial programs take staff nursing positions in hospitals not only because they are needed there but because most initial programs provide more hospital nursing experience than any other kind, and graduates from them feel more comfortable nursing inside than outside hospitals. It is also true that many new graduates believe they profit by additional experience in giving nursing care in hospitals, even the fundamentals of care, and by more practice in the basic skills.

The rising rate at which nurses with baccalaureate degrees are entering and graduating from master's programs and later doctoral programs indicates an established demand in the United States for nurses with more thorough preparation for their work.

Nursing, like all new professions, has found it difficult to provide its schools with faculties whose educational preparation was comparable to that of faculties in the established professional schools and, therefore, to establish graduate programs. Of the 28,820 nurses employed in schools of nursing in 1972, 7128 (24.7 percent) had less than a baccalaureate education; 8953 (31.1 percent) had a baccalaureate degree; 9810 (35 percent) had a master's degree in nursing or another field and 601 (2.1 percent) had a doctoral degree.[1] In 1974 there were 7924 students enrolled in master's programs and 312 in doctoral programs.[2]

Until nurses on the faculties of college and university schools of nursing have master's or doctoral degrees, there will be a crying need for nurses with graduate degrees, and until nurses in administrative positions, in research and in specialized clinical practice have master's or doctoral degrees, opportunities for graduate study should be increased; Rozella Schlotfeldt[3] would say until all "professional" nurses can study in a graduate program leading to a doctoral degree, they should be increased. Margaret A. Newman[4] takes the same position.

The Purpose and Nature of Master's Programs

In 1972, there were 86 colleges and universities in the United States offering master's programs for graduate nurse students.[5] The evolution of master's programs for graduate nurses before the late 1940s did not differ very much from the baccalaureate programs for graduate nurses. Both offered preparation for teaching or administration or for public health nursing, and in some cases school or industrial nursing. There were a few postbasic programs offering courses on nurse midwifery, and later still, nursing of children, medical and surgical nursing, tuberculosis and cancer nursing. If the graduate nurse student had earned a baccalaureate nursing degree, the clinical courses might be built into a master's program, but they might also be part of a baccalaureate program. Until midcentury, advanced preparation in clinical nursing was far less common than advanced preparation for the functions of teaching and administration.

In the late 1940s, the NLN issued a series of publications on advanced clinical courses, stressing the need for them and suggesting the form they might take. By 1969, the ANA gave as the "major purpose of graduate . . . study in nursing":

> . . . the preparation of nurse clinicians capable of improving nursing care through the advancement of nursing theory and science. . . . Traditionally, graduate education in nursing has been considered as preparation for particular functions and positions—primarily teaching and administration. This emphasis unfortunately has tended to devalue nursing care and practice by suggesting that there is no more nursing knowledge than can be encompassed in the initial, undergraduate preparation.[b]

The following statement by the NLN in 1974 emphasizes advanced clinical courses and preparation for research in both master's and doctoral programs:

> Graduate study is education pursued beyond the baccalaureate degree in an institution of higher learning. The characteristics of graduate education in nursing include specialization in a clinical area of interest, mastery of knowledge in that area, freedom of inquiry in the pursuit of knowledge and the acquisition of skills, and competence in research. The programs are organized according to a conceptual scheme and culminate in the awarding of a master's or a doctoral degree in a chosen area of study. . . .[c]

While the current need is for nurses who are able and accountable in specialized clinical nursing, master's programs for graduate nurses in the United States offer a wide variety of courses. The University of Maryland in 1974–75, for example, offered more than 50 courses; the University of Texas in 1975–76 offered more than 40 courses.[6,7] Some programs offer courses in nursing history, nursing concepts, and nursing process on a graduate level. Not every master's program has developed all the clinical specialties—maternal and infant health, child health, medical-surgical nursing, and psychiatric nursing, but the current bulletins examined indicated that the trend was in this direction. Some programs offered developmental nursing, or study of the nursing care of infants, children, young adults. the middle-aged, and the aged. "Intradisciplinary nursing" and "liaison nursing" are courses providing opportunity to study the mental health aspects of nursing in any clinical department or health service.

Courses in nursing according to the setting in which the nurse functions were uncommon except for community health nursing, which may still be called public health nursing and which is sometimes called family health nursing.[d] In describing the "practicum" or the experience offered in connection with the various clinical specialties, there was the implication in some bulletins that students might elect to have it in a wide variety of health institutions and agencies.

Community health nursing included nursing in industry and schools and might include nursing in penal institutions. Study of nursing in these settings, however, tends to be neglected, although the ANA reports that of the 308 master's programs in public health nursing, nine "focused" on school nursing.[8] Community health programs emphasized the function of the nurse in state, county, and city health departments and in visiting nurse agencies. If there was a school of public health in the university, its courses were available to students in master's programs in nursing, or the nursing school might itself offer such courses as epidemiology and public health administration.

While few master's programs were focused on the functions of teaching, administration, or research, many offered courses in educational and managerial theory and systems analysis and some offered experience in teaching or administration, or both. As indicated earlier, employers expect nurses holding master's degrees to be familiar with the scientific method of investigation, to be able to read research reports, and to apply the findings of research. Most master's programs include experience in conducting a study of some sort, usually leading to a master's thesis. Courses in statistics and the use of computers are common.

Master's programs studied included a wide variety of electives. Graduate nurse students were urged to take courses in other schools or departments in the university—the schools of public health, education, medicine, law, or management, and the departments of biologic and physical sciences and social sciences. If and when the United States develops out of the present chaos a well-defined and effective pattern of health service, all universities may develop interdisciplinary courses in those aspects of the service that can be studied profitably by all health professionals.

The Purpose and Nature of Doctoral Programs

The purpose and nature of doctoral programs in nursing have been and remain controversial. As noted, the first nurse from the United Slates to earn a doctoral degree is believed to be Edith S. Bryan, who earned a Ph.D. in psychology. Her dissertation, submitted to Johns Hopkins University in 1928, is titled "A Psychological Study of the Reactions of the Newborn."[9] It was not until 1946 that nurses were offered an opportunity in two universities to get doctoral degrees in nursing; before 1946, they were obliged to get a doctorate in education, philosophy, law, a biologic or physical science, public health, or some other area of study. Simmons and Henderson found that of the 80 doctoral degrees earned by nurses (other than M.D.s earned by nurses) between 1928 and 1955, there were four types distributed as follows: Ed.D. 46; Ph.D. 32; Jur.D. 1; and Sci.D. 1.[e,10] When the U.S. Department of Health, Education, and Welfare reported the *Conference on Future Directions of Doctoral Education for Nurses*, it showed that in 1969, 25 kinds of doctoral degrees were being awarded nurses, which included Doctor of Nursing (D.N.), Doctor of Nursing Science (D.N.Sc. or D.N.S.), Doctor of Public Health Nursing (D.P.H.N.), and Doctor of Nursing Education (D.N.Ed.).[11]

Publications of the NLN and ANA, cited earlier, encourage graduate nurse students to take programs leading to doctoral degrees in nursing, although few question the value of advanced study in related fields. Susan Taylor and her associates, reporting on nurses with earned doctoral degrees by 1971, gave the following figures: 47 percent held degrees in the behavioral sciences, 33.8 percent in education, 8.3 percent in the biological sciences, 6.4 percent in nursing, 1.9 percent in epidemiology and public health, and 2.6 percent in other fields.[f]

For both master's and doctoral students, the NLN in 1974 gave the following characteristics as cited by Kelly:

> The nurse in the advanced professional program (1) pursues an area of clinical specialization; (2) elects an area of role development: (3) develops and tests nursing theories; (4) advances knowledge in the field through systematic observation and experimentation; (5) relates basic science theories to the development of knowledge in the clinical and functional areas; (6)

identifies and implements nursing's leadership role within the health care delivery system; and (7) engages in a collaborative role with others interested in health care.[8]

Rozella Schlotfeldt[12] and Margaret A. Newman[13] maintain that the nurse is the worker most available to the public and most interested in and able to give primary health care, particularly the service directed toward health promotion and disease prevention. They believe preparation on a doctoral level is needed to qualify nurses for this function and to give them the public recognition and authority of other major health professionals.

The assumption that professional nurses are particularly interested in "care," in the psychosocial problem of patients, as opposed to "cure" and the technical aspects of treatment said by some to be typical of the associate degree graduate and/or the practical nurse, seems to be borne out by a number of recent studies. However, Bonnie Bullough and Colleen Sparks[14] questioned the "care-cure dichotomy." They think this distinction, expressed in the ANA's position paper of 1965, may be creating a difference in initial nursing programs "contrived" by nurse educators or theorists. They suggested that by creating two types of graduates who function differently, upward mobility for the "cure" nurse may be blocked and the nurse who is primarily concerned with "care" may be frustrated in real life situations where the nurse is expected to function in both capacities. Marlene Kramer[15] questioned whether professional nurses are being prepared in present-day schools to meet the public's expectations and to satisfy their own desire to practice effectively. Dorothy A. Mereness[16] suggested that "evidence of ability to practice professionally" be a prerequisite to acceptance of nurses as candidates for master's degrees.

The effort in Canada to identify specific functions that nurses in each clinical area should learn to perform, the competences they should demonstrate in an educational program is one practical approach to the question of whether care and cure can or should be separated, and whether the preparation of professional nurses should be comparable in length, depth, and breadth to that of physicians and dentists.

William K. Selden, who has directed educational research in various fields, says that problems in graduate nursing education are not unique. He made the following observation:

As nursing fosters and supports more educational offerings in academic institutions in contrast to education in service agencies, it should be more discriminating than it appears to have been in adopting the pedagogical mores of higher education. It should select only those educational practices that will assist its practitioners to improve their competencies in the delivery of health care.[h]

Selden applauded one institution's "lucid and direct . . . statement of philosophy" from which the following was excerpted: "The primary purpose of the doctoral program is the enhancement of clinical competence through the development of a body of nursing knowledge upon which a sound practice of nursing is based."[i]

Regional commissions on higher education have for decades promoted graduate programs for nursing. Interstate planning has resulted in less duplication of programs and the development of better programs. Funds from private foundations and the USPHS have supported a variety of projects. Cooperative graduate education in nursing, in which twelve universities in California and Nevada are participating, was in progress under a 5-year US-PHS grant (1971–1976). This has demonstrated the feasibility of a master's student taking courses in several universities simultaneously.[17]

Patricia A. Moxley and Dorothy T. White[18] discussed "Fitting the Graduate Program to the Student" at the School of Nursing, Medical College of Georgia, and "removing barriers to admission." A volume, *Open Learning and Career Mobility in Nursing*, edited by Carrie B. Lenburg, asks for "diversity for a learning society." She reviewed the current efforts to fit initial and graduate programs to the needs of the people. She noted that "Open learning is not a phenomenon unique to the United States; it is an international movement, with institutions around the globe. . . ." She noted that "The University of London developed an external degree program in 1836 and has been meeting the education needs of working students for more than 138 years."[j]

A doctoral degree is now awarded in the United States by the Union Graduate School—a union for experimenting colleges and universities, which had 31 member institutions in October, 1975. The Ph.D. program (a non-campus graduate program initiated in 1969) "now enrolls over 300 students and has more than 200 graduates."[k]

While graduate programs of study in nursing in the United States do not seem to the writer to present as confused a picture as do initial programs, they are far from stable, and the developments just mentioned suggest some of the differing directions they are taking. Depending on what happens in the development of health service and the role nurse practitioners play in it, graduate education may continue to change drastically, as it has throughout this century.

Postbasic education at the beginning of the century consisted at first of blocks of experience in hospitals and health agencies that differed little from the experiences of nurses employed in them except that the "postgraduate student" was paid little or nothing. The program for hospital nurse administrators established at Teachers College, Columbia University, New York City, was at the time a great innovation. This program for administrators was duplicated for teachers. Soon, programs were developed to prepare graduate nurses to function in special settings. Finally, programs were designed to prepare clinical specialists and researchers. In one setting, the latter includes research historians.[19,20] Today, the major emphasis in graduate education is on the preparation of clinical specialists.

While the preceding pages have stressed the development of opportunities for graduate study in nursing in the United States, opportunities in Canada are also increasing. There were, in 1969, eight institutions offering master's degrees, with 18 graduations[21]; in 1972, there were eleven institutions offering master's degrees, with 45 graduations and 159 students enrolled;[22] in 1974 the number of master's programs increased to sixteen.[23] In 1954, the Florence Nightingale International Foundation published an international list of advanced programs in nursing education and has since brought out supplements.[24]

Study beyond the initial nursing program may take many forms. All major nursing investigations have stressed the need for nurses with broad social experience and higher degrees. The report of a 1973 conference is entitled *Redesigning Nursing Education for Public Health* (Division of Nursing, Public Health Service, Health Resources Administration, US Department of Health, Education, and Welfare, Bethesda, Md., [1975] (DHEW Pub. No. [HRA] 75-75). Conferences on education in other fields might properly suggest comparable changes.

Summary

Nursing is shown in this chapter to be an essential health service that attracts increasing numbers of men and women, although women still dominate the profession and, in the United States, minorities do not have proportionate representation in nursing. Types of nursing personnel continue to increase, with numbers of "allied" or "auxiliary" workers exceeding registered nurses in number in this and some other countries. One authority on international standards for health workers is quoted as saying that 400 categories are involved. Coordination of health care is increasingly difficult, with fragmentation and impersonalization of care common complaints of the public.

Because the roles of health workers overlap and vary from place to place and from one era to another, an understanding of the development of nursing depends upon some knowledge of the development of medicine. And since health workers share with other general educators the responsibility for health education of the public, this relationship must be recognized. Health education is especially pertinent today when the loudest critics of health care stress putting more emphasis than there is at present on prevention and the development of self-help, or self-reliance, in matters of health.

The role of the registered nurse has unquestionably "expanded," but there is currently more recognition than in the past of the extent to which registered nurses have always been "extenders of medical care"—a role now shared with feldshers in Russia and physician's assistants in this and some other countries.

While nurses, physicians, special therapists, medical social workers, and all health personnel have the same goal in raising health standards and reducing unnecessary suffering, each category has a function or role in which it is most proficient. Various definitions of the nurse's function are recognized and have been noted, but the concept dominating this book is stressed—namely, that nurses are uniquely qualified to help people perform those functions (related to health) that they would perform unaided if they had the strength, the will, or the knowledge, and to give people this help in such a way that they gain their independence as soon as possible, learn to cope with a health handicap that cannot be eliminated, or die in dignity when death is inevitable.[1] When physicians are unavailable, and just as in emergencies when any citizen may treat the victim, nurses may prescribe therapy; they regularly help patients with the therapeutic regimen prescribed by physicians. The extent to which nursing is a profession is examined in this chapter, the independent nurse practitioner is recognized, and the conclusion is reached that all registered nurses are legally accountable for their acts.

If nursing is studied as an occupation, it is seen in most countries to be the largest in the health field. Certain social scientists have noted that the public image and self-image of nurses are different and that there is a lag in the public's understanding of the role nurses are playing in health care. Whether or not there is a national (tax-supported) health service available to all citizens or a mixture of private and public services, there is a pervasive feeling in many countries that the cost of health care is too high. In the United States, current studies are in progress to establish quantitative and qualitative standards to facilitate planning and act as controls on health care, although some critics say the present system in the United States is beyond salvage with any contemplated controls. While the cost of health care in the United States, Canada, Great Britain, Sweden, and other countries is burdensome for the taxpayer or the individual (according to the system), international and national studies show that there is less economic reward for nursing than for other occupations, such as teaching, with which it might be compared.

Registered nurses who graduate from initial or basic programs may hold diplomas in nursing, or associate, baccalaureate, or master's degrees in nursing. In a postbasic program, registered nurses earn baccalaureate degrees, and in graduate programs, they earn master's and doctoral degrees. Allied or auxiliary nursing personnel are prepared in a variety of programs and function under a variety of titles. Some reasons why nursing education is said to be "chaotic" are shown in this chapter.

While the emphasis is on the role of the registered nurse in the United States and Canada, there are many references to related health personnel and to health care in other parts of the world.

The work of nurses is vital and varied in its character, because of its variety and impelling interest, it appeals to many different natures. A study of successful nurses seems to show they have a number of common characteristics, but this does not mean that the successful nurse is "a type." There is the science of nursing, but equally important, there is the art of nursing. In its highest form, nursing calls for the same qualities that are found in most persons who work successfully in other professional fields—sensitiveness to people and their moods, insight into human nature, an ability to distinguish what is true from what is false, the capacity for sustained effort, and the mastery of the techniques involved.

Notes

---

[a]Beginning in 1974, the Yale University School of Nursing, New Haven, Connecticut offered an initial 3-year master's program for college graduates that prepares these men and women to give generalized primary care, to function as specialists in a field of their choice, and "to gain basic skills in research in nursing practice." This was said, in 1974, to be the only such program in existence.

[b]American Nurses' Association: *Statement on Graduate Education in Nursing*. The Association, Kansas City, Mo., 1969, p. 2.

[c]National League for Nursing: *Characteristics of Graduate Education in Nursing*. The League, New York, 1974.

[d]The terminology is questionable when it only applies to extra-hospital nursing, since, ideally, nurses in all health services, including those in hospitals, clinics, and nursing homes, work with patients as members of a family.

[e]The holders of these doctoral degrees were at the time, or afterwards became, citizens of the United Slates.

[f]Taylor, Susan, et al.: "Doctoral Degrees," *Nurs. Res., 20:*415, (Sept.–Oct.) 1971.

[g]Kelly, Lucie Young: *Dimensions of Professional Nursing*, 3rd ed. Macmillan Publishing Co., Inc., New York, 1975, p. 179.

[h]Selden, William K.: "Are Problems in Graduate Nursing Education Unique?" *Nurs. Outlook, 23:*622, (Oct.) 1975.

[i]Ibid.

[j]Lenburg. Carrie B. (ed.): *Open Learning and Career Mobility in Nursing*. C. V. Mosby Co., St. Louis, 1975.

[k]The Union Graduate School consists of The Union Graduate School—I, The Center for Minority Studies, The Union Graduate School—Elementary and Secondary Education, The Union Research Institute, and The Union Graduate School—West. [Prospectus 1975.]

[l]The fact that the ICN uses this definition makes it of special interest.

References

1. American Nurses' Association: *Facts About Nursing 72–73*. The Association, Kansas City, Mo., 1974, p. 10.

2. National League for Nursing. Division of Research: "Educational Preparation for Nursing—1974." *Nursing Outlook 23:*578, (Sept.) 1975. (Report prepared by Walter L. Johnson).

3. Schlotfeldt, Rozella: "Can We Bring Order Out of the Chaos of Nursing Education?" *Am. J. Nurs., 76:*105, (Jan.) 1976.

4. Newman, Margaret A.: "The Professional Doctorate in Nursing: A Position Paper," *Nurs. Outlook, 23:*704, (Nov.) 1975.

5. American Nurses' Association: *Facts About Nursing 72–73*. The Association, Kansas City, Mo., 1974, p. 116.

6. University of Maryland: *School of Nursing, University of Maryland at Baltimore, 1974–1975.* The University, Baltimore, p. 27.

7. *University of Texas System School of Nursing: 1975–1976 Catalogue.* The University, Austin, El Paso, Forth Worth, etc., p. 52.

8. American Nurses' Association: *Facts About Nursing 72–73.* The Association, Kansas City, Mo., 1974, p. 119.

9. Simmons, Leo W., and Henderson, Virginia: *Nursing Research: A Survey and Assessment.* Appleton-Century-Crofts, New York, 1964, p. 4.

10. *Ibid.,* p. 124

11. US Department of Health, Education, and Welfare: *Future Directions of Doctoral Education for Nurses. Report of a Conference.* US Government Printing Office, Washington, D.C., 1971, p. 6.

12. Schlotfeldt, Rozella: *op. cit.*

13. Newman, Margaret A.: *op. cit.*

14. Bullough, Bonnie, and Sparks, Colleen: "Baccalaureate vs. Associate Degree Nurses. The Care-Cure Dichotomy," *Nurs. Outlook, 23*:688, (Nov.) 1975.

15. Kramer, Marlene: *Reality Shock Why Nurses Leave Nursing.* C. V. Mosby Co., St. Louis, 1974.

16. Mereness, Dorothy A.: "Graduate Education, As One Dean Sees It," *Nurs. Outlook, 23*:638 (Oct.) 1975.

17. Chater, Shirley S.: "COGEN: Cooperative Graduate Education in Nursing," *Nurs. Outlook, 23*:630, (Oct.) 1975.

18. Moxley, Patricia A., and White, Dorothy T.: "Fitting the Graduate Program to the Student," *Nurs. Outlook, 23*:625, (Oct.) 1975.

19. Roberts, Mary M.: "The Story of the Department of Nursing and Health, Teachers College, New York," *Am. J. Nurs., 21*:518, (May) 1921.

20. "The Contribution of Teachers College to Nursing Education," *Teach. Coll. Rec., 16*:71, (May) 1915.

21. Canadian Nurses' Association: *Countdown 1970.* The Association, Ottawa, 1970, p. 79.

22. Canadian Nurses' Association: *Countdown 1972.* The Association, Ottawa, 1972, pp. 84, 89.

23. Personal communication, Aug. 25, 1976, Canadian Nurses' Association.

24. Florence Nightingale International Foundation: *An International List of Advanced Programmes in Nursing Education, 1951–1952.* International Council of Nurses, Geneva, 1958.

Chapter 12

The Nursing Process—Is the Title Right?

Use of Words

Discussion of the nursing process immediately raises two questions: Is it *the* nursing process (in other words, has it the same meaning as nursing); or is it the *nursing* process (or is it a process peculiar to nursing)?

There was at the University of Virginia around 1900 a professor named Noah K. Davis. Although officially he taught the history of religion, unofficially, and more passionately, he taught the exact use of words. As a child I heard impersonations of Noah K. by my uncle who would stand before an imaginary class in an imaginary classroom and declaim in stentorian tones:

> 'The Acts of the Apostles! Title's wrong! It's not *all* the acts of *all* the apostles but *some* of the acts of *some* of the apostles!'

Professor Davis's presumption in criticizing the language of the Bible amazed the students of his day. My presumption in the following criticism of a widely accepted substitute for the term nursing may equally amaze the readers of the *Journal of Advanced Nursing*. In a report of the 1981 Congress of the International Council of Nurses it is said that in the 36 concurrent sessions from all parts of the world "nursing process and primary nursing care emerged as the development seen as most important to improving care world wide." The implication in this statement is that the nursing process and primary nursing care are interdependent. While this question is not debated here I question whether such a relationship is valid.

In the following pages I will explain why I believe the nursing process, as commonly defined, is neither *the* nursing process nor the *nursing* process, but rather an analytical process that should be used by all health care providers when their intervention, or the help they offer, is of a problem-solving nature. Even then I believe the process should be modified. I will define the process and trace the development of the concept of the nursing process, as I've observed its evolution, over more than 50 years and I will point out certain differences in the way the term has been used.

A Present-Day Definition of "The Nursing Process"

In a publication of the Nursing Theories Conference Group (1980), nursing is said to be, "the process. . . . of determining the client's problems, making plans to solve them, initiating the plan or assigning others to implement it, and evaluating the extent to which the plan was effective in resolving the problems identified."

In 1979 Karen C. Sorensen and Jean Luchmann, in an American textbook, described the nursing process in essentially these terms, as did Charlotte R. Kratz (1979) in a British text. For purposes of discussion in this paper it seems fair to assume that the nursing process is now defined in the established steps of problem-solving. In fact, the chapter on the nursing process in the Sorensen & Luchmann (1979) text gives problem-solving as the subtitle of the chapter. The authors tell readers that they should be able to define 53 related terms after studying the chapter. Charlotte Kratz's (1979) text eliminates what has been called the metalanguage or the jargon of the American theorists, but her presentation differs in style rather than in meaning.

Evolution of the Nursing Process

During my life in the nursing occupation, which spans more than 60 years, nurses have been on the move, searching for an effective and satisfying role in promoting health, preventing disease, caring for the sick and helping people to die a peaceful death. The emphasis has changed from one decade to another with ever wider swings of the pendulum which, with the influences of the UN, WHO, ILO, and the ICN, affect nursing worldwide. While I do not presume to be able to encapsulate the history of nursing during most of this century I will suggest that the nursing process has evolved largely from the following movements to:

1. individualize nursing care;
2. identify and help people with their psychosocial as well as their physical problems;
3. emphasize the science of nursing as opposed to the art of nursing;
4. establish the right of the nurse to an independent, professional, and unique role.

The effort to *individualize or personalize the care of the client or patient* may go back to the beginning of nursing as we know it. Ever since men and women learned within hospitals how to practice, the hospital nursing role has dominated the nurse's role in other settings. Nurses have therefore tended to fit patients or clients into institutional routines rather than to promote programs of care that suit the specific needs and desires of patients, or clients or their families. Hospital nursing has been influenced by militaristic, religious and governmental regulations and by industrial management principles that stress efficiency. Task assignment or assembly-line methods have been used to speed up production. Now the health care industry is big business and some international firms are taking over the management of hospitals, the limit of whose sophisticated technology cannot be anticipated nor can its standardizing and depersonalizing effect be estimated.

Those of us who have seen patient assignment, rather than task assignment in hospitals and those who have nursed patients in their homes have been convinced that the best health care is patient-focused; better still, family-focused. Since World War One this has been demonstrated par excellence in rehabilitation centers where the plan of care is based on the amount of help the client needs in performing daily activities. Such plans of care have of necessity been individualized.

Rehabilitation

Believing that the aim of nursing is rehabilitation when partial or total recovery is possible, those of us responsible for the revision of the National

League of Nursing Education's proposed curriculum in 1937 introduced a unit on *planning patient care*. Case study as a basis for planning was included. Soon after this, nursing texts began to present these concepts and forms were suggested that showed plans incorporating the prescribed treatment in hospitals and at home (Harmer & Henderson, 1939). Such plans usually coordinated treatment and care by all health care providers. The importance of planning *with* rather than *for* the patient and the family was stressed. During the 1940s there were demonstrations of family-centered health care, such as the Peckham Experiment in England (Pearce & Crocker, 1944) and the experiment at the Community Service Society of New York City in the United States (Shetland, 1943). Both showed the value of individualized plans and family health guidance with stress on self-help.

While in practice, depersonalized care is today the commonest criticism of health service, in principle an individualized plan is now accepted as a criterion of the quality of health care in hospitals. The (US) Joint Commission on Hospitals puts so much emphasis on nursing care plans that some critics believe that hospital staff nurses who do not see the value of written plans, prepare them before a visit from the Commission for the sole purpose of a favorable evaluation.

Marie Manthey, the hospital nurse administrator who has so successfully promoted patient assignment here and abroad (calling it *primary nursing*), made the following observation on hospital nursing care plans.

> No other single issue, thought, technique, problem, or phenomenon in nursing has received as much attention, has been as much written about, taught, talked about, worked at, read about and cried over, with so little success. No other issue in nursing has caused so much guilt—energy to be misspent. Yet, no other piece of paper in a hospital system is as devoid of information as that entitled *nursing care plan* unless Joint Commission (on Hospitals) is coming or students have recently worked on the floor. (Manthey, 1980)

Nurses in community health agencies, in homes, schools, industries and other settings keep records that may include something in the nature of a plan of care, as may the records of nurses in private practice. But whether or not they do, nurses are aware that one measure of excellence in nursing is the extent to which they help patients and their families plan and follow a regimen that is healthy for *them*. It is possible that written plans are unnecessary; it is more likely that realistically useful written plans of care have not been designed and that practicing nurses, as they assume more accountability for patient care, *will* see their value. A written plan that also serves as a record of care has been suggested as a *time-saving version of the plan of care* (Harmer & Henderson, 1955).

Patient Assignment

Patient assignment, or "primary nursing" is spreading rapidly in the United States and elsewhere. Individualized care is almost impossible without it as is the optimum satisfaction of the persons served and the care givers. The nursing process presupposes patient- rather than task-assignment and some written plan of care that informs all health providers who collaborate with each other, the client and the family in implementing the plan.

Identifying and helping people with their psychosocial as well as their physical problems has been the goal of nurses, in varying degrees, from one country to another and from age to age. In some countries and in some institutions, social workers have also been nurses. However, the emphasis on psychiatry and psychiatric nursing in the last 40 or 50 years, and especially the stress on the interdependence of mental, emotional, and physical well-being has tended to make all health care providers and the public, aware of the importance of psychosomatic illness. The importance of treating the whole man is now evidenced by frequent reference to "holistic medicine." (The open sesame for those who want current recognition in health circles!)

Of all the clinical nursing studies conducted in this century, those in psychiatric services have predominated. Social scientists, more than any others, have worked with nurses and have of course, studied nurses and their work. Higher degrees of many nurses both in the USA and in the UK have been earned in social science departments of universities. There has been a public demand for the upgrading of psychiatric institutions and psychiatric services in general hospitals. Experience in psychiatric services has been made part of the basic nursing programme in numerous countries, with emphasis on the psychosocial aspects of nursing throughout the basic curriculum. Psychiatric nurses have been appointed to nursing faculties and as consultants to nursing services.

At Yale University, Ida Orlando, a psychiatric nurse, conducted a study of the psycho-social content of general nursing. She reported it in 1961 under the title *The Dynamic Nurse Patient Relationship*. In this publication Miss Orlando (now Mrs. Robert Pelletier) says:

The purpose of nursing is to supply the help a patient requires in order for his needs to be met. The nurse achieves her purpose by initiating a *process* which ascertains the patient's immediate need and helps to meet the need directly or indirectly (emphasis added).

She then goes on to say that the nurse must be able to validate how her actions and reactions help or fail to help the patient. Florence Wald, a psychiatric nurse, then Dean of the Yale School of Nursing, and Robert Leonard, a sociologist on the faculty of the school, discuss the nursing process as then interpreted at Yale in an article entitled 'Toward development of nursing practice theory' (Wald & Leonard, 1964). The same subject was pursued by Ernestine Wiedenbach, a nurse member of the Yale Faculty, with two philosophers, Patricia James and William Dickoff, also of this faculty (Dickoff et al. 1963). A later work, Miss Wiedenbach's (1969) *Clinical Nursing—A Helping Art*, gives in detail the kind of communication between patient and nurses that Miss Orlando (1961) saw as the essential part of the nursing process. Such exchanges revealed the perception, thoughts and feelings of patients and nurses. As then interpreted the nursing process incorporated the reflective technique of Carl Rogers (1950) and certain concepts of L. Thomas Hopkins (1954).

A survey of nursing research made during the 1950s shows a number of nursing faculties caught up in studies of interpersonal relations (Simmons & Henderson, 1964). Some critics of present day nursing education say that there remains today too much emphasis on what nurses *say* to their clients, or patients, too little on what they *do* for them. (A current joke is about the student nurse who draws up a chair to the bedside of a hemorrhaging patient asking her if she wouldn't like to talk about how it feels to be bleeding to death.)

In spite of Florence Nightingale's example of basing recommended changes in health care systems on statistical evidence, nurses have been slow to develop the scientific aspect of nursing or to accept the idea that their work should be based on research. Few nurses held this view until recently, but M. Adelaide Nutting (1927) recognized Miss Nightingale's contribution as a statistician.

Research Developments

Isabel M. Stewart tried in the late 1920s to establish a research institute at Teacher's College, New York City. Although the dream was not realized until after her death, during Miss Stewart's administration, the faculty was encouraged to conduct studies and most students were required to take a course that introduced them to a scientific method of investigation. The purpose of the course was not only to give them an opportunity to use this method, but to help these graduate nurses to learn to find research reported in the literature and to relate these findings to their practice. Students were persuaded that "we've always done it this way" was not the best reason for using any procedure, nor was it acting responsibly to depend always on the opinions of experienced nurses and doctors as authority for practice. As post-basic nursing programs developed in American universities, they all included some training in research and theses were required of master's as well as doctoral candidates.

At no centres was the emphasis on research more pronounced than at Catholic University of America, at Teachers College and at the Yale University School of Nursing where Dean Annie W. Goodrich had an abiding faith in the benefits of medical science. The effect on faculty and students in these centres was to develop a habit of inquiry, an analytical approach to nursing practice and the rejection of traditional practices, as a basis for responding to human needs. And these developments were paralleled in other countries, as for instance in the UK where a nursing research unit was established within the University of Edinburgh and the Dan Mason Research Committee was established in London and a series of nursing care research studies financed by the Department of Health and Social Security were conducted within the Royal College of Nursing. By 1951 the International Council of Nurses held an International Conference on the Planning of Nursing Studies (1957). During the 1950s and 1960s nursing research flourished so that by 1967, when the first conference on the nursing process was held, the idea of nursing science was in the ascendancy. The interpretation of the nursing process as a problem-solving procedure akin to research almost immediately met with wide acceptance.

Nursing's Unique and Interdependent Role

To *identify a unique professional and independent role for nursing* has been a goal of some nurses throughout the existence of nursing as a paid occupation. With the passage of nurse practice acts in this century, definitions of nursing were essential. Written into the laws governing nursing practice, up until very recent times, however, has been the implication that nurses could not (legally) function independently of physicians; they could not admit people to the health care system and could not diagnose or treat disease. In other words, nurses were not providers of primary health care.

Now, with recognition that nurse-midwives and other nurses in regions unsupplied with physicians have been giving health care, and with the recognition that few, if any, countries can afford to prepare enough physicians to provide primary health care for all the people, there has come to be acceptance of the nurse as one who does give, and should be adequately prepared to give, primary health care.

Since the World Health Organization proposes to make health care available to all people by the year 2000, new ways must be found to provide this care and the functions of health workers must depend to a large extent on the numbers available, their preparation and the potential value of their services. Overlapping of functions is admitted, boundaries between fields of service are shifting and few would question the statement that nurses are expected to take more and more responsibility in both critical and chronic illness, as well as in prevention of disease and in health promotion. Economically feasible health programs in most countries, if they are to be successful, include the education of the public in self-help, in health maintenance and disease prevention. Health science libraries are being opened to the public and physicians required to get informed consent for treatment.

The nursing process is seen by many nurses as describing an independent role for nursing that parallels the role of the physician but is different from that role: the nursing history parallels the medical history; the nurse's health assessment, the physician's medical examination; the nursing diagnosis corresponds to the physician's diagnosis; nursing orders correspond to medical orders; the plan of nursing care to the plan of medical management and nursing evaluation to medical evaluation. It seems as if the medical model has been followed but with a modification in language that makes it possible to legally justify the role of the nurse in therapy.

Lawrence Weed (1971), a physician, has also promoted the identification of patients' problems and medical management focused on them, rather than on a single diagnosis. What I have seen of his work leads me to believe that he treats the nurse as a coworker and that, with other health professionals, they collaborate on identifying the patients' problems and on helping patients cope with them. Barbara Bates (1970) is another physician who sees the current overlapping of medicine and nursing but thinks collaboration is the answer, rather than competition. Some physicians and some nurses have come to believe that the clinical nurse specialist in all fields of practice could function in relation to physicians as does the nurse-midwife of the UK, where the majority of births are attended by nurse-midwives, rather than obstetricians.

But as long as nurses are the only health workers offering a 24-hour service to clients or patients their position as the alter ego of those they serve remains unique no matter whether they assist physicians, collaborate with them or compete with them.

A Critique of "The Nursing Process" as Currently Defined

On purely semantic grounds the nursing process is a debatable term. "The" makes it so specific that activities outside those in the problem-solving steps of the process cannot be peculiar to or characteristic of nursing.

Activity analyses made during the 1950s show nurses performing more than 400 tasks in hospitals and a different set of activities in other settings. Granting that many of these were non-nursing tasks that should have been performed by non-nurses, many, presently considered legitimate functions of the nurses would be hard to fit into the problem-solving steps of the nursing process.

Clinical Judgment

It is possible that the majority of nurses' responses to human needs require instant decisions. This would certainly be true in emergency departments or critical care units. These responses are dictated by what might be called clinical judgment. This may be derived from theoretical knowledge or from experience but it is also intuitive. To some extent clinical judgment is mysterious since health care providers with the same opportunity to develop it vary so greatly in the degree to which they demonstrate it. Nor can nursing interaction be divorced altogether from the emotional, or very subjective response of the nurse to the behavior of the patient. It may be dictated by the nurse's past experience or value system. Nurses are not free from prejudices. Their immediate response to a disoriented person, for example, may differ according to the patient's age, sex, race, color, religion, or the suspected cause of the disorientation, as for instance a fever, an injury, alcoholism, or senility.

A cartoon in a recent *New York Times* shows Rodin's The Thinker in duplicate. One thinker is sitting on a DNA double helix, the other on the tower of a university(?) building. The figures are of equal size. The implication is clear that the thinker's conclusions are based on what he derives from his genes, or his inherent humanity, as well as from his schooling.

Carl Sagan (1978) says, writing on the evolution of human intelligence that man is born with the knowledge stored in a very large library. City dwellers are constantly reminded that the cockroach with only its genetic endowment and the lessons of experience has eluded mankind's effort to exterminate it. Even the simpler forms of life, as for example, pathogenic bacteria, have little understood powers of adaptation that make the eradication of the diseases they cause a complex and unending task.

The point has perhaps been made that reducing the nurse's function to an analytical, more or less objective process divorces it from the intuitive, subjective response. While there are people who object to almost any categorization, most of us see science and art as different: one as objective with the mysterious element reduced to a minimum; the other as subjective with qualities that are mysterious, hard to define or that even defy description. The nursing process now weighted so heavily on the scientific side, seems to belittle the intuitive, artistic, side of nursing. The process depends to a large extent on the knowledge that the nurse has acquired, but the intuitive intervention of the nurse depends upon the kind of a person he or she is. To use an old fashioned term, upon character. A. Vassiliki Lanara's recent book (1981), *Heroism as a Nursing Value* suggests the importance some critics of nursing attach to the inherent qualities of the nurse.

And, while nursing decisions based on authority are rarely stressed now as the basis for practice, they are inevitable in a law-abiding and orderly world. All health care providers, including nurses, operate within some sort of an establishment that puts limitations, or boundaries, on their practice. It is undesirable to be ignorant of these limitations as for example, the laws affecting health care. While nurses should be in the vanguard of those that promote just laws governing health services, knowledge of, and regard for, the law are part of a complete concept of nursing.

Opinions of Experts

I believe that nurses must often base their actions on the opinions of experts. It is not possible for nurses to find answers to all the questions they may face through a time-consuming, analytic process. Client–nurse association is often too brief for these problem-solving steps. If nursing students are taught that this is *the* nursing process they will feel guilty and inadequate when they don't use it. Quite often because of the time factor, if for no other reason, the best and only available guide for the nurse's intervention is the opinion of the more experienced.

Nurses should certainly be more able and willing than they presently are to find and apply related research before embarking on their own investigations. This, too, is a very important aspect of any nursing process which the current definition, in my opinion, fails to stress sufficiently.

But assuming that the nursing process as currently described is practicable and effective, does it not ascribe to the nurse an unduly omnipotent role? I question the nurse's identifying a patient's problem and making a plan to solve it, although he or she can *help* the patient and the family do both, just as he or she can help them implement and evaluate the program. The contemporary play, *Whose Life Is It Anyway*, suggests how aware the public are of the failure of health care providers to realize that the choice should always be the client's or the family's. Self-help agencies on the order of Alcoholics Anonymous (AA), that operate on this assumption, are eminently successful.

The resiliency of the human mind and body is a theme that runs through the writings of medical philosophers such as Lewis Thomas and René Dubos. The latter stresses the conflict arising out of current values based on technology and the more enduring ones that stem from the genetic endowment. Charles Lewis, an American physician, speaking at the 1981 ICN Congress in a session on "Nurses As Partners in Developing Future Health Care," said that doctors were "poorly educated in the giving of human service; better educated in the arrogance of science." In nursing's zeal to base its practice on research it must avoid the danger of de-emphasizing humanistic care (personal communication).

Frederick Leboyer is said to have delivered about 10,000 babies. His picture books with an accompanying story in elegant prose have radically changed conditions surrounding childbirth in many countries. He denies being a scientist, saying rather that he is a poet. When asked the source of his ideas on birth without violence he claims that the infant taught him. He likes to use the expression, "the infant knows" (personal communication). The induction of labor in an otherwise normal birth might be an ultimate form of intervention based on the arrogance of science.

Habit of Enquiry

The nursing process has served a useful purpose in reminding nurses that they should practice the habit of inquiry throughout their life in nursing practice. However, as long as it is synonymous with problem-solving in the service of the client, it is no more peculiar to nursing than to medicine, dentistry, social work or physiotherapy. And in no field of applied or even pure science should research be thought of as yielding immutable truths. I am told that the inspired insight of Albert Einstein modified or discredited laws of physics based on what was *thought* to be excellent research.

But even if the nursing process is interpreted to include the range of activity that, realistically or idealistically, characterizes nursing, the use of the term remains debatable. Can we further the understanding of nursing, medicine, dentistry, or social work by preceding these words with the process of?

Conclusion

The nursing process is now often used as a substitute for nursing. It is described as:

1. determining the client's problems;
2. making plans to solve them;
2. implementing the plans;
4. evaluating the success of the plans.

In this paper questions are raised as to whether problem-solving is all there is to nursing (so that it can be called *the* nursing process) and whether problem-solving is peculiar to nursing (or whether it can be called the *nursing* process)?

Use of the term nursing process, as I have known it, is traced from the 1950s, when I heard it discussed as a way of describing client–nurse communication conducive to mutual understanding, until the present when it is used to mean problem-solving by the nurse for the benefit of the patient. As usually interpreted, the term involves a nursing history, a nursing diagnosis of physical, but particularly psychosocial, problems, a plan for nursing intervention and evaluation of its effect. These steps seem to be taken independently of comparable activities by other health professionals, most notably physicians, with the nurse in an independent rather than an interdependent relationship with other health care providers.

While the nursing process recognizes the purpose of the problem-solving aspects of the nurses' work, a habit of inquiry and the use of investigative techniques in developing the scientific basis for nursing, it ignores the subjective or intuitive aspect of nursing and the role of experience, logic and expert opinion as bases for nursing practice. In stressing a dominant and independent function for the nurse, it fails to stress the value of collaboration of health professionals and particularly the importance of developing the self-reliance of clients.

References

1. Bates, B. (1970) Doctor and nurse: changing roles and relations. *New England Journal of Medicine 283*, 129–134.

2. Dickoff, J. James P. & Wiedenbach E. (1963) *Theory in a Practice Discipline*. Yale University School of Nursing, New Haven.

3. Harmer, B. & Henderson V. (1939) *The Principles and Practice of Nursing*, 4th edn. The Macmillan Company, New York.

4. Harmer B. & Henderson V. (1955). *The Textbook of the Principles and Practice of Nursing*, 5th edn. The Macmillan company, New York.

5. Hopkins, L. T. (1954) *The Emerging Self in School and Home*. Harper and Brothers, New York.

6. International Conference on the Planning of Nursing Studies, Sevres, France (1957) November 12–14 Proceedings. International Council of Nurses, London.

7. International Council of Nurses (1981) Congress. *American Journal of Nursing 81*, 1664–1671.

8. Kratz C. R. (1979) *The Nursing Process*. Balliere Tindall, London.

9. Lanara V. A. (1981) *Heroism as a Nursing Value: A Philosophic Perspective*. Publications: Sisterhood Evniki, Athens.

10. Manthey M. (1980). *The Practice of Primary Nursing*. Blackwell Scientific Publications. Boston.

11. National League of Nursing Education (1937). *A Curriculum Guide for Schools of Nursing*. The League, New York.

12. Nursing Theories Conference Group (1980) *Nursing Theories. The*

Base for Professional Nursing Practice. Prentice Hall Inc., Englewood Cliffs, N.J.

13. Nutting M. A. (1927) Florence Nightingale as a statistician. *Public Health Nurse 19*, 207–211.

14. Orlando I. (1961) *The Dynamic Nurse Patient Relationship*, pp. 8–9. G. P. Putnam's Sons, New York.

15. Pearse I. & Crocker L. H. (1944) *The Peckham Experiment—A Study of the Living Structure of Society.* Yale University Press, New Haven.

16. Rogers, C. R. (1950) *Client-Centered Therapy.* Houghton Mifflin Co., Boston.

17. Sagan C. (1978) *The Dragons of Eden: Speculations on the Evolution of Human Intelligence.* Random House, New York.

18. Shetland, M. (1943) *Family Health Service: A Study of the Department of Educational Nursing of the Community Service Society.* The Service, New York.

19. Simmons L. & Henderson V. (1964) *Nursing Research—A Survey and Assessment.* Appleton-Century-Crofts, New York.

20. Sorensen K. C. & Luchmann J. (1979) *Basic Nursing—A Psychophysiologic Approach.* W. B. Saunders Co., Philadelphia.

21. Wald F. & Leonard R. (1964) Toward development of nursing practice theory. *Nursing Research 13*, 309.

22. Weed L. L. (1971) *Medical Records Medical Education and Patient Care.* Press of Case—Western Reserve University, Cleveland (distributed by Year Book Medical Publishers, Chicago).

23. Wiedenbach E. (1969) *Clinical Nursing—A Helping Art.* Springer Verlag, New York.

Chapter 13

The Nature of Nursing

It is self-evident that an occupation, and especially a profession whose services affect human life, must define its function. Nursing's attempt to do so has a long, and still unfinished, history.

While official statements on nursing may serve the purpose for which they are intended, there is abundant evidence that they have not satisfied everyone. And, in recent years, with the development of varying types and grades of nursing personnel, the difficulty of defining function has been compounded. Probably the effort of organized nursing to formulate a statement of its function will always be unfinished business since conditions change from one era to the next and with the culture or nature of a society. But so long as available definitions are unsatisfying to nurses, or too general to guide practice, research, and education, individuals will continue to search for statements that fulfill their needs.

Development of a Concept

My interpretation of the nurse's function is the synthesis of many influences, some positive and some negative.

My basic training was largely in a general hospital where, for the nurse, technical competence, speed of performance, and a "professional" (actually an impersonal) manner were stressed. We were introduced to nursing as a series of almost unrelated procedures, beginning with making an unoccupied bed and progressing to, say, aspiration of body cavities. In this era, ability to catheterize a patient seemed to qualify a student for "night duty" where, without any previous experience in the administration of a service, she might have the entire care of 30 sick souls and bodies.

An authoritarian type of medicine and nursing were practiced in this hospital. Teaching was based on the textbook. Not even lip service was given to "patient centered care," "family health service," "comprehensive care," or "rehabilitation."

But there was, for me, an influence in these early student days that tended to negate this mechanistic approach to patient care. Annie W. Goodrich was dean of my school, the Army School of Nursing, and whenever she visited our unit she lifted our sights above techniques and routines. She saw nursing as a "world-wide social activity," a creative and constructive force in society, and, having a powerful intellect and boundless compassion for humanity, she never failed to infect us with "the ethical significance of nursing."[1] It is to her that I attribute my early discontent with the regimentalized patient care in which I participated and the concept of nursing as merely ancillary to medicine. But while Miss Goodrich presented us with the highest aim for nursing she left us to translate it into concrete acts. I needed someone to "show me"—as Eliza Doolittle sang, when work had ceased to be enough for her. I seldom, if ever, saw graduate nurses practice nursing; never my teachers. Their teaching was in a classroom.

A positive nursing experience, however, was a summer spent, when I was still a student, with the Henry Street Visiting Nurse Agency. Here I began to discard the formal approach to patients approved in the general hospital. In fact, I acquired a skepticism of medical care in hospitals that remains with me. Seeing the sick return to their homes following hospitalization, I began to realize that the seemingly successful institutional regimen nevertheless often failed to change the factors in the patient's way of living that had hospitalized him in the first place. Even today I question whether our traditional hospital routines and practice can really prepare a patient for a return to health. Nowhere during my entire student experience, it seems to me, did I have the opportunity to see or practice individualized care—to acquire the human relations skills that I needed. My psychiatric nursing affiliation concentrated on disease entities and their treatment, not on how the nurse might help the individual patient. And although, during my pediatric nursing affiliation, I first experienced the satisfaction—and saw the superiority—of a "case" as opposed to a "functional" assignment, the care was too mechanistic to teach me the true value of patient-centered care.

With this background and after a year of visiting nurse work I became the only full-time instructor in a school of nursing. Here I was forced to learn as

I taught. I at least sensed the need for more knowledge and clarification of my ideas and, fortunately for all concerned, I went back to school.

Except for a brief period of clinical supervision and teaching at the Strong Memorial Hospital, I remained at Teachers College, Columbia University—as student and teacher—for some 20 years, and during this time my concept of nursing was not so much changed as clarified. It is impossible to identify all the persons and experiences that brought this about, but a few stand out.

Caroline Stackpole based her teaching of physiology on Claude Bernard's dictum that health depends upon keeping the lymph constant around the cell.[2] This emphasis on the unit structure taught me relationships in what were, up to that time, unrelated laws of health.

Now, as I read reports of malnutrition from therapeutic diets, emotional and physiological crises from endocrine therapy, drug-induced skin lesions, and the varied complications from cortisone administration, I think to myself: "the constancy of the intercellular fluids has been dangerously reduced." Ever since I grasped this danger I have believed that a definition of nursing should imply an appreciation of the principle of physiological balance. It makes so vivid the importance of forcing fluids, of feeding the comatose or of relieving oxygen want.

Dr. Edward Thorndike's work in psychology, also at Teachers College, provided some parallel generalizations, or fixed points, in the psychosocial realm. His study of the fundamental needs of man made me realize that illness all too often places a person in a setting where shelter from the elements is almost the only fundamental need that is fully met. In most hospitals, the patient cannot eat as he wishes, his freedom of movement is curtailed, his privacy is invaded; he is put to bed in strange nightclothes, making him feel as unattractive as a punished child; he is separated from the objects of his affection; he is deprived of almost every diversion and of his work, and is reduced to dependence on persons who are often younger than he is, and sometimes less intelligent and courteous.

From the time I saw hospitalization in this light I have questioned every nursing routine or restriction that is in conflict with the individual's fundamental need for shelter, food, communication with others, and the company of those he loves; for opportunity to win approval, to dominate and be dominated, to learn, to work, to worship, and to play. In other words, I have since conceived it to be the aim of nursing to keep the individual's day as normal as possible—to keep him in "the stream of life" to the extent that is consistent with the physician's therapeutic plan.

My participation in preparing the 1937 *Curriculum Guide*, in the work of the NLNE's special committee on postgraduate clinical courses, and regional conferences associated with Miss Esther Brown's study, all forced me to express in writing these evolving concepts of nursing. It was not until the 1940s, however, that I could test my ideas in actual practice, when we developed at Teachers College a unique—at least, for that time—type of advanced study in medical-surgical nursing.

This course was unique because it was organized around nursing problems rather than medical diagnoses and diseases of body systems. The associated field experience gave the graduate nurse student an opportunity, for example, to increase her competence in helping a patient to cope with such problems as long-term illness, impending surgery, the relative isolation necessitated by a communicable disease, or the depression following the loss of an arm or a leg. It was one of the first advanced clinical courses where students actually nursed patients and conducted nursing clinics and interdisciplinary conferences around the care of the patients they nursed.

Unique Function

In 1958 the Nursing Service Committee of the International Council of Nurses asked me to describe my concept of basic nursing. The resulting statement published in pamphlet form by the ICN in 1961, was an adaptation of the definition of nursing in Harmer and Henderson and represented the final crystallization of my ideas on the subject.[3]

It is my contention that the nurse is, and should be legally, an independent practitioner, so long as she is not diagnosing or treating disease or making a prognosis, for these functions fall in the physician's realm. But the nurse is *the* authority on basic nursing care. And, by basic nursing care, I mean helping the patient with the following activities or providing conditions under which he can perform them unaided:

1. Breathe normally.
2. Eat and drink adequately.
3. Eliminate body wastes.
4. Move and maintain desirable posture.
5. Sleep and rest.
6. Select suitable clothes—dress and undress.

7. Maintain body temperature within normal range by adjusting clothing and modifying the environment.
8. Keep the body clean and well groomed and protect the integument.
9. Avoid dangers in the environment and avoid injuring others.
10.Communicate with others in expressing emotions, needs, fears, et cetera.
11.Worship according to one's faith.
12.Work in such a way that there is a sense of accomplishment.
13.Play, or participate in various forms of recreation.
14.Learn, discover, or satisfy the curiosity that leads to "normal" development and health and use the available health facilities.

In helping the patient with these activities the nurse has infinite need for knowledge of the biological and social sciences and of the skills based on them. There are few more complex arts than that of keeping a patient well-nourished and his mouth healthy during a long comatose period; or of helping the depressed, mute psychotic re-establish normal human relations. There is no worker but the nurse who can and will devote herself so consistently day and night to these ends.

This unique function of the nurse I see as a complex service. But, in emphasizing this basic function, I do not mean to disregard the nurse's therapeutic role. She is in most situations the patient's prime helper in carrying out the physician's prescriptions.

If we put total medical care in the form of a pie graph we might assign wedges of different sizes to members of what we now refer to as "the team." The wedge must differ in size for each member according to the problem facing the patient; in some situations certain members of the team have no part of the pie at all. The patient always has a slice, although that of the newborn infant or the unconscious adult is only a sliver; his very life depends on others, but most particularly on the nurse.

In contrast, where an otherwise healthy adult is suffering from a skin condition such as acne, he and his physician compose the team and they can divide the whole pie between them. If the problem is an orthopaedic disability, the largest slice may go to the physical therapist; when a sick child is cared for at home by the mother, then the latter's share may be by far the largest. But of all the members of the team, excepting the patient and the physician, the nurse has most often a piece of the pie and, next to theirs, hers is usually the largest share.

In talking about nursing we tend to stress promotion of health and prevention and cure of disease; we rarely speak of the inevitable end of life. Critics of our culture say we are prone to shrink from the thought and sight of old age and death. The nurse, however, cannot do this if she is to fulfill her unique function as I see it. There is a great deal that the nurse can do to keep the environment in which death occurs an aesthetic one, and to relieve the patient's discomfort with nursing measures. Even more important, in my concept of nursing, is the nurse's effort to assist the patient toward a "peaceful death" by facing it with him honestly and courageously, thus lending it dignity and even an awesome beauty.

In essence, then, I see nursing as *primarily complementing the patient by supplying what he needs in knowledge, will, or strength to perform his daily activities and also to carry out the treatment prescribed for him by the physician.* What are the implications of such a concept for nursing practice, research, and education?

Nursing Practice

The nurse who sees herself as reinforcing the patient where he lacks will, knowledge, or strength must make an effort to know him, to understand him, to "get inside his skin," as we have said. She will listen to him, his family, and his friends with interest. She will be especially aware of her relation with the patient and will try to make it a constructive, or therapeutic one realizing that this demands self-understanding. Finally, and most important, she will give of herself to the patient.

She will be willing, even anxious, to help the patient perform the functions we have just enumerated. In cooperation with the patient, his family, and other members of the health team, and according to the situation, she will make some sort of individualized plan, or a daily regimen that meets the whole range of human needs. She will not be satisfied to provide merely shelter, sanitary facilities, three meals a day, and the treatments prescribed by the physician.

But just as the nurse seeks to meet the patient's needs during a period of dependency, so she also tries to shorten this period. Before she commits any act for the patient, she asks herself what part of it he could himself perform. If he is unable to act at all, she identifies what he lacks and she helps to supply this lack as rapidly as she can. She evaluates her success with each patient according to the degree to which he establishes independence in all the activities that make up for him, a normal day. The rehabilitation of *all* patients, in the hands of such a nurse, begins with her first service to them.

This primary function of the practicing nurse must, of course, be performed in such a way that it promotes the physician's therapeutic plan. That means helping the patient carry out prescribed treatments or administering the treatment herself. Again, she will consider herself more successful if she assists the patient than if she acts for him.

Now, in certain situations, the nurse may find it necessary to assume the role of a physician—in hospitals with no resident physician, for instance, or in emergency conditions. First aid, which has elements of diagnosis and therapy, is expected of all informed citizens under certain circumstances.

As long as nurses are better prepared than any other member of the health team to act as a physician surrogate they will be tempted, in the interests of the patient, to assume this role. But it is not, in my judgment, their *true role*. In assuming it they not only practice skills in which they are ill prepared but rob themselves of the time needed for the performance of their primary role. Inevitably it forces nurses to delegate their primary function to inadequately prepared personnel. In my opinion, the social pressures that have called for a phenomenal increase in nurses has also demanded a proportionate increase in doctors.

This brings us to the question of the coordinating, managerial, and teaching functions that now consume so much of the professional nurse's time. Nurses must, of course, administer nursing services and teach nursing, but whether they should co-ordinate the services of the entire medical team is questionable.

The nurse who sees her primary function as a direct service to the patient will find an immediate reward in his progress towards independence through this service. To the extent that her practice offers this reward, it will be satisfying; to the extent that the situation deprives her of it, she will be dissatisfied. And she will use whatever influence she possesses to foster conditions that make the social rewards for practice at least commensurate with those for teaching and administration.

Nursing Research

When a nurse operates under a definition of nursing that specifies an area in which she is pre-eminently qualified, she automatically imposes on herself the responsibility for designing the methods she uses in her area of expertness. Studies of nursing functions have shown that, of the hundreds of specific acts performed by nurses, many are non-nursing in nature and could be assigned to other personnel; others are medically prescribed procedures for the design of which the physician is partially responsible. But if the nurse carries out the latter procedures and is liable, in the legal sense, for harmful effects on the patient, then she *must* share the responsibility for the design of the procedure with the physician.

The activities with which I am mainly concerned, however, are those having to do with nursing care itself. Most of these procedures—in fact, most aspects of basic nursing, including the nurse's approach to the patient and what she may and may not say or do for him—are based on tradition or authority, learned by imitation, and taught with little, if any scientific backing. It is my contention that methods in this all-important area will remain static and invalidated if the nurse fails to study them.

In a survey and assessment of nursing research, Leo W. Simmons and I have pointed out the preponderance of education and occupational studies over clinical investigations.[4] We tried to identify the conditions that discouraged patient-centered research and found: that the major energies of the occupation have gone into improving preparation for nursing and into learning how to recruit and hold sufficient numbers of workers in the occupation; that the demand for administrators and teachers almost exhausts the supply of degree holders, with the result that nurses with a university background tend to study administrative and educational problems; and that those few nurse practitioners prepared to study nursing practice often fail to get the support they need from hospital administrators, nursing service administrators, and physicians.

But if, by definition, nursing has an area of independent professional practice, is not clinical nursing research as necessary, if not more so, than research into other professional problems? Do we not deny our function when we fail to investigate it?

It is my belief that on every clinical service of a hospital a medical research committee and a nursing research committee are needed—both devoted to the ultimate and common goal of improving patient care. The medical research committee would study those problems lying wholly in the realm of medical practice; the nursing research committee would investigate procedures or problems that lie wholly within the realm of nursing practice. But still another committee—a joint one which would include not only doctors and nurses but other specialists as indicated—is also needed to study such treatments or diagnostic tests as are prescribed by the physician and carried out entirely or partially by the nurse.

In this era, research is the name we attach to the most reliable type of analysis. It is based on the full use of scientific findings and is the most reasonable approach man has invented to the solution of his problems. No profession, occupation, or industry can, in this age, adequately evaluate or improve its practice without research. Nursing, if it is truly to represent an area of independent practice, must therefore assume responsibility for validating and improving the methods it uses.

Nursing Education

A definition staking out an area of health and human welfare in which the nurse is the expert and an independent practitioner calls for education rather than training; a liberalizing education, a grounding in the physical, biological, and social sciences, and the ability to use analytic processes. The curriculum must be organized around the nurse's major function rather than that of the physician, as it has been in the past.

Early emphasis must be given to fundamental human needs, to patients' daily activities, and to the development of the nurse's ability to assess them properly and help the person meet them. In the next stage of the professional curriculum the student might then be introduced to the modifications in nursing care demanded by chronological and intellectual age, sex, emotional balance, state of consciousness, nutritional balance, and other conditions common to all patients and found on any clinical service. This content might constitute the core of the clinical curriculum. Finally, the student would be helped to study the particular needs of each patient, both in relation to these more general conditions and to those stemming from his specific disease, handicap, or condition.

Since the turn of the century, prominent American nurses—conspicuous among them, Miss Goodrich and Miss Nutting—and physicians have said that nursing schools should be developed within the educational system—not within the service institutions—of this country. But it is not only in this country that this need has been recognized. Informed physicians and educators throughout the world expressed this opinion.

A revision of established patterns of nursing education calls for strong leadership. At a meeting 20 years ago when someone was bemoaning the fact that there were no leaders in nursing coming along to take the place of our great women of the past, Miss Goodrich rose to protest. She said that the conditions were passing that demanded the militant personalities of earlier years; the idea—not the individual—should lead, she said. She believed firmly that what she called "the complete nurse"—the woman with social experience and a thorough education—had proved her worth, not only as administrator and teacher but more particularly as a practitioner. Therefore she saw as inevitable, rather than as something we must fight for, the preparation of nurses, within the colleges and universities.

I think that the professional quality of nursing service and the appropriateness of a professional preparation have been grasped in many countries, but the means by which these ideas can be implemented are slow in developing. It is up to us who share this faith in the social value of nursing to speed this process.

The function we believe the nurse performs is primarily an independent one—that of acting for the patient where he lacks knowledge, physical strength, or the will to act for himself. We see this function as complex and creative, as offering unlimited opportunity for the application of the physical, biological, and social sciences, and the development of skills based on them. We believe society wants and expects this service from the nurse, and no other worker is as able, or willing, to give it.

If a nurse believes that she is pre-eminent in an area of health practice, she will try to develop a working milieu in which she can realize her potential value to the person served. She will also recognize her responsibility for the validation and improvement of methods she uses, or for clinical nursing research.

In order to practice as an expert in her own right and to use the scientific approach to the improvement of practice, the nurse needs the kind of education that, in our society, is available only in colleges and universities. Educational programs operated on funds pinched from the budgets of service agencies cannot provide the preparation she needs. Her work demands self-understanding and a universal sympathy for and understanding of, diverse human beings. The "liberalizing" effect of a general education must be recognized, for the personality of the nurse is possibly the most important intangible in measuring the effect of nursing care. As Clare Dennison herself once said, "Finally and fundamentally the quality of nursing care depends upon the quality of those giving care."[5]

References

---

1. Goodrich, Annie W. *The social and ethical significance of nursing.* New York, Macmillan Co., 1932.

2. Kimber, Diana C., and others. *Anatomy and physiology* (14th ed.). New York, Macmillan Co., 1961.

3. Henderson, Virginia. *Basic principles of nursing care*. London, International Council of Nurses, 1960.

4. Simmons, L. W., and Henderson, Virginia. *Nursing research: A survey and assessment*. New York, Appleton-Century-Crofts, 1964.

5. Dennison, Clare. Maintaining the quality of nursing service in the emergency. *Amer. J. Nurs., 42*:774–784, July 1942.

PART III

Nursing Research

Introduction

Miss Henderson was a consummate nurse researcher. While she performed clinical research herself, she advanced the research of all nurses by being the driving force in creating the four-volume *Nursing Studies Index*. The *Index* project followed a study of nursing research undertaken with Leo Simmons at Yale University. Miss Henderson went to New Haven in 1953 from New York where she had just completely revised her textbook, Harmer and Henderson's *Principles and Practice of Nursing*. Their book, *Nursing Research: Survey and Assessment*, was the first to fully document the state of nursing research, concluding that studies of nurses outnumbered studies of nursing care ten-to-one. One impediment to research in nursing was the ineffective dissemination of previous studies, upon which new research was to build.

Miss Henderson set out to remedy the absence of an index to nursing studies by organizing and directing a team of nurses, librarians, and scientists who compiled the *Index*. Almost immediately after the Simmons and Henderson critique was published, nursing research shifted toward studies of nursing care. At no place was this more apparent than at the Yale School of Nursing. Faculty and students there influenced a generation of nurse researchers by using sophisticated methods and research designs like randomized controlled clinical trials, and building their research on a sound theoretical base. Yale led these research efforts for over two decades until doctoral programs in nursing became more common.

A classification scheme for nursing studies was created for the Nursing Studies Index and later abandoned for the topical listing in *Index Medicus*. These Medical Subject Headings or MESH were adopted to classify nursing studies so they could be co-mingled with medical studies in *Index Medicus*; this way nurses and physicians would have immediate access to each other's literature on the same topic. Unfortunately, computer searches now separate journals into medical and nursing categories before listing titles, so the intent of the *Index* study team has been foiled. Nurses have also renamed subjects so that literature searches are even more difficult. For example, constipation is alternately a nursing diagnosis or an alteration in bowel function, which hampers the location of relevant literature.

One selection in this section (Chapter 17) on nursing research was co-authored with Dr. Faye Abdellah. It is the chapter from *Principles and Practice of Nursing* (6th edition), which introduced the section on therapeutic measures, procedures or techniques (interventions?) and implies that research is the preferred method for selecting a technique. What works? How simple and elegant is the question implied in the placement of the research chapter in the procedures section. The chapter is subtitled "Research as a Means of Improving Nursing Practice." My colleague, Dr. Janice Janken, RN of the Presbyterian Hospital and the University of North Carolina at Charlotte, uses a single criterion when she engages in nursing research with her hospital nurse colleagues: "How will this research change your practice?" If no practice changes are anticipated, she declines participation, suggesting the research is not nursing. Studies of lactation, ear wax and hearing, flatulence, falls, and constipation have been undertaken at Charlotte and at Rhode Island Hospital where she developed the innovative model for research by hospital nurses.

In the Preface of *Principles and Practice of Nursing* (6th edition), Miss Henderson says that the book is drawn from the research and expert opinion literature. Few would not be intimidated by the sheer volume of literature cited in this work. I have seen no work in any professional field that covers such a diversity of topics and is so well tied to the research literature; there are tens of thousands of references and footnotes. The 6th edition flows directly from her work on the *Nursing Studies Index* but also articulates with all previous editions of the Harmer and Henderson textbook, dating from 1922. In spite of the remarkable changes in health care in the 56 years between the book's first and most recent editions, there is a reassuring continuity in nursing. So many of us are immersed in the here and now and the newest; it seems as if what we deal with changes so quickly and constantly confronts us with new situations. Miss Henderson's writings, structured around principles, reveal strong links with our predecessors. Her recommendations for research on nursing practice also connects us to the future.

References

Henderson, V. (1963, 1966, 1970, 1972). *Nursing studies index*. New York: Lippincott.

Henderson, V., & Harmer (1955). *Principles and practice of nursing*. New York: Macmillan.

Simmons, L. & Henderson, V. (1964). *Nursing research: Survey and assessment*. New York: Appleton-Century-Crofts.

Chapter 14

Research in Nursing Practice—When?

If research in any occupation were divided into two categories: (1) studies of the workers, and (2) studies of their work, which type would usually predominate? Would we find more research on lawyers or the law; on engineers or engineering; on cleaners or cleaning? In all these occupations, be they so-called "professions" or "vocations," the conclusion is the same—that there has been more research on practice than on the practitioner.

Why is it, then, that in our field, studies on the nurse outnumber studies on the practice of nursing more than ten to one? (To define our terms, we should say here that we consider research on the nurse to include: studies of motivation, selection, and education of the nurse; needs and resources; the nurse's intellectual, social, and economic status, and her function or role in society; her satisfactions or dissatisfactions; her working and living conditions; the ways in which nurses are organized; and the laws affecting them. In contrast, studies on nursing practice are mainly concerned with the persons the nurse serves—the patient and his family—or at least with the equipment and materials used in giving the nursing care or treatment.

It can, of course, be argued that any study leading to improvement in recruitment, selection, preparation, and distribution of nurses; to better administration of nursing services; and to clarification of the nurse's role or function automatically affects practice. However, an even stronger argument might be made in the reverse—that research in the practice of nursing might even more substantially affect recruitment, role, status, preparation, needs, and working conditions.

Perhaps a wiser reaction to the undeniable fact that the bulk of nursing research deals with the worker rather than the work is to wonder why. Has society's demand for more and more nursing care made it necessary for the occupation to emphasize numbers, recruitment, and job satisfaction? Has the apprenticeship mold in which the nurse's preparation has been cast forced the occupation to confine its principal investigations to education of the nurse? Is the discrepancy between supply and demand responsible for the continuing studies of nursing resources, of patterns of nursing service, and of functional analyses in the major fields of nursing?

Another explanation of the focus of attention on the nurse rather than on nursing may lie in the sources of support received by nurses in advanced education where much of the research originates. University nursing programs, if not independent, are often associated with the university's school of education; sometimes the association is with the department of social sciences, occasionally with the department of biological and physical sciences, and in many cases with the schools of medicine. Is it possible that educators and social scientists have been more inclined to help nurses with their research than have the physical, biological, or medical scientists?

Do those in the latter categories tend to regard the nurse who participates in clinical research as a technician rather than as a partner, and have they discouraged the initiation of clinical research by the nurse? Is it also possible that it is easier to study the nurse than the patient? Is the study of the behavior of the sick so complex and so difficult that the research experts to whom nurses have turned for help have been afraid of it? Or is it the nurse who shies away from studies that necessitate observation of the patient's reaction?

Another explanation of the paucity of clinical nursing research may lie in the pull of the well-prepared nurse toward administration or teaching. Since less than 10 percent of the "professional" nurses hold degrees of any kind, the supply of qualified administrators and teachers is inadequate to meet the demand. The well-educated nurse is pressured into teaching and administration, partly by the need for such services and partly by the fact that economic advancement and improvement of status are not generally available to the nurse who remains a practitioner. Clinical nurses whose collegiate training might prepare them to develop clinical research are rarely left to practice nursing.

It is not surprising that more than half of the 80 or more doctoral dissertations by nurses deal with education, and less than 15 percent with nursing care. The emphasis in master's theses follows somewhat the same pattern. Analyzing the contents of *Nursing Research* from 1952 to 1955 we note that more than half of the studies published relate to administration and education, while a little less than half relate solely or in part to clinical nursing. It is encouraging, on the other hand, to find some light thrown on a few basic nursing techniques, on health teaching, and on the patient's reaction to illness. In addition, interaction between nurses and patients is under investigation in many psychiatric hospitals. Judging by the number and excellence of such studies, it would seem that psychiatric nurses, more than those in any other field, are learning how to study nursing care.

Responsibility for designing its methods is often cited as an essential characteristic of a profession. Whether or not nurses achieve full professional status is unimportant, however, unless this development results in, or is accompanied by, improvement in nursing care in all its physiological and psycho-social aspects.

Chapter 15

An Overview of Nursing Research *

T his review of studies on nursing and nurses is mainly derived from the Survey and Assessment of Nursing Research, a project initiated in 1953 by the National Committee for the Improvement of Nursing Services, and carried out, with Leo W. Simmons as director, under the auspices of Yale University. Generally referred to as the Yale Survey, the project's original and basic purpose was to find, classify, and evaluate the research in nursing during the past decade.

This present review of nursing research could be approached from several different standpoints: for instance, according to sponsorship, methodology, or content. The last approach—from the standpoint of *content*—is the one that will be followed here, with individual studies presented in rough chronological order.

The Yale Survey staff has developed what we have found to be a workable content classification as follows:

A. Historical, philosophical, and cultural
B. Occupational orientation and career dynamics
C. Specialties in nursing by occupational categories
D. Organizations for nursing—professional and vocational
E. Administration of nursing services

*The paper by Virginia Henderson published here served as introduction to a group of shorter project reports, presented at the same program session during the 1957 NLN convention. These latter project reports were not intended as full accounts of research studies, but rather as brief summaries of representative research in progress or recently completed.

F. Nursing care
G. Patients' reactions to identifiable variables related to their illnesses
H. Interaction patterns between nurse, patient, patients' families, other nurses, physicians, and other members of the health team
I. Education for nursing.

These are the categories to which reference will be made, with some telescoping for expediency. Studies under the "B" and "C" headings are discussed together since all are occupational research. Studies filed under "H" on the relationship between nurses, between nurses and other medical personnel, and between nurses and the public are grouped with those in the "E" category—administration and nursing services. Studies in the "G" category that directly involve the patient are discussed with the research on nursing care.

No cut-off date is observed in this paper. A current study may be something like a third story on a house built 20 years ago. To talk about current investigations without mentioning their forerunners seems as inappropriate as to describe the third story without reference to its foundation.

Historical, Philosophical, and Cultural Research

There are relatively few studies on nursing or by nurses that are primarily historical, philosophical, or cultural, according to our criteria. And—as one might suspect—there is more historical than philosophical or cultural research.

Some nurse leaders believe a knowledge of the past is essential to effective planning for the future. This may explain why many national, state, and local organizations and various other agencies have commissioned historical studies, or have published student theses of this nature. Sometimes the history is focused on the sponsoring organization or agency and sometimes it is the history of an epoch, or a time period, of nursing in an area, or of a particular kind of service such as Army or Red Cross nursing.

Biographical research has been encouraged by the *American Journal of Nursing* but there are only a few full-length published life histories—those of Florence Nightingale, Lillian D. Wald, and Annie W. Goodrich—and only one of these biographies is exhaustive. The current collection of Nightingaliana is of particular interest. The directors of this project from the sponsoring agencies, the Florence Nightingale International Foundation and the

Wellcome Historical Medical Library of London, believe the catalogue when completed may prove to include the largest known collection of letters—over twenty thousand.[5]

The student of research cannot help but be arrested by the fact that Florence Nightingale was an expert statistician on whose studies were based important changes in the domestic and colonial British health services in the 19th century. Although she herself was very largely self-taught, it is ironic that she is represented as the founder of the current hospital nursing school system which has upheld tradition and discouraged inquiry. Few realize that Miss Nightingale proposed independence for nursing schools, a proposal that few founders adopted.

Studies centered on a definition of function, or a statement of values (as in a code of ethics), might be considered philosophical, and the American Nurses' Association has spent more than half a million dollars in the past five years on studies of the nurse's function. Their nature is such, however, that they fall primarily under the category of occupation and nursing service research and will be discussed under these headings. Clara A. Hardin entitled her last year's progress report on this research: *Nurses Invest in Patient Care.*[6]

Nurses have participated in, but rarely initiated, studies of health needs and practices in ethnic or cultural regions. Gladys Sellew might be cited as an exception and her study as an example of the kind of investigation to which reference is made here.[7] In 1938, Miss Sellew lived on a subsistence level in one of Washington's worst alleys; her purpose was to identify with the residents so that she could study their health needs and practices.

As the social sciences are strengthened in basic and graduate programs, research in this category will almost certainly increase. Recently appointed national committees on "the future," on "long-term goals," and on "early source materials" will certainly foster philosophical and historical studies.

Occupational Research

In the United States the demand for the services of the graduate or so-called "professional nurse" has exceeded the supply, except during the last economic depression. At the same time, most of the men and women who have chosen this vocation have been forced to work their way through training programs owned and administered by hospitals, which are essentially service agencies.

These two facts—the demand exceeding the supply and the discrepancy between the preparation nurses have wanted and the kind available to them—must account for the two major emphases in nursing research

A glance at the Yale Index of nursing studies shows two types predominating: occupational and educational. Not only are the items most numerous in these categories, but in them fall the majority of the studies to which full-time workers have been assigned and large grants made.

During two world wars the great demand for nursing service stimulated surveys of needs and resources and the development of inventories. The American Red Cross, the military and civil federal nursing services (particularly the U.S. Public Health Service), the American Nurses' Association, the National Organization for Public Health Nursing, the National League of Nursing Education, war councils and a manpower commission, the Department of Labor, the Bureau of Census, and state and local nursing organizations all have cooperated in this type of research which continues in peacetime. Figures published in the ANA's annually revised *Facts About Nursing* are increasingly reliable as statistical methods are refined.[8]

Since 1945, most states have estimated their nursing needs and resources, usually with expert help from the Public Health Service. Under the editorship of Margaret Arnstein, the latter's Division of Nursing Resources has prepared a guide for such surveys.[9]

Irwin Deutscher, of Community Studies, Inc., in Kansas City, Missouri, has reported what is possibly the most refined canvass of nurses to date.[10] This investigation is a state sponsored, ANA financed study, with the emphasis on the development of method. The report states that our present national estimates may give a distorted picture. This is borne out by a recent New York state analysis which shows a very wide discrepancy between nurses registered in the state and those believed to be active. Possibly present figures underestimate both the actual and potential nurse power. The problem of holding personnel in the occupation may deserve more attention than that of attracting potential candidates.

Motivation for nursing, the satisfactions and dissatisfactions within it, the effect of role and status have all been investigated within the ANA program of function studies.[11] A promising study on the relationship of role concept to satisfaction and success is now in progress at the University of Minnesota.[12]

In 1955, Frances Payne Bolton initiated a survey of public opinion on health care, which included nursing. The report can be read in the *Congressional Record*.[13]

Other related and earlier studies are the Grading Committee's report, *Nurses, Patients, and Pocketbooks* (1928), the public opinion poll on nursing conducted by Edward L. Bernays in 1948, and the economic studies made by the ANA in collaboration with the U.S. Bureau of Labor Statistics, also published during the last decade.[14,15,16]

The ANA's research and statistics unit, through *Facts About Nursing*, publishes annual summaries of the economic data on nurses. Some of this is collected by this unit, some by state nurses associations, and some is taken from the Bureau of Labor Statistics occupational wage surveys. All told, these data give a fairly accurate picture of the economic status of the professional nurse. For some groups within the nursing occupation economic studies are badly needed—investigations as thorough as, for example, the ANA's hospital staff nurse salary study in 1943, or the NLN's recent salary study for public health nurses.[17,18]

In 1937, the U.S. Office of Education studied the economic status of college alumni, including nurses, and the U.S. Woman's Bureau reports a similar study for 1955.[19,20] These two studies make it possible to generalize tentatively on the relationship of earnings and education in nursing.

While the material reward for service is a major vocational incentive or deterrent in a money-conscious culture, nurses, in the studies to date, have not given it first place. Edward A. Suchman is presently investigating, under a USPHS grant, the reasons why those eligible for enrollment are selecting or rejecting nursing as a career.[21] It will be interesting to see what he learns about the money motive.

In addition to the studies that have been mentioned (most of which relate to all professional nurses) there are many that focus on a special group. Examples are studies of nurses in a clinical field, such as psychiatry; of those who hold a particular position, such as head nurse; and of those employed in a type of agency such as a public health department, or a health service, like the Army Nurse Corps. In addition, nurses have been studied according to characteristics of sex, age, marital status, race, educational achievements, social status, geographic background, health indices, and status of employment.

The spotlight was first turned on the public health nurses with Isabella M. Waters' study in 1909.[22] After the First World War an exodus from the private duty field brought special attention to these practitioners, while the depression stimulated what was then called "experimentation" with the use of the graduate nurse for bedside nursing in the hospital.[23,24] At the moment, psychiatric nurses seem to occupy a major share of the limelight. A review of the studies on special groups of nurses shows that few are altogether neglected.

The comment is often made by persons from other professions that none of the occupations has been studied more thoroughly than nursing. Whether or not this be true, nurses have never before had so much factual material on which to base their plans and with which to answer their critics.

Surveying the "conspicuous research" in this category leaves certain clear-cut impressions.

Nurses are unevenly distributed but the ratio of nursing personnel to the population has steadily increased, while the ratio of physicians and dentists has remained almost constant during the past 50 years. The most rapid rate of increase is presently in the subprofessional nursing group. Estimates of nursing needs are still rough. Those based on present *demands* are believed to be almost if not quite unattainable.

Motivation for nursing is widespread among very young females but decreases from the first years of high school on. Motivation is higher in rural than in urban populations. For the population as a whole teaching is the only occupation that rates higher for women than nursing.

Satisfactions in nursing outweigh dissatisfactions. Attrition in nursing as compared with other occupations has not been measured, so it is difficult to say whether the occupation "should" or "should not" hold more of its members. Some believe that the better the preparation the lower the attrition rate, but proof of this is needed.

The service motive ranks high in such studies as have been made; but economic security is a factor, particularly with the better prepared worker. College-educated nurses averaged the third highest salaries in the 1955 study of women college graduates, and even higher in the 1937 study; the average income of the diploma-holding nurse is very much lower. Subprofessional nursing personnel can look forward to steady employment but an economic dead end, unless some plan for their educational progression materializes.

The public appears to value nurses but to be increasingly critical of all who give medical service. Some of this is due to overcrowded facilities, short-term hospitalizations, and the fractionalization of care that has impersonalized service. The elaboration of nursing personnel makes a clear-cut picture difficult but a few studies seem to indicate that public evaluation *is* related to the time spent by the practitioner in his or her preparation. The static doctor-population ratio coupled with the phenomenal rise in public demand for medical service and ability to pay for it has greatly affected the function of the graduate nurse. To meet the public demand for service it has been necessary to keep shifting functions to less highly qualified groups within the nursing categories; and these groups continue to elaborate amid mounting confusion as to how they can best be utilized.

In spite of the research and the remarkable accomplishments within the ANA's sections, where statements of functions have been laboriously forged, the identification of functions according to qualification and preparation, and based on patient-worker welfare, is still the major occupational problem.

Organizational Research

Organizational research occupies a relatively small space in a file of studies on nursing but this does not mean that nursing leadership has underestimated the value of organization. The International Council of Nurses antedated the international hospital and medical associations, and in 1950 it was the largest international organization of women in the world.

National nursing organizations have been handicapped financially. A Rockefeller endowment enabled the National Organization for Public Health Nursing to establish a headquarters office with a salaried full-time secretary in 1912, but the ANA and the NLNE functioned without either until 1920 when a joint headquarters office for these three major nursing organizations was made possible by a grant from the American Red Cross.

From that time on the committees appointed to consider organizational structure worked more competently until, in 1952, a plan was implemented for the amalgamation of the five major national organizations into two organizations. The rapid development of the ANA and the NLN in the past four years is a tribute to the structure committee and its consultants.[25] A study of the annual reports of the organizations shows that analysis of structure and function continues.

Another example of productive organizational research is the amalgamation in 1949 of the Florence Nightingale International Foundation with the ICN, following a study of the former by R. H. Hamley and Muriel Uprichard of Canada, and a study of the latter by a committee of which Alma H. Scott of the United States served as chairman.[26,27]

Through what might be termed action research, nurses have evolved highly successful ways of working toward a common goal with other occupational groups. Some significant developments along these lines are the relationships of organized nursing to the World Health Organization, the United Nations, the National Council of Social Agencies, and the National Society for Medical Research; or with other clinical workers as, for example, in the International Clinical Conference on Pediatrics or Midwifery. The nursing seminar under the Southern Regional Education Board, nursing participation in the Western Interstate Commission for Higher Education, and the current seminars on psychiatric nursing under a grant from the National Institute for Mental Health are interesting experiments in regional organization. On the state level mention might be made of the decision in Mississippi to transfer the accreditation of schools from the State Board of Nurse Examiners to the State Education Department's Division of Institutions of Higher Learning. Nurses are currently participating in the National Social Welfare Assembly's pilot study of the relationships of locals to their national organization.[28]

Perhaps the most important organizational development toward which nurses have contributed so largely is the joint committee to discuss problems of patient care, made up of representatives of the consumers and major groups who give medical services. The National Committee for the Improvement of Nursing Service was a 5-year experiment financed by the Kellogg Foundation.[29] Its accomplishments have helped stimulate the formation of joint state and local "Commissions on Improvement of the Care of the Patient." In 1955, 18 states had such commissions.[30] Hopefully, this type of organization will spread to all states and finally be adopted by individual health agencies.

Research units were established within the NLNE in 1930 and within the ANA in 1945. These units and the new American Nurses' Foundation represent, to date, successful organizational experimentation in promoting and conducting research.

In summary, nurses are demonstrating an ability to criticize their established organizational patterns; their resistance to change is not so strong as it was. Their lack of preparation for research has been converted from "loss" to "gain" since it has forced them into collaborative research. This, in turn, has been made possible through new cooperative organizations.

Administration of Nursing Services

Under this heading are included studies on how services are organized; studies of facilities; personnel practices; leadership; public relations; cost analyses; teamwork; activity analyses; functions of workers; operational standards; and appraisals of service. The research in this category is so interesting and important that its summarization is particularly difficult.

From 1909 until 1952, when its program was absorbed by the National League for Nursing, the NOPHN used research methods to establish public health nursing service standards. From 1930 to 1952 the NLNE conducted comparable investigations in hospital nursing service. The ANA, and often the American Hospital Association, collaborated with the NLNE. In the past few years the ANA and the NLN have been deeply involved in nursing service research. The Kellogg Foundation has sponsored administrative exploration and experimentation, and a considerable number of recent and current USPHS grants have been given to university centers and research institutes for nursing service investigations. Studies made within various divisions of the Public Health Service fall under this heading. Other federal agencies that should be mentioned in connection with service research are the Veterans Administration and the Army Nurse Corps.

Public health studies were first designed to establish standards of practice, since such nursing agencies were cropping up all over the country with wide variation in the services they offered and in personnel practice. The first study, in 1909, sponsored by the Rockefeller Foundation, has been mentioned. Later there were activity analyses, studies to establish nurse-population ratios, studies to develop staffing formulae and case load standards. Katharine Tucker, Hortense Hilbert, Sophie C. Nelson, Alma Haupt, Pearl McIver, and Marion Ferguson all contributed to this type of research, which was sponsored by the NOPHN and often financed by the Commonwealth, Rockefeller, or Milbank Foundations. Health demonstrations of the 20's and 30's established the value of the public health nurse beyond any gain-saying, but they were not set up to measure the nurse's contribution as distinct from that of other medical workers.

As the philanthropic concept of community nursing service has waned and the extension of tax-supported health service has been accepted, public health nursing has undergone an administrative revolution. One study of combination services in public health nursing agencies was made and reported under Dorothy Rusby's leadership in 1951.[31] A progress report of the current study was published in 1955. The combining of the public and private agency almost necessitated the current cost and activity analyses.[32,33] A study of income and expenditures in public health nursing agencies was reported in 1954. A comparative cost study of 11 public health nursing agencies was reported in 1956 and a salary study this year (1957).

On the basis of a study, the inclusion of nursing in prepayment health plans was recommended by a joint committee of the NOPHN and the ANA in 1950.[34,35,36] A pilot study of home nursing benefits under the Associated Hospital Service of New York in 1955 is an example of the kind of experimentation needed in many centers.[37] The way in which the cost of public health nursing should be met is part of the larger problem of financing health service.

Besides these types of investigation in the generalized public health services, there are studies in related fields, as—for example—school and industrial nursing, and in clinical specialties such as material and child care, but space does not permit discussion of them.

Public health nurses are increasingly critical of their service and are wondering whether the public's more general knowledge of health, the changing standards of living, and the greater availability of health service have not materially altered the kind of help the average person in his home wants from the nurse. With other medical workers, nurses are sponsoring a study on health attitudes and practices in a large sampling of the citizenry. The National Opinion Research Center of Chicago, under a grant from the Health Information Foundation, is making the investigation. Under a grant from the USPHS, Ruth B. Freeman is developing a method of matching public health nursing service to community needs.[38] Marion Ferguson and her associates are studying the function of the public health nurse, with special reference to what the consumer wants from her.[39] Some of the less obvious needs of the patient will show up, it is believed, in the current American Nurses' Foundation's study of the professional nurse's function in public health.[40]

There is a wealth of data on hospital nursing service; its synthesis or interpretation is in itself a major piece of research. Here is where we see the greatest elaboration of nursing and related personnel and possibly the most striking change in nursing function. One hospital nursing staff, studying its service during the past 20 years, found the average census increase only 6.4 percent but the admission rate increased 37.2 percent. Use of oxygen increased 900 percent and intravenous injections 177 percent. Paid nursing personnel increased 54 percent, but full-time professional personnel decreased by 37 percent. The head nurse, instead of being responsible for 10 patients, directed the care of 33 patients.[41]

It is commonly thought that patients in general hospitals are more acutely ill, are receiving more concentrated treatment, and need more nursing care now than they did 20 years ago. Comparison of the findings of two studies by Blanche Pfefferkorn of the NLNE in 1937 and 1948, with the findings of a recent study by Faye G. Abdellah and Eugene Levine of the USPHS, indicate that *more* care *is* available to patients.[42,43,44] If it is true, as if often stated, that patients are less satisfied with hospital nursing care now than 20 years ago, the Abdellah-Levine study contains a clue: in their investigation of 60 hospitals, patient satisfaction was high in relation to the proportion of professional nursing care available. "The patient wants and is demanding more professional nursing time," they state. "The nurses too want to be with the patient."

Evaluation studies in nursing service and in patient care overlap and are indistinguishable very often. Reference is made to investigations similar to the one just mentioned in the next section of this overview. The Division of Nursing Resources of the USPHS has been especially interested in evaluative research. A number of its recent grants have been made to centers attempting to find better ways of utilizing presently available nursing service personnel as measured by patient satisfaction and recovery. In others the research team is trying to find an optimum pattern of service that might be a goal in the future.[45,46,47]

In summary it would seem that the recent activity analyses, utilization, and personnel-interaction studies give a fairly clear picture of what nursing service is like in representative agencies and institutions. The chief sources of satisfaction and dissatisfaction among the workers have perhaps been identified. Social scientists, as if holding up a mirror, have enabled hospital workers to see themselves. A few psychiatric hospitals have developed radical change in their patterns of service through the cooperative experimentation of staff and patients. There is reason to believe that general hospitals will in the near future evolve equally striking changes that will prove their worth through greater continuity of service, a more rapid rehabilitation of the sick, and in a higher rate of patient-worker satisfaction.

The emphasis in nursing service research is shifting from quantitative to qualitative studies. There is a demand for criteria by which to evaluate service. Many persons believe that these criteria are most likely to be sound if arrived at through the combined efforts of the persons who give and those who receive the service.[48–61]

Research on Nursing Care

In the index developed for the Yale survey, studies under this heading have been subdivided into five types: (1) those in a particular clinical field as, for example, child care, geriatrics, or surgery; (2) studies focused on a condition the nurse might encounter in any field as, for example, the person under stress, the unconscious, or the dying; (3) special aspects of nursing care applicable to most patients, such as teaching and rehabilitation, or nutrition; (4) studies of a specific technique such as an ear irrigation, an intramuscular injection, or a surgical dressing; and (5) evaluation of nursing care. Under the general heading of clinical research might also be catalogued such investigations as nurses have made on the reaction of patients to identifiable variables related to illness, and studies of nurse-patient relationships. Miss Roberts in *American Nursing* comments on the difficulty of getting nurses to write for the *Journal* "on the actual practice of nursing." However, she points to a report in 1902 by Jane E. Hitchcock on "Five Hundred Cases of Pneumonia" and several other articles of an investigative nature written by nurses who were then on a 72-hour work week.[62]

Nurses have seldom been recognized by physicians as partners in clinical research. Dr. Bayne-Jones, referring to the nurse's contribution to medical research, says that the laboratory technician's part is more likely to be acknowledged by physicians.[63] All too often, it must be admitted, the nurse neither initiates nor designs the study, nor is she prepared to write a report of it for her professional journals. Until such time as nurses can and will "defend" and report clinical findings there will be no way to assess the joint studies in which they participate. It is encouraging, however, to find nurses included among the authors of reports on recent research in cardiac catheterization, treatment of ringworm and syphilis, epidemiological studies of influenza, and alcoholism.[64–69]

Nurses have, however, initiated and reported some independent clinical research. There are interesting studies in certain aspects of maternal and child care; two of these major studies were sponsored by the Children's Bureau and one by the ANA.[70–77]

It is intriguing to find a nurse during the 20's setting up a "therapeutic environment" in a foster home to see whether she could control asthma in children when removed from the stress present in their homes. However, this experiment was never systematically reported, and it was only by chance that we learned of it.[78]

The national nursing organizations, in collaboration with the National Tuberculosis Association, have sponsored some studies in tuberculosis nursing, but the League's consultant service has been largely educational. The National Institutes of Health in the USPHS have reported studies in cancer nursing and in neuropsychiatric nursing research.[79,80,81]

In the Yale survey, more major clinical studies have been found in psychiatric nursing than in any other specialty. Generous grants have been made by the National Institute for Mental Health of the USPHS; other sources of funds are private foundations and the ANA. There is a concerted effort in this country to improve psychiatric care, in which the NLN is deeply involved. The clinical psychologists in hospitals for mental diseases, well trained in research, have provided leadership, and psychiatrists seem to be more inclined than other physicians to treat the nurse as a partner in research.

Psychiatric nursing research is often of the interaction type. Some workers have now reported nurse-patient behavioral activity in detail over a long enough period of time to demonstrate the therapeutic value of the nurse's role—for instance, Gwen E. Tudor, Harriet M. Kandler, June Mellow, Alice M. Robinson, and Francoise Morimoto.[82-86] Florence Burnett, in association with Dr. Maurice Greenhill, has helped through experimentation to develop the mental hygiene approach in general nursing.[87]

Few published studies have been found on conditions that cut across all clinical fields. Examples of such research are two unpublished investigations on the nurse's concept of death (one made by students at Teachers College under a grant from the Kellogg Foundation) and a published study by Catharine T. McClure on measurement of hearing loss.[88,89]

Special aspects of nursing, such as teaching and rehabilitation, are rarely the subject of reported studies. There has been an investigation of body mechanics in nursing and some experimentation with teaching programs for patients.[90,91]

Methods analysis has interested nurses for many years. Isabel M. Stewart in 1919, sensing the significance of the standardization and simplification process in industry, wrote an article for *Modern Hospital* that has furnished the profession with what she called a "yardstick" for evaluating a nursing procedure.[92] Soon afterwards Mary Marvin Wayland and Martha Ruth Smith developed a course at Teachers College that was in effect the application of the scientific process to the study of nursing procedure.[93]

Courses such as the one just mentioned were later started at the Universities of Minnesota, of Washington, and of Pittsburgh, and at many other centers for graduate nurse study. In such university nursing departments are files of studies on nursing techniques. Most of them are too limited to be of much value, but the making of each helped a graduate nurse develop an objective, analytical approach to nursing methods as contrasted with the authoritarianism on which nursing practice was based in the past. These are the baby studies from which has grown the substantial research on disinfection of thermometers, the use of masks, and the preparation of hypodermics. Other techniques on which there are reported studies include care of the body after death, nasal gavage, use of the oxygen tent, and wet packs.[94-100]

Management engineers and bacteriologists are among those who have worked with nurses to improve their methods. A major study of the hospital bed is in progress at the University of Pittsburgh School of Nursing, and a study of records used by nurses is under way at the University of Arkansas. For both, grants have been awarded by the USPHS.[101,102]

Study of nursing methods has been for some time a regular part of the program of the federal nursing services. Full-time nurses have been assigned to methods analysis in the Army Nurse Corps. Before a new item of equipment is adopted, nurse analysts may experiment with such factors as its use, durability, and therapeutic effectiveness.

No question is more persistently raised in the field than "How can nursing care be evaluated?" Educators want to know whether the graduate of one program nurses the patient more or less effectively than another; employers are seeking guides for employment and for staffing schedules; and nurse practitioners want the satisfaction that comes through success that is identifiable by themselves and others.

Occupational competence can best be measured by the quality of the product the worker produces; when the product has not been identified, evaluation is likely to depend solely upon the opinion of the worker's associates.

If the product of nursing is some alteration in patient status or behavior, these alterations have not yet been established on a measurable scale. Possibly this is because in most situations an alteration in a patient's behavior cannot be attributed to any one nurse or type of nurse since so many individuals and so many types serve him, and since the nurse's contribution to patient welfare is still confused with that of the physician and other medical workers.

There is almost a concerted effort in the current nursing studies to solve this problem. Again the sponsorship for most of the investigations comes from the USPHS. A number of studies have been mentioned under evaluation of nursing service. Others are listed in the references to this section.[103-109] Marguerite Kakosh is carrying on a study in the Veterans Administration which is ultimately to focus on evaluation.[110] A member of the staff of the Institute for Research and Service in Nursing Education at Teachers College is preparing a bibliography on evaluation which should prove very valuable when it is made available.

Summarizing the studies on nursing care, the conclusion is inescapable that nurses, by and large, are not yet at home in clinical research. Unlike workers in most occupations, nurses have spent more time studying the worker than the work. Various explanations can be offered. One obvious conclusion is that until society offers the college-prepared nurse adequate inducement to stay in the practice field, she will inevitably be drawn into teaching and administration. And this means that the only nurses prepared to carry on research will become involved in teaching and administrative problems.

An encouraging number of well-prepared psychiatric nurses are staying close to practice and are producing interesting clinical research. Some critics of the scene believe that in all areas there is more emphasis on nursing care studies. Nurses are finally realizing, as they assume other professional obligations, that they are responsible for the methods they use.

Nursing Education

From 1900 to 1930 the major energies of the profession went into organizing, administering, and teaching in the hospital schools. By the second decade professional leadership was well aware of the weaknesses in the hospital school system. Among the writings of Miss Nutting and Miss Goodrich are early reports of fact-finding studies showing how economically and educationally unsound were these so-called schools.[111,112] Their findings agreed with the views of outstanding leaders in the health field such as Dr. William H. Welch, Dr. Richard Olding Beard, Dr. C.-E. A. Winslow, and Dr. Milton J. Rosenau. From such men came support for the movement to put nursing schools into the colleges and universities.

Between the first and second world wars and again in 1950, national studies of nursing education were made.[113,114,115] The conclusions of each have coincided with Dr. Welch's publicly expressed statement in 1903 that nurses could not know too much and that nursing education should have the same public support accorded other professions.[116]

In spite of the encouragement given the collegiate school movement by the Goldmark-Winslow-Rockefeller report and subsequent studies, the majority of nursing schools remain in service agencies and are uniquely outside the regular educational channels. In 1931, Dean Lyon of the University of Minnesota said, "These two facts—that nurses do not control their educational institutions and that hospitals do control them and run them to save money—are the basis of nearly all that is wrong with nursing."[117]

But nurses have had to prove with repeated fact-finding studies what Dean Lyon said so confidently. An administrative cost study was made in 1940 and, more recently, one confined to a few collegiate schools, or order to develop a sound method of cost accounting.[118,119] Nursing education has been so inextricably bound up with service that cost analyses are complex, to say the least.

These major studies, national in scope and dealing with the larger issues, are only one type of educational research. Even while these investigations were going on, most nurses were busy making the best of a very faulty system and trying, very successfully, to upgrade it by studies on policy, administration, recruitment, and qualifications of faculty and students; by studies on curriculum, methods of teaching, and testing; by the accreditation of schools and evaluation of programs; and by studies related to student welfare, health, recreation, counseling, and rates and causes of attrition.[120-137]

Elsewhere mention has been made of the public demand for increasing numbers of trained nursing personnel. To meet this demand and, at the same time, to continue the upgrading of schools for the graduate (or "professional") nurse, educational programs have been multiplied so that candidates for the occupation from grammar school to college graduates could be accommodated.

It is remarkable that the chaos in nursing education is as well organized as it is, to use a phrase overheard in a college cafeteria after an examination. Such order as exists can be attributed largely to the guidance of the NLNE, the NOPHN, the ACSN, and the present NLN.

Individually or collectively, these organizations have assumed responsibility for all types of programs. There is understandably more research on the hospital-diploma schools, but many of the recent studies have been focused on the basic collegiate program, the basic junior college program, the programs for advanced study in universities, the schools for practical nurses, and the training programs for attendants and aides.[138-154]

The foundations have sponsored major investigations or experimentation in all these programs. As in most categories of research, the U.S. Public Health Service has furnished leadership and financial support. While great progress has been made in nursing education, the problems seem to multiply. Differentiation of objectives for the various nursing curricula is most pressing, though a good start has been made in this direction. Demonstrations are badly needed of the relative effectiveness, or social value, of the graduates of the major educational programs.

Medicine turns away from its schools thousands of gifted college graduates every year. The occupation of nursing, in contrast, sets up an ever larger number of training programs, with entrance requirements ranging from a grammar school education to a baccalaureate degree so as to accommodate all who are motivated to nurse.

In 1948 the President's Commission on Higher Education recommended that the professional nursing schools be placed in universities and that vocational (or practical) nursing schools be within the junior college system. Under such circumstances the conferred degrees would signify in nursing, as they do in other occupations, the thoroughness of the holder's preparation for his work. At present this is a distant goal.

When standards of nursing education really parallel those of other medical groups it may be possible for the leaders to plan, and get public support for, programs that will accommodate within the health occupations all of the most highly qualified candidates so that elimination may come at the lower rather than at the upper end of the scale of potential competence.

The complete change from apprenticeship program to real schools can only come through an evolutionary process, but evolution can be speeded or retarded. Research, with effective publicizing of the findings, can act as a powerful catalyst.

Summary

An overview of nursing research during the first century of what was called "trained" and is now called "professional" nursing shows that relatively few studies were made before 1930. Beginning with Miss Nightingale, who was skilled in certain kinds of research, the top-ranking nurses have been aware of its value; but only within the last decade has the rank and file been made aware of a profession's responsibility for basing practice on the results of scientific analysis.

The weakness in the training programs and yet the growing demands for their products have made nurse leaders acutely aware of educational and occupational problems. Until very recently investigations of such problems have predominated. In the past decade the emphasis has changed. The elaboration of nursing personnel and educational programs into many categories of workers and schools, and the shifting relationships of all workers within the health field have resulted in a confusion of function. Studies designed to clarify function and to provide some guides for the utilization of nursing personnel have occupied the spotlight in the nursing research of the past decade. As a result of the accumulated findings, we know a good deal about the service given in the nursing occupation and about nursing schools.

Now there is an insistence on the evaluation of service. Many studies in progress are attempts to measure the effectiveness of nursing care in terms of the patient's satisfaction, in improvement in his health status, and in terms of nurse-satisfaction to some extent. There is also a demand for the evaluation of educational programs as measured by the relative effectiveness of the graduates in the practice of nursing. But some nurses ask, "Is it not time to place our emphasis in research on investigations of the service itself—on nursing methods?" They ask, "Can we contribute effectively to the present concept of comprehensive care until, as a member of the so-called medical team, we accept a professional responsibility for research in our own specialty? Can we be effective on the team until we can participate as partners in joint clinical research and understand the common goal for the patient through an appreciation of all research in the field of health?"

Acknowledgement

Limitation of time forces us to generalize but it seems ungrateful not to acknowledge specifically the debt we owe in this country to M. Adelaide Nutting, Lavinia L. Dock, and Isabel M. Stewart for the historical research done in their so-called "spare time."[1,2,3] To Mary M. Roberts we are greatly indebted for her interpretive study, *American Nursing*, sponsored by the American Journal of Nursing Company.[4]

References

1. Nutting, M. Adelaide, and Dock, Lavinia L. *A History of Nursing*. New York, G. P. Putnam's Sons, 1937. 4 vols.

2. Dock, Lavinia L., and Stewart, Isabel M. *A Short History of Nursing*. 4th ed. New York, G. P. Putnam's Sons, 1939.

3. Seymer, Lucy R. *A General History of Nursing*. 2d ed. New York, Macmillan Co., 1949.

4. Roberts, Mary M. *American Nursing*. New York, Macmillan Co., 1954.

5. Florence Nightingale bibliography. *Nursing Research,* 5:87, Oct. 1956.

6. American Nurses' Association. *Nurses Invest in Patient Care.* New York, The Association, 1956.

7. Sellew, Gladys. *A Deviant Social Situation—a Court*, (Ph.D. Dissertation, Catholic University of America, School of Social Services, Washington, D.C., 1938)

8. American Nurses' Association. *Facts About Nursing.* New York, The Association. (annual)

9. U.S. Public Health Service, Division of Nursing Resources. *A Design for Statewide Nursing Surveys, a Basis for Action.* Washington, D.C., U.S. Government Printing Office, 1956.

10. Deutscher, Irwin. The identification of the complement of graduate nurses in the metropolitan area. *Nursing Research* 5:65, Oct. 1956.

11. American Nurses' Association. *Nurses Invest . . . Op. cit.*

12. Taves, Marvin J. *The Influence of Role Conception on Vocational Choice and on Satisfaction and Success in Nursing.* Minneapolis, Minn., University of Minnesota Department of Sociology and School of Nursing, 1957.

13. Bolton, Frances P. Survey of health care situation in America. In *Proceeding of the 83rd Congress of the United States*, Washington, D.C., 1955.

14. Burgess, Mary Ayres, *Nurses, Patients, and Pocketbooks, Report of a Study of the Economics of Nursing.* New York, Committee on the Grading of Schools of Nursing, 1928.

15. Bernays, Edward L. America looks at nursing. *Am. J. Nursing 48*:45, Jan. 1948.

16. U.S. Bureau of Labor Statistics. *The Economic Status of Registered Professional Nurses, 1946–1947. (Bulletin No. 931).* Washington, D.C., Government Printing Office, 1948.

17. American Nurses' Association. *Annual Salaries and Salary Increases and Allowances Paid to General Staff Nurses.* New York, The Association, 1943.

18. National League for Nursing, Department of Public Health Nursing. *Salaries of Public Health Nurses.* New York, The League, 1953.

19. U.S. Office of Education. *Economic Status of College Alumni*, by W. J. Greenleaf. Washington, D.C., Government Printing Office, 1937.

20. U.S. Women's Bureau. *Employment After College; Reports on Women*

Graduates, Class 1955. Washington, D.C., Government Printing Office, 1956.

21. Suchman, Edward A. *Why is Nursing Selected or Rejected as a Career or Omitted Completely from Consideration by Those Eligible for Enrollment?* Ithaca, N.Y., Cornell University Department of Sociology and Anthropology, 1956. (In preparation)

22. Waters, Isabella M. *Visiting Nursing in the United States.* New York, Charities Publications Committee, 1909.

23. Geister, Janet M. Hearsay and facts in private duty. In *Proceedings of the American Nurses' Association, 24th Annual Convention*, 1924, p. 35–37.

24. National League of Nursing Education. *A Study of the Use of the Graduate Nurse for Bedside Nursing in the Hospital.* New York, The League, 1933.

25. Nelson, Josephine, ed. *New Horizons.* New York, Macmillan Co., 1950.

26. Hamley, R. H., and Uprichard, Muriel. *A Study of the Florence Nightingale International Foundation.* London, Welbeeson Press, Ltd., 1948.

27. Scott, Alma H., Chairman, *The Structure, Function, and Relationships of the International Council of Nurses.* A report of a Special Committee to the Board of Directors and Grand Council of the I.C.N., 1947.

28. (The Utica Study, *Memo to Member Agencies.* National League for Nursing, Department of Public Health Nursing), September 25, 1956.

29. National Committee for the Improvement of Nursing Services. *Final Report.* December 1953.

30. Eighteen states have joint commissions. *Am. J. Nursing* 55:89, Jan. 1955.

31. Rusby, Dorothy. *Study of Combination Services in Public Health Nursing Agencies.* New York, National Organization for Public Health Nursing, 1951.

32. National League for Nursing, Department of Public Health Nursing. *Nursing Activities of Public Health Nurses, a Statistical Analysis of the Activities of 513 Public Health Nursing Agencies.* New York, The League, 1955.

33. _____. *Cost Analysis for Public Health Nursing Services.* New York, The League, 1952.

34. Joint Committee of the ANA and NOPHN on Nursing in Prepayment Health Plans. Report in *Proceedings of the American Nurses' Association, 35th Biennial Convention*, 1946, vol. 1, p. 112.

35. National Organization for Public Health Nurses and American Nurses' Association. Committee on Nursing and Medical Care Plans. *Guide for the Inclusion of Nursing Service in Medical Care Plans.* New York, 1950.

36. Haupt, Alma C., and Conners, Helen. Nursing in Medical care plans. *Am. J. Nursing 51*:357, June 1951.

37. Associated Hospital Service of New York. *Blue Cross Pilot Study of Home Nursing Benefits.* Prepared in collaboration with the Visiting Nurse Services of New York, Brooklyn, and New Rochelle. New York, 1956.

38. Freeman, Ruth B. *How to Match Public Health Nursing Service to Community Needs, the Development of a Method.* Baltimore, Johns Hopkins University, 1957.

39. Ferguson, Marion, and others. What does the consumer want? *Nursing Outlook 2*:257, Nov. 1954.

40. Public health nursing study entering second phase. *PHNS Newsletter.* (American Nurses' Association, Public Health Nurses Section.) November 1956, p. 1.

41. University Hospitals of Cleveland Nursing Staff. *Changes in Nursing from 1930 to 1953.* (Unpublished report)

42. National League of Nursing Education. *Nursing Service in Fifty Selected Hospitals.* New York, The League, 1937.

43. _____. *Study of Nursing Service in One Children's and 21 General Hospitals.* New York, The League, 1948.

44. Abdellah, Faye G., and Levine, Eugene. Developing a measure of patient and personnel satisfaction with nursing care. *Nursing Res. 5*:100, Feb. 1957.

45. Kitchell, Myrtle E., and Tener, Marie. *Ways in Which Various Amounts and Kind of Nursing Services Affect the Speed With Which Patients Recover.* Iowa City, State University of Iowa, 1957.

46. Bryant, W. D. *Nursing Resources on the Ward and Nurse–Patient Relationships.* Kansas City, Mo., Community Studies Inc., 1957.

47. Howland, Daniel. *Development of a Methodology for the Evaluation of Patient Care Within a Hospital in Terms of the Restrictions Imposed on the Hospital Operation by the Limitations and Financial Reasons*, Plan, Equipment and Manpower Utilization. Columbus, Ohio State University, 1957.

48. American Nurses' Association. *Patients Invest in Nursing Care.* New York, The Association, 1956.

49. Barnowe, T. J., and others. *A Study of Human Relations Involved in*

Administering Nursing Service in a Modern Hospital. Seattle, University of Washington, 1956.

50. Bordue, Ruth, and others. *Analysis of the Provision for Continuity of Medical Care from the Records of a Public Health Service.* Syracuse, N.Y., Council of Social Agencies, 1952.

51. Burling, Temple, and others. *The Give and Take in Hospitals; a Study of Human Organization,* New York, G. P. Putnam's Sons, 1956.

52. George, Frances L., and Kuehn, Ruth P. *Patterns of Patient Care.* New York, Macmillan Co., 1955.

53. U.S. Public Health Service, Division of Nursing Resources. *The Head Nurse Looks at Her Job,* by Ruth Gillan, and others. Washington, D.C., Government Printing Office, 1952.

54. Hagen, Elizabeth. *Development or Selection of Instruments Designed to Identify or Select Persons for Leadership Positions in Nursing.* New York, Institute of Research and Service in Nursing Education, Teachers College, Columbia University, 1957.

55. LeMat, Aline, and others. *Evaluation of Service to 658 Families.* New York, Community Nursing Service Society, 1951.

56. Reisman, Leonard, and Rohrer, John H., eds. *Change and Dilemma in the Nursing Profession; Studies of Nursing Services in a Large Urban Hospital.* New York, G. P. Putnam's, 1957.

57. Simmons, L. W., and Wolff, H. G. *Social Science in Medicine.* New York, Russell Sage Foundation, 1954.

58. Tannenbaum, Robert. *Interpersonal Influences and the Nursing Function.* Los Angeles, School of Nursing, University of California, 1956. (In preparation)

59. Waterhouse, Alice M. and others. *A Study of Selected Home Care Programs.* Washington, D.C., U.S. Public Health Service, 1955.

60. Whiting, Frank, and others. *Study of Nurse-Patient Relationship, Rutland Heights Veterans Administration Hospital, Mass. 1957. (In preparation)*

61. *Wright, Marion, T. Improvement of Patient Care.* New York, G. P. Putnam's Sons, 1954.

62. Hitchcock, Jane E. Five hundred cases of pneumonia. *Am. J. Nursing* 3:169, Mar. 1902.

63. Bayne-Jones, Stanhope. The role of the nurse in medical progress. *Am. J. Nursing 50:*601, Oct. 1950.

64. Gray, Florence I. The nurse participates in cardiac catheterization research. *Am. J. Nursing 50:*771, Dec. 1950.

65. Barnett, I. P., and Shannon, Emma G. Tinea capitus and its management. *Pub. Health Nursing 44*:187, April 1952.

66. Rivers, Eunice, and others. Twenty years of follow-up experience in a long range medical study. *Pub. Health Rep. 68*:391, Apr. 1953.

67. Wright, John J. Obstacles to eradicating congenital syphilis. *Pub. Health Rep. 67*:1179, Dec. 1952.

68. Philip, R. N., and others. Epidemiological studies on influenza in familial and general population groups. 1. Preliminary report on studies with adjuvant vaccines. *Am. J. Pub. Health 44*:34, Jan. 1954.

69. Lisansky, Edith S., and others. Relationship of personality adjustment to eating and drinking patterns in a group of Italian-Americans. *Quart. J. Stud. Alcohol 15*:545, Dec. 1954.

70. Blackburn, Laura. To bathe or not to bathe the baby. *Am. J. Nursing 40*:767, Sept. 1940.

71. Etherington, Judy. Old wives on new lives, a study of pre-natal superstitions. *Pub. Health Nursing 44*:557, Oct. 1952.

72. Godfrey, Anne Elizabeth. A study of nursing care designed to assist hospitalized children and their parents in the separation. *Nursing Res. 4*:52, Oct. 1955.

73. Hyder, Kate. *Experimentation with Nurse Midwives as Clinical Nursing Specialists in a Teaching Hospital—Johns Hopkins and Teachers' College, Columbia University.* 1955. (Unpublished report)

74. Iffrig, Sister Mary Charitas. Nursing observations of one hundred premature infants and their feeding problems. *Nursing Res. 5*:71, Oct. 1956.

75. Lesser, Marion S., and Keane, Vera R. *Nurse-Patient Relationships in a Hospital Maternity Service.* St. Louis, C. V. Mosby Co., 1956.

76. Pfefferkorn, Blanche. *A study of Pediatric Nursing,* prepared for The National League of Nursing Educators and U.S. Children's Bureau. New York, The League, 1947.

77. Rohrer, John, and Walker, Virginia. *Studies in the Premature Nursery at Charity Hospital, New Orleans.* New Orleans, Urban Research Institute, Tulane University, 1954.

78. Reiley, Margaret. (Personal communication)

79. A study of the nursing care of tuberculosis patients. *Am. J. Nursing 38*:1021, Sept. 1938.

80. Peterson, Rosalie I. Study of a cancer caseload; an analysis of the 1948 cancer caseload in the Visiting Nurse Society of Philadelphia. *Pub. Health Nursing, 45*:566, Oct. 1951.

81. Nursing care in epilepsy. *Nursing Res. 4*:134, Feb. 1956.

82. Tudor, Gwen E. A socio-psychiatric nursing approach to interaction in a problem of mutual withdrawal on a mental hospital ward. *Psychiatry 15*:193, May 1952.

83. Kandler, Harriet M. *Psychiatric Nursing Studies*. (In preparation).

84. Mellow, June. Research in psychiatric nursing: Part 2. Nursing therapy with individual patients. *Am. J. Nursing 55*:572, May 1955.

85. Robinson, Alice M. A study of twelve negative elements common to patients and non-patient groups. *Nursing Res. 2*:141, Feb. 1954.

86. Morimoto, Francoise R. Favoritism in personnel-patient interaction. *Nursing Res. 3*:109, Feb. 1955.

87. Burnett, Florence, and others. Learning the mental health approach through the chronic medical patient. *Pub. Health Nursing 43*:319, June 1951.

88. Bregg, Elizabeth A., and others. *A Study of the Nurse's Concept of Death*. New York, Columbia University, Teachers' College, Nursing Education Division, 1953.

89. Doefleur, Leo G., and McClure, Catherine T. The measurement of hearing loss in adults by galvanic skin response. *J. Speech and Hearing Disorders 2*:184, June 1954.

90. Winters, Margaret C. *Protective Body Mechanics in Daily Life and in Nursing: a Manual for Nurses and their Co-workers*. Philadelphia, W. B. Saunders Co., 1952.

91. Wandelt, Mabel A. Planned versus incidental instruction for patients in tuberculosis therapy. *Nursing Res. 2*:52, Oct. 1954.

92. Stewart, Isabel M. Possibilities of standardization in nursing techniques. *Mod. Hosp. 44*:46, Oct. 1946.

93. Marvin, Mary M. The place of experimentation and research in improving the nursing care of patients. *Am. J. Nursing 27*:529, May 1927.

94. Welsh, Margaret, and Erdman, Martha E. Studies in thermometer technique. In *Nursing Education Bulletin*, Bureau of Publications, Teachers' College, Columbia University, New York, 1929, No. 11.

95. Ryan, Elizabeth, and Miller, Virginia B. Disinfection of clinical thermometers. *Am. J. Nursing 32*:197, Feb. 1932.

96. Notter, Lucille E. Disinfection of clinical thermometers. *Nursing Outlook 1*:569, Oct. 1953.

97. Sommermeyer, Lucille, and Frobisher, Martin J. Laboratory studies on disinfection of oral thermometers. *Nursing Res. 1*:32, Oct. 1952, and Rectal thermometers. *Nursing Res. 2*:85, Oct. 1953.

98. McNett, Esta H. The face mask in tuberculosis. *Am. J. Nursing 49*:32, Jan. 1949.

99. Dodds, Thelma, and others. Simplifying hypodermic injections. *Am. J. Nursing 40*:1345, Dec. 1940.

100. Baer, Marjorie Helfers, and others. Are organisms introduced into vials containing medication when air is injected? *Nursing Res. 2*:23, June 1953.

101. Smalley, Harold, *Study of the Hospital Bed.* Pittsburgh, University of Pittsburgh, School of Nursing, 1957. (In preparation)

102. Stewart, Donald D., and Needham, Christina E. *Study of Records Used by Nurses in Clinical Practice with the Aim of Simplification.* Fayetteville, Ark., University of Arkansas, 1957. (In preparation)

103. Corley, Catharine. Study of the results of public health nursing procedures as judged by infant welfare records. *Nursing Res. 3*:92, Oct. 1954.

104. Forrer, Gordon R., and Hawkins, Christy. *Relationship of Patient Improvement to the Use of Available Psychiatric Nursing Service Time for Direct Patient Care in a Progressive Setting.* Northville, Mich., 1957. (In preparation)

105. Institute for Human Relations. *A Design for the Study of Nursing Care and Patient Welfare*, by M. D. Havron, and Douglas Courtney for the Division of Nursing Resources, U.S. Public Health Service, Washington, D.C., 1951.

106. Kogan, Leonard, and Weber, Beatrice. *A Followup Study of Patients Given Health Examinations in the Department of Educational Nursing.* New York, Community Service Society, 1951.

107. O'Malley, Martha, and Kosock, Carl F. A statistical study of factors influencing the quality of patient care in hospitals. *Am. J. Pub. Health 40*:958, Nov. 1950.

108. Swartz, Doris R. Nursing care can be measured. *Am. J. Nursing 48*:3, Mar. 1948.

109. Yankauer, Alfred, and others. *A Preliminary Evaluation of Group Classes for Expectant Parents in a Suburban Community.* Albany, N.Y., New York State Department of Health, 1953.

110. Kakosh, Marguerite. *A Method for Studying the Utilization of Nursing Personnel in Veterans Administration Hospitals.* (In preparation)

111. Nutting, M. Adelaide. *A Sound Economic Basis for Schools of Nursing.* New York, G. P. Putnam's Sons, 1926.

112. Goodrich, Annie W. *The Ethical Significance of Nursing.* New York, Macmillan Co., 1932.

113. *Nursing and Nursing Education in the United States*. Report of the Committee for the Study of Nursing Education and Report of a Survey by Josephine Goldmark. New York, Macmillan Co., 1923.

114. Committee on the Grading of Nursing Schools. *Nursing Schools Today and Tomorrow*. New York, 1934.

115. West, Margaret, and Hawkins, Christy. *Nursing Schools at the Midcentury*. New York, National Committee for the Improvement of Nursing Services, 1950.

116. Welch, William H. Address to the graduating class of the School of Nursing, Johns Hopkins Hospital, 1903.

117. Lyon, E. P. Taking the profit out of nursing education. *Modern Hosp.* *37*:122, Nov. 1931.

118. *Administrative Cost Analysis for Nursing Service and Nursing Education*, sponsored by American Hospital Association, National League of Nursing Education, and the American Nurses' Association under the direction of Blanche Pfefferkorn and Charles Rovetta. New York, National League of Nursing Education, 1940.

119. *Cost Analysis for Collegiate Programs in Nursing. Part I, Analysis of Expenditures*, prepared under the joint direction of the National League for Nursing and the U.S. Public Health Service. New York, National League for Nursing, Division of Nursing Education, 1956.

120. U.S. Public Health Service, Division of Nursing Resources. *Appraising the Clinical Resources in Small Hospitals*, by Faye G. Abdellah and Eugene Levine, Washington, D.C., Government Printing Office, 1954.

121. American Nurses' Association, Special Committee of State Boards of Nursing. Studying state board test scores. *Am. J. Nursing 55*:1093, Sept. 1955.

122. Couey, Fred. *Curriculum Study of the Hospital School of Nursing*. Montgomery, Ala. 1957. (In preparation)

123. Dunn, M. J. Public health nursing curriculum study. *Pub. Health Nursing 33*:13, Jan. 1941.

124. Fox, David J. *Stress Patterns as Related to Selected Socio-psychological Factors in Basic Students and Faculty and Graduate Registered Nurses on General Hospital Duty*. New York, Teachers' College, Columbia University, 1957. (In preparation)

125. National League for Nursing, Division of Nursing Education. *Toward Better Nursing Care of Patients with Long-Term Illness*. A project developed by the Cornell University-New York Hospital School of Nursing in co-

operation with the National League for Nursing, under the direction of Edna L. Fritz. New York, The League, 1956.

126. Jones, Walter B., and Iffert, R. E. *Fitness for Nursing—a Study of Student Selection in Schools of Nursing*. Pittsburgh, Pa., Bureau of Educational Records and Research, 1953.

127. National League of Nursing Education. *Standard Curriculum for Schools of Nursing*, 1917, and *Curriculum Guide for Schools of Nursing*, 1937.

128. National League for Nursing, Division of Nursing Education. *Objectives of Educational Programs in Nursing*. New York, The League, 1955.

129. National League for Nursing, Department of Public Health Nursing. Field instruction for students in 200 health nursing agencies. *Nursing Outlook 3*:90, Feb. 1955.

130. National League for Nursing, Division of Nursing Education. *Study of Basic Professional Education in Psychiatric Nursing*. New York, The League, 1954.

131. *Public Health Nursing Curriculum Guide*, prepared by a Joint Committee of the National Organization for Public Health Nursing and the U.S. Public Service. New York, 1942.

132. The NLN graduate nurse qualifying examination. *Nursing Res. 3*:21, June 1954.

133. Education programs in nursing accredited by the National League for Nursing, 1956. *Nursing Outlook 4*:112, Feb. 1956.

134. Shields, Mary R. A project for curriculum improvement. *Nursing Res. 1*:4, Oct. 1952.

135. Sleeper, Ruth. A study of audio-visual teaching aids. *Nursing Outlook 2*:205, Apr. 1954.

136. Taylor, Ella A. *Withdrawal of Students*. New York, National League of Nursing Education, 1951.

137. Triggs, F. C., and Bigelow, E. B. What student nurses think about counseling. *Am. J. Nursing 43*:669, July 1943.

138. Preliminary report on University Schools of Nursing. *Am. J. Nursing 21*:620, 1921.

139. Boyle, Rena. A study of programs of professional education for teachers of nursing in nineteen selected universities. *Nursing Res. 2*:98, Feb. 1954.

140. Bridgman, Margaret. *Collegiate Education for Nursing*. New York, Russell Sage Foundation, 1953.

141. Florence Nightingale International Foundation. *An International*

List of Advanced Programmes in Nursing Education, 1951–52. (Report I) London, International Council of Nurses, 1954.

142. Hall, Bernard, and others. *Psychiatric Aide Education.* New York, Grune and Stratton, 1952.

143. Hullerman, Hugo V., and Cathcart, Robert H. Junior college pilot study, a hospital school experiment. *Hospitals 30:*28, Mar. 1956.

144. Montag, Mildred L. Experimental programs in nursing. *Am. J. Nursing 55:*45, Jan. 1955.

145. Moore, Louise. *Practical Nurse Training Comes of Age.* Washington, D.C., U.S. Office of Education, 1954.

146. Pros and cons of progression in nursing education. *Nursing Outlook 1:*358, June 1953.

147. Factors in the success of students in schools of practical nursing. *Nursing Outlook 2:*423, Aug. 1954.

148. Practical nurse education. *Nursing Outlook 3:*366, July 1955.

149. National League for Nursing, Department of Hospital Nursing, American Hospital Association and U.S. Public Health Service. *The Nursing Aide In-Service Project, 1954.* (In preparation)

150. National League for Nursing. *Educational Programs for the Preparation of Public Health Nurses for Beginning Public Health Nurse Positions.* New York, The League, 1956.

151. National League of Nursing Education, Department of Studies. Some data from a questionnaire to schools of practical nursing. *Am. J. Nursing 49:*604, Sept. 1949.

152. Sand, Ole. *Curriculum Study in Basic Nursing Education.* New York, G. P. Putnam's Sons, 1955.

153. Sand, Ole, Ed. *Evaluation of Practice Nursing Education Programs* sponsored by the Kellogg Foundation. 1957. (In preparation)

154. Theilbar, Frances C. Administrative organization of collegiate schools of nursing. *Nursing Res. 2:*52, Oct. 1953.

Chapter 16

We've "Come a Long Way," But What of the Direction?

My experience with *Nursing Research* goes back to its first issue—so proudly hailed by its founders 25 years ago; my experience with "nursing research" goes back to the 1920s, when, as a student at Teachers college, I was exposed to the questioning spirits of Jean Broadhurst, a bacteriologist, Caroline Stackpole, a physiologist, and Isabel M. Stewart, the head of the Nursing Department. They taught us (the students) to answer our own questions by searching for reliable evidence, by conducting experiments, or by studying the findings of other experimenters. A modest investigation of medical and surgical asepsis conducted during a master's program involved me in daily care of laboratory animals and the tedium of examining mountains of Petri dishes. Both made me respect scientists who spend uncomplaining years in monotonous tasks punctuated only rarely by the thrill of discovery. The difficulty I had in growing spores under laboratory conditions has, ever since, made me skeptical of all amateurish studies of asepsis—and all studies that claim too much.[1]

In the 1920s I learned that Miss Stewart was trying to establish an institute of nursing research in the Department of Nursing Education at Teachers College and I was impressed. I also saw her support a course taught by Martha Ruth Smith in which students were introduced to the scientific method of investigation and encouraged to question all aspects of nursing practice. Later I was delighted to be asked to help Miss Smith teach this course.

When Miss Smith went to Boston University (where she continued to promote the investigation of nursing practice), I fell heir to the courses she taught. The particular course that introduced students to what might be called nursing research (if it didn't sound too pretentious) was eventually called "Comparative Nursing Practice." All graduate nurse students who were planning to be teachers or supervisors were required to take this course. Between 1932 and 1947 I worked with hundreds of them from this country and abroad.

This association with graduate nurse students at Teachers College left me amazed at the fierce and unquestioning loyalty they showed for methods, they had been taught in their initial programs—methods for making beds, bathing patients, irrigating body cavities, giving parenteral injections, helping patients in body casts to manage their daily activities, or any other aspect of what was then considered nursing. Demonstrations of procedures led to class discussions where there was far more heat than light. As a structure for these discussions, students learned to use the criteria first enunciated by Miss Stewart in 1919.[2] She said that nurses should have a "yard stick"—that nursing methods should be therapeutically effective, safe, as comfortable and as aesthetic as possible, and economical of time, effort, and materials. The two methods demonstrated by small groups in the course, "Comparative Nursing Practice," were actually scored on these points. Demonstrators and viewers alike came to recognize the shaky ground on which the scores were based so the discussions gave rise to lists of unanswered, or inadequately answered, questions, The remainder of the course was devoted to individual or small-group investigations of these questions, or problems. The investigations often took the form of laboratory experiments, as, for example, measuring the oxygen content of the air in an oxygen tent during a bed bath to see whether it dropped below a therapeutic level; or determining a person's subjective and objective responses to body "packs" or to eye irrigations at currently prescribed temperatures. Investigations also included questionnaire studies in which patients were respondents. They might, for example, be asked to describe the discomforts of a body cast. Other studies might take the form of cost analyses or library investigations of pertinent research.

Students submitted oral and written reports of their investigations and, by the end of the course, they had a critical, questioning audience. All the reports were filed and the students in the course had access to this file; occasionally one was published in the *American Journal of Nursing*.[3]

Enthusiasm over "the scientific method of investigation" ran high among the students with whom I worked, and many of them left Teachers College with a declared determination to continue the improvement or validation of nursing practice through research. Remembering those ardent young researchers who looked forward so zealously to improving nursing practice has, ever since, left me wondering why so few persisted in this intent. Many of them later earned advanced degrees, but any research conducted as part of their programs was more likely to focus on the function of teaching or management than the practice of nursing.

I am aware that surveys of doctoral dissertations written by nurses during this century show that they increasingly focus on nursing practice. I am also aware that certain service agencies, notably Veterans' Administration hospitals, employ nurses who devote full time to research and that in recent years it has been easier to get funds for the investigation of problems related to practice than to problems of education or management. And analysis of the content of *Nursing Research* shows an increasing number of clinical investigations. So, the emphasis *is* changing, but it does seem to me that nurses are still loathe to take responsibility for designing the methods they use; for undertaking studies that, if the findings were applied, might revolutionize practice. They are, perhaps, less comfortable in collaborating with physiologists and physicians than with social scientists, less likely to expect or ask for a colleague relationship if they work with physicians on questions of health care. In my judgment, nurses have scarcely begun to appreciate what Annie W. Goodrich[4] called the "Social and Ethical Significance of Nursing"—the extent to which they might better the lot of mankind; the extent to which they might change health care in this, or any other, country.

The great clinician, George D. Deaver, working with Mary E. Brown[5] and other physical and occupational therapists, introduced a systematic approach to rehabilitation after World War II that has affected rehabilitation worldwide. The process of reducing to a minimum the help a person needs with the activities of daily living has been universally adopted in rehabilitation units. This system *might* have been developed by a nurse, Sister Kenny,[6] who did modify the care of polio victims, demonstrated that a nurse could get a hearing worldwide. "Dr. Bill,"[7] the founder of Alcoholics Anonymous, whose particular form of group therapy is conceded to be the single most effective approach to the arrest of alcoholism and a prototype for all self-help, *might* have been "Nurse Bill" (or "Nurse Bell"). Frederick Leboyer,[8,9] a French obstetrician, is now revolutionizing the management of deliveries to reduce the trauma of birth; nurse-midwives *might* have introduced his methods. The qualities all these clinicians have in common are sensitivity to human suffering, the courage of their convictions—a determination to give the kind of help they believe is needed, and ability to describe their methods simply and clearly.

It is often said that nurses are handicapped by the superficiality of their scientific training, but many nurses now have as thorough a preparation in the sciences as these physicians had or have. When I asked Dr. Leboyer for a bibliography of his scientific publications, he said he had not published in scientific journals, "I am a poet, not a scientist." Most nurses of today have a broader knowledge of the health sciences than Nightingale demonstrated, but she, as much as anyone, affected worldwide changes in health care.

I am sure that colleagues everywhere rejoice in the research competence demonstrated by so many nurses in the United States; they rejoice in the quality of this journal and the progress in nursing research outlined by Susan R. Gortner and Helen Nahm.[10] Few nurses of today, who never experienced its lack, can appreciate what it means to have a journal committed to the publication of nursing research. Before the establishment of *Nursing Research* it was hard to find a publisher for reports of studies on nursing and nurses. It was assumed that few readers of nursing journals would find them interesting. During its short life *Nursing Research* has demonstrated that there are nurses throughout the world who read, value, and use reports of research. In my opinion this publication has not only filled the need for periodic publication of research, but it has raised the standards of writing for all nursing journals.

While I too rejoice and too applaud our progress and our present emphasis on "sound research," on studies that can compete for a part of the $2,910 million budget of the Department of Health, Education, and Welfare (1977 estimate)[11] for development and research, I also hope that future health-related research has humane goals. I hope that the hypotheses it tests are worth testing, that nurse researchers are more interested in improving practice than in academic respectability. I hope they are more interested in writing understandable reports than in using the latest jargon of the social or medical scientists. While it may be tiresome to hark back to Nightingale's work, one reason she was so effective was the clarity of her writing, the universality of its appeal.

I hope most ardently that in nursing we cherish the "poets" among us—the visionaries—those sensitive to universal needs as well as those who are the technically proficient—and I hope that we encourage the research that is most likely, if applied, to result in the greatest good for the greatest number. In saying this I do not mean to denigrate technical competence (or to suggest that the visionary may not also be a great technician). Whenever Dr. Edmund Pellegrino[12] discusses the humane practice of medicine, he stresses the inhumanity of technically incompetent practice. By the same token, I would stress the immorality of incompetent, misleading, and wasteful research.

Notes

---

[1]I could not claim that a method destroyed spores unless I could demonstrate their presence in the contaminants I used on the materials "sterilized."

[2]Stewart, I. M. Possibilities of standardization in nursing technique. *Mod. Hosp., 12*:451, June 1919.

[3]It was not easy in the 1930s to find a publisher for reports of studies. Perhaps for this reason Miss Stewart, as its editor, devoted most of the *Bulletin* of the Nursing Education Department to reports of "research" by students and faculty. The publication of this journal was, however, at irregular and infrequent intervals.

[4]Goodrich, A. W. *Social and Ethical Significance of Nursing.* New York, Macmillan Co., 1932.

[5]Brown, M. E. Daily activity inventory and progress record for those with a typical movement. *J. Occup. Ther., 4*:195, Oct.–Nov. 1951 and *5*:23, Jan.–Feb. 1952.

[6]Kenny, Sister Elizabeth. *And They Shall Walk*, written in collaboration with Martha Ostenso. New York, Dodd, Mead and Co., 1943.

[7]Bill, W. *Three Talks to Medical Societies.* New York, Alcoholics Anonymous General Service Congress, 1955.

[8]Leboyer, Frederick. *Birth Without Violence.* New York, Alfred A. Knopf, 1975.

[9]Trotter, R. J. Leboyer's babies. *Sci. News 3*:59, Jan. 22, 1977.

[10]Gortner, S. R., and Nahm, Helen. An overview of nursing research in the United States. *Nurs Res., 26*:10–33, Jan.–Feb. 1977.

[11]Transition budget: Steady growth for R & D. (Science News of the Week) *Sci. News 3*:52, Jan. 22, 1977.

[12]Pellegrino, E. D. Educating the humanist physician. *JAMA 227*:1288–1294, Mar. 18, 1974.

Chapter 17

Basis for the Selection of Method: Research as a Means of Improving Nursing Practice

T his chapter is devoted to therapeutic measures, procedures, or techniques. Every profession embodies method as well as theory, and the competence of its practitioners can be measured by their mastery of method as well as their knowledge of underlying principles. Creativity, a quality characteristic of those who practice, not only competently but imaginatively, is hard to measure but is perhaps the most important quality in a rapidly changing environment.[a]

Nursing is both a science and an art. Those who practice it are urged to be scientists, which means a lifetime of study, for without it they may be implementing discredited data[b]; but they are also urged to be creative in their practice. Painters respond to an inner prompting that says this is "true" or "beautiful," but without a knowledge of technique they cannot make their inner vision a reality or paint a picture whose colors remain unchanged; architects may design a beautiful house, but if it is to withstand the elements they must know the science of building.

The science of nursing is ultimately as useful as it is effective in helping people achieve a higher standard of health. Since each person is unique, his or her plan of care and the way it is implemented must be unique to some extent; therefore, the methods in this chapter are "suggested procedures," modifiable as the situation demands.

The suggested procedures are based on all that the writers have learned. People learn in various ways and base their conclusions, or judgments, on intuition, authority, tradition, inductive and deductive reasoning, random and planned experience, and on scientific investigation, or research. These processes range from the most inborn, or universal, to the most learned, selective, or sophisticated. They include the chief bases for action among primitive peoples, the Socratic method of reasoning—which put the classical Greek intellectually ahead of his contemporaries—and the process of research, which is modern man's approach to solving problems of education, industry, government, and all professional practice, including that in the field of health.

Before presenting a suggested procedure, pertinent research or the conflicting views of experts in the field found in the literature are cited. Basic nursing curricula in the universities of the United States included the widest range of physical, biologic, and social sciences. The position was taken that all health workers are dependent on the knowledge developed in these fields and that "medical science" and "nursing science" are questionable entities since the boundaries between them and between each with other sciences are constantly shifting. So it will not surprise readers to find that the research cited is drawn from many fields; it may or may not surprise them to see that a small proportion of the investigations cited were conducted by nurses. The fact that there is comparatively little research on nursing practice is explained in the following pages.

The Development of Nursing Research

Nursing, which as someone has said, was born in the church and bred in the military, has relied heavily on authority and tradition, not to mention intuition. There is evidence, however, that some "professional" nurses in every decade since 1860 have used the approach of a researcher in seeking solutions to problems. Florence Nightingale spent many more years in research on health problems than in administering nursing services—the work for which she is famous. She was an expert statistician who persuaded the British Government to make changes in the military and colonial health services because she collected, reported, and interpreted the facts about current practices so thoroughly and effectively that she could show the advantage of change over the status quo.[1]

The system of nursing in our Western culture derives from the practices Florence Nightingale advocated in *Notes on Nursing* and other publications on nursing education written before 1900. These works and the Nightingale pattern of nursing have been widely acclaimed; few people seem to have recognized and emulated Miss Nightingale's ability to conduct investigations and use the findings as leverage for social action or as a basis for nursing practice. While certain British nurses, such as Ethel Gordon Fenwick, may have appreciated the full range of Florence Nightingale's accomplishments, M. Adelaide Nutting and Isabel M. Stewart in the United States were certainly aware of the importance of her research as well as her revolutionary concepts about health promotion and the care of the sick. They showed this awareness in their writings and they followed her example to some extent.

In 1907, Nutting[2] conducted a survey of nursing schools addressed to the U.S. Office of Education. It is often referred to as the first full-scale investigation in nursing. Stewart and other outstanding nurses of that period, as, for example, Annie W. Goodrich, continued to use surveys and statistical reports to demonstrate the need for change in nursing education and administration. In 1909 a national survey of public health nursing showed the wide variety of practice and administrative policy.[3] It introduced a new era in this type of nursing which soon attracted independent and well-prepared nurses who continued to rely on surveys of practice.

During the twenties and thirties there was a movement toward standardization in industry, education, and health agencies.[c] Frank Taylor and Frank Galbraith conducted many highly publicized industrial studies and Lillian M. Galbraith (wife of Frank) continued this work after his death up until recent times.[4]

The American Hospital Association, seeing in the operation of hospitals many parallels with industry and education, set up a Simplification and Standardization Committee whose recommendations soon influenced working conditions, hospital structure, furnishings and supplies.[5] The committee worked closely with the U.S. Bureau of Standards and non-governmental agencies set up to protect and inform consumers. In this era, industries created research units that resulted in standardized products and processes. Labor shortage in World War I (and later in World War II) intensified the search for uniform and reliable machine-made products. Supplies that were once made by nurses, as, for example, dressings and solutions, were replaced by commercially prepared supplies. Time, motion, and cost studies were instituted in this period. Ralph M. Barnes[6] gives the history of these processes and the related aspects of industrial management. Blanche Pfefferkorn and Marion Rottman's *Clinical Education in Nursing*[7] was actually an activity analysis and time study.

But even earlier, Stewart realized the applicability of time, motion, and cost studies to nursing. She also sensed the limitation and possible danger of the standardization movement. She pointed out the difference between industry, where the goal is a uniform product, and a health service, where the product must not be standardized because the needs of each person served are unique. In an article titled "Possibilities of Standardization in Nursing Technique,"[8] she emphasized the importance of using what she believed were "flexible" standards. She said, in effect, that the reliability of each procedure should be judged on the following basis.

1. Does it provide maximal *safety* for the patient, the nurse and other persons involved?
2. Is it *therapeutically effective*?
3. Does it provide the greatest degree of *comfort and happiness (or least amount of pain) for the patient* that is consistent with accomplishing the therapeutic aim?
4. Is it as *economical* of time, effort, and materials as it can be made without sacrificing the first three factors?
5. Does the equipment present a pleasing appearance and [does] the performance give an impression of finished workmanship?
6. Is the procedure as *simple* as it can be made without destroying its therapeutic effectiveness, safety, and comfort, and is it *adaptable* to hospital and home nursing?

Had she added the questions Does it take into consideration the patient's wishes? and Does it provide for optimum patient independence, participation, and learning? the Stewart criteria would be as acceptable today as they were in 1919. Her article was the cornerstone for a course initiated at Teachers College, Columbia University, about 1930 that was later called "Comparative Nursing Practice." It introduced students to the research process. Nursing procedures or techniques were evaluated for their safety, therapeutic effectiveness, comfort, economy, and aesthetic appeal. Each student, either alone or with others, conducted a library investigation, an interview or questionnaire survey, and a laboratory experiment or some other kind of study.[d]

Stewart and her associates, appreciating the importance of research, proposed in 1930 the establishment of an institute for nursing research within the Department of Nursing Education at Teachers College.[9,10] Jean Broadhurst, a bacteriologist there, strongly supported this position. Her support is evidenced by the number of bacteriologic studies made by graduate nurse students under her direction in the 1920s and 1930s.[e] With Martha Ruth Smith of the Nursing Faculty, Broadhurst edited a text on the principles of nursing care[11] which dealt with the science underlying nursing rather than its techniques. During the publication of the *Nursing Education Bulletin* at Teachers College, it carried very little except the reports of studies by students and faculty. An Institute of Research and Service in Nursing Education was finally established at the college in 1953 (and was the first such institute in a university), but the studies conducted under its sponsorship since have rarely been directly related to nursing practice.[f] In fact, until this decade, nursing research has focused on educational or occupational problems. Leo W. Simmons and Virginia Henderson showed this clearly in their 1964 report, *Nursing Research—A Survey and Assessment.*[12g] Because so many studies were focused on the nurse rather than nursing, the second author, while making this survey, was moved to write an editorial in *Nursing Research*, the journal initiated in 1952, "Research in Nursing—When?"[13]

For the first three or four decades of the twentieth century, studies focused on practice were designed chiefly to make a nursing procedure, or specific activity, more valid; just as most medical research was designed to make a laboratory test more reliable, an operation or a drug safer and more effective. Research in the health field was more likely to be technical rather than philosophic. The virtue of the health system had not come under such a barrage of criticism as it has in this era. It was generally assumed that if the parts of which it was composed were each more reliable, the system as a whole might meet the needs of man. However, some persons in every decade *were* doubtful about the health care system. Some nurses, and others too, questioned the way students were selected for nursing, the way they were prepared, the conditions under which they worked, and in general, the utilization of the services they were prepared to give. In the survey of research reported by Simmons and Henderson in 1964, the most persistent question asked by approximately 500 persons interviewed was, "What is the [proper] function of the nurse?"

In 1950, the American Nurses' Association instituted a 5-year program to study the function of the nurse. By 1957, $400,000 had been spent on 21 separate studies conducted in 17 states and reported in 1958 by Everett C. Hughes et al. in *Twenty Thousand Nurses Tell Their Story*.[14] While this momentous nationwide effort failed, apparently, to give a final and satisfactory answer to the question, "What is the function of the nurse?" it provided an enormous amount of information about nursing. One study, for example, showed the wide range of nursing activities (more than 400) for hospital nurses in one statewide investigation and other studies threw considerable light on the concepts held about nurses and nursing and on many occupational problems.[15] This investigation is one of six or more nationwide studies that, made periodically during the twentieth century, have identified and focus attention on occupational problems. Some of the data collected in such studies is now kept current in the United States by the ANA's annual publication, *Facts About Nursing*.[16] The Canadian Nurses' Association publishes a comparable annual publication titled *Countdown*.[17] National nursing organizations around the world are committed to occupational research but they are also beginning to promote research on nursing practice..

In 1953, the major national nursing organizations in the United States implemented the recommendations of their Structure Study begun in 1948 and research units were created in each.[h] In 1956, the American Nurses' Foundation was established as an independent agency to accept funds, make grants for, and conduct research. It maintains a directory of nurses with earned doctoral degrees.[18] Generally speaking, most graduate programs now offer or require clinically oriented research experience. Educational programs for graduate nurses were first nothing more than post-basic experience in hospitals. However, a midwifery program based at Teachers College was developed during the 1930s, and in the next decade, programs in pediatric, psychiatric, and medical-surgical nursing were developed. Other programs in general public health, school nursing, or industrial nursing at Teachers College offered field experience with emphasis on practice. After World War II the national nursing organizations began to emphasize the importance of post-basic, collegiate study of clinical nursing. Presently, this is the emphasis in most graduate programs rather than the functions of teaching, supervision, and administration. The fact, however, that so many degree-holding nurses were then and still are fully occupied in teaching, supervision, and administration has undoubtedly led graduate students to investigate nonclinical questions. The current preoccupations with recognizing, legalizing, and preparing the nurse for an expanding clinical role, eliminating non-nursing functions, and reducing the administrative super-structure in health service, have created an insistent demand for research centered on nursing practice.

Many of the national nursing investigations, as, for example, that directed by Esther Lucile Brown,[19] reported in 1948 under the title, *Nursing for the Future*, stressed the importance of research. The latest study by the National Commission for the Study of Nursing and Nursing Education, reported as *An Abstract for Action*,[20] gives the most persuasive argument for the research approach in dealing with all aspects of nursing—practice, administration, and education.

Nurses employed in the national, state, provincial, and local governments of many countries, most particularly in the United States, have made signal contributions to the development of nursing research. For example, Marion Ferguson and Pearl McIver of the U.S. Public Health Service began, even before World War II, to foster nursing investigations. During World War II, with the creation of the Cadet Nurse Corps in 1943 and the Division of Nursing of the USPHS in 1949, nursing research was seen as essential to the development of nursing. Faye G. Abdellah, Margaret Arnstein, Ava Dilworth, Lucile Petry Leone, Jessie Scott, and Ellwynne Vreeland are among those who have fully appreciated the importance of research. Studies conducted or sponsored by the Division were, at first, surveys of nursing needs and resources. In 1954, Abdellah reported that since 1947, "thirty-seven states, the District of Columbia, and the Territory of Hawaii have used the nursing survey as a tool for identifying the most important community nursing problems which demand action and about which something can be done."[i] During the last and the current decade the national nursing agencies and health agencies of which nursing is a part in the United States tend to encourage other types of studies and particularly clinical investigations.

Since the creation of the Division of Nursing in the USPHS, grants totaling approximately $39 million (fiscal years 1956–June 1976)[21] have been made for all kinds of nursing studies. Nurses in these agencies have worked with the ANA's Research and Statistics Unit and have played important roles in the creation of the Journal *Nursing Research* and in international, regional, state, and local conferences devoted to discussing and promoting nursing research. The National Center for Health Services Research and Development, established in 1968, and reorganized as the Bureau of Research and Evaluation in 1973, is said by Faye G. Abdellah, the former Deputy Director, to have as one of its primary goals the evaluation of new types of health manpower vital to the improved delivery of health services."[j] Rita K.

Chow, a former member of the Bureau's staff, has reported a method for identifying and categorizing nursing action in the care of patients with cardiac surgery that has general application. Reviewing current proposals for reducing the roadblocks in the delivery of health care, she says, "There is urgent need for increased efforts by all health professionals to analyze and synthesize more efficient modes of organizing and delivering health services research."[k]

While it is not possible to discuss even the high points in the development of nursing research around the world, we might mention that the Canadian Nurses' Association publishes an annual list of nursing studies, *Index of Canadian Nursing Studies*[22]; the Finnish Foundation for Nursing Education's *Yearbook of Nursing* is a collection of study reports[23]; there is an international journal devoted to research, the *International Journal of Nursing Studies*.

Professional nurses have always been involved in the physician's clinical research but they have, for the most part, played a passive and relatively uninformed role. Stanhope Bayne-Jones,[24] a physician writing in 1950, said that the role of a laboratory technician was more likely to be recognized in written reports of research in medical journals than that of the nurse. However, today, interdisciplinary research (but with the nurse as full partner) is more likely, in some quarters, to find a sponsor than research devoted to the concern of one discipline. Research-conscious and often knowledgeable nurses are working closely with physicians, statisticians, physical, biologic, and social scientists in such agencies in the United States as the National Center for Health Services Research and Development, and the National Institutes of Health, as well as in many health organizations and foundations. Nurses in some states have, with physicians, social scientists, and others, designed and carried out interdisciplinary studies under the sponsorship of regional medical programs.

Vernon W. Lippard, in *A Half Century of American Medical Education: 1920–1970* (Josiah Macy, Jr. Foundation, New York, 1974, p. 73), showed the expansion of federal funds for medical research. He noted that 1930 legislation changed the name of the Hygienic Laboratory, established in 1887, to the National Institute of Health. Its appropriation in 1931 was $43,000. The National Cancer Institute was created in 1937. The establishment of the Office of Scientific Research and Development in the 1940s led to large-scale appropriations. The National Science Foundation was established in 1950. The P.H.S. Omnibus Act this same year empowered the Surgeon General to establish separate institutes to support research in neurologic diseases and blindness, arthritis, and metabolic disease, allergy, and infectious diseases. Within 20 years the total dollars for medical research increased 24 times.

While physicians may have been slow to collaborate with nurses as full partners in clinical research, many social scientists seem to have embraced the opportunity. These circumstances and the current and growing emphasis on the psychosocial aspects of health and disease may account for the fact that most of the clinical nursing research lies within this area.

Since 1958, a number of volumes devoted to nursing research have been published. Some are surveys, others are source books, and others are on method; some serve many purposes.[25-31] The authors of these works are nurses and social scientists. A 1970 publication by three sociologists (all of whom are members of the faculties in university schools of nursing) is titled *Behavioral Science, Social Practice, and the Nursing Profession*.[32] The authors accept the position (which they seem to think is held by most nurses) that the physician's goal is cure or "the more or less permanent correction of the patient's diagnosed pathology" and "The goals of nursing treatment [meeting the patient's 'situationally derived needs,' including his response to the biophysical treatment] are usually short-term and palliative rather than curative." The writers say that the boundaries of research in any profession are set by the limits of its responsibility for prescribing action and they suggest that it is only within the realm of social science (or human interaction) that the nurse is free to prescribe. Hence the supposition that finding the rational bases for nursing practice through research is largely a task for nurses in collaboration with social scientists. Robert Leonard, the third author of this monograph, with Florence Wald[33] published an often-cited article "Toward Development of Nursing Practice Theory" in which they follow this same line of reasoning—that nursing contribution is largely one of interaction. The authors suggest that research methods used in the physical and biologic sciences aren't appropriate for the study of nursing practice.

The term "nursing science" is not different from medical, or health, science; nor are these independent or different from the biologic sciences. In other words, a rational practice for any health practitioner depends on research that may take the researcher into the field of the physicist, the chemist, the microbiologist, the physiologist, the psychologist, the anthropologist, the sociologist, the lawyer, or the economist. The nurse is presently, and within the legal meaning of nursing as defined by nurse practice acts (and statements of official nursing organizations), initiating or prescribing treatments or protective measures that relate to all these fields. Nurses, for example, decide how to keep the mouth of an unconscious patient clean, how to prevent pressure sores, or when the comatose are sufficiently recovered to be safely fed by mouth, just as they initiate measures to persuade the mute to talk or the agitated and anxious to express their fears. Even though a treatment, such as an enema, may be prescribed by physicians, nurses select the equipment, often the injected liquid, and they help the patient take the treatment so that the therapeutic purpose is accomplished. While physicians prescribe and sometimes (but not always) start an intravenous feeding or medication, its safe and effective administration is largely dependent on nurses. Some procedures, as for example lumbar punctures, are prescribed and carried out by physicians but nurses work with them in preparing patients, giving the treatment, and giving aftercare. Whether or not nurses play a major or minor role in prescribing, initiating, and carrying out a treatment, they have a professional responsibility for validating, or rationalizing through research, what they do and how they do it.

Tracing the development of nursing research from the time of Florence Nightingale to the present, we find an uneven progression with changing emphases: In the nineteenth century Nightingale's studies using such data as morbidity and mortality statistics to persuade a national government to alter health services; in the first decades and throughout the succeeding decades of the twentieth century, periodic nationwide educational and socioeconomic surveys; in the third and fourth decades, a number of studies designed to make specific procedures more valid, especially as related to medical and surgical asepsis or the control of infection; in the fourth and fifth decades, surveys of nursing needs and resources and studies of the role and function of the nurse; in the sixth and seventh decades, the emphasis on interaction between nurse and patient—or client—and on studies aimed at the validation or improvement of nursing practice. There is at present a high priority on research and especially on evaluation of nursing care, either alone or as an aspect of health service. In some cases the research attempts to relate the value of care to the type of preparation for nursing. Presently, there is considerable preoccupation with the development of nursing theory, with assessing the quality of nursing care, and particularly the care given by nurses with special preparation for assuming more than the usual responsibility for clinical management.

Criteria for Evaluating Method or Assessing the Quality of Care

The difficulty of measuring the effect of nursing as distinct from the effect of care by other health workers, most notably treatment by the physician, is obvious. Louis I. Dublin,[34] in 1932, evaluated frontier nursing and midwifery services to the Kentucky mountains and was able to show that their first 1000 deliveries were almost totally free from morbidity or mortality. This compared most favorably with mortality rates in the United States or any other country. Nurse-midwifery is, however, atypically independent of medicine in its practice.

The survey and assessment of nursing research by Simmons and Henderson[35] attempts to identify types of evaluative studies through 1963, to give outstanding examples, and to list the research methods or techniques used in making judgment about, or measuring, quality.[1]

Quality assessment is believed by many persons to be essential in substantiating the claims of professions (including nursing) that the kind (length, content, and methods) of learning in the educational process affect the kind of care graduates give. While patient opinion polls, such as that by Abdellah and Eugene Levine[36] in 1957, indicate that patients rate the services of better-prepared nursing personnel higher than those of less well-prepared ones, the issue is still alive and the search for criteria in measuring quality goes on.

Since the roles of nurses, physicians, physical therapists, social workers, and others often overlap, and since what each health worker does affects the total outcome of care, evaluation of any system of care is really a joint responsibility. Paul J. Sanazaro and his associates[37] note that all medical and health care professions and the federal government are involved. Professional Standards Review Organizations (PSRO) composed of physicians have been established in many states and in two states (Utah and Hawaii) include nurses. In 1970, legislation was introduced in the U.S. Congress to establish such organizations in each state for the purpose of monitoring all medical services reimbursed under provisions of the Social Security Act (P.L. 92–603).[m]

Effective nursing has always been dependent on the nurse's knowledge of the treatment plan. As nurses assume more responsibility for therapeutic management and as the patient-problem-oriented system of health care spreads, it will be increasingly necessary to make interdisciplinary evaluations.[n]

Avedis Donabedian,[38–41] discussing the evaluation of medical care between 1966 and 1969, distinguished between assessing the process of care, the organizational structure under which it is given, and the outcome. The Donabedian model provides a basis for an assessment of total quality of care.[o]

John W. Williamson[42–43] in 1968 and 1971 discussed priorities and a strategy for relating outcome and process in assessing quality of patient care. This is akin to the Donabedian model.

Another investigator, Beverly C. Payne,[44] developed in 1966 an extensive set of process criteria by which care for in-hospital patients could be assessed.[p] At best, assessment of the quality of care given by physicians is complex; it may be equally so for all health professions.[q]

Measuring the Quality of Nursing

Attempts to answer the question "What is good nursing care?" are as old as professional nursing. The remarkable reduction in the death rate among British soldiers in the Crimean hospitals after the arrival of Florence Nightingale and the nurses associated with her gave some sort of measurement because she described the nursing care given and provided before-and-after statistics.[45] Jane E. Hitchcock's[46] report in 1902 of 500 cases of pneumonia was not so much a report on this disease as a comparison between the effectiveness of nursing care given in hospitals and by Henry Street visiting nurses. Dublin's report on the first 1000 deliveries of the Frontier Nursing Service, mentioned earlier, was a form of measurement. The Stewart "yardstick" was an attempt to provide specific criteria for measuring the reliability of a single activity. In reviewing the literature it is clear that these attempts have steadily increased. In 1950, Frances Reiter and Marguerite E. Kakosh[47] identified the following 12 components of nursing care: control of environment; mental adjustment; condition of skin and mucous membranes; elimination; posture, position, and exercise; rest and sleep; nutrition; observation of signs and symptoms; administration of laboratory tests; administration of medicines; administration of treatments; and teaching health. Each component was defined in operational terms. An observational guide was developed. The six following qualitative categories were defined as criteria that might be quantitatively scaled: *Dangerous*: The patient's health or welfare is endangered by the nursing care he received; *Safe*: No harm comes to the patient for having had nursing care; patient's life and values are protected; *Adequate*: To the extent that it is possible, the patient's standards and customary way of living are kept as normal as possible; that he recovers to the greatest extent his former state of health at his own rate of recovery; *Optimum*: The patient's integrity is respected and he is helped to improve his state of health and is better able to care for himself; *Maximum*: The design of patient care is based on the best known scientific advances to date; *Ideal*: Patient care is examined and evaluated for the purpose of improvement through controlled research in nursing.

Kakosh,[48] in a doctoral dissertation that took the form of a film script, tried to show the "differentiating characteristics of professional nursing care." In 1955, Myrtle Kitchell Aydelotte and her associates[49] initiated a long-range study using skin condition, mental attitude, and mobility of patients as criteria. In 1964, Gladys Nite and Frank Willis[50] reported a 4-year study of hospitalized patients with myocardial infarction, identifying "measuring rods" that could be used in evaluating care given to such patients. They concluded that nursing practice is therapeutic when in each case patients' problems are correctly identified and nursing care is directed toward resolution of these problems (a very close parallel with the Weed approach). Nite and Willis identified specific criteria to measure the progress of cardiac patients. Some examples are the following: patients will gradually show less apprehension toward pain as they gain an understanding of the physiologic process causing pain; patients permit the nurse to perform necessary activities for them; patients will tend to sleep during the day after major activities and during the entire night without medication.

A number of attempts have been made to compare the effect on patients of a traditional (less analytic) type of nursing with a deliberate (more analytic) process as described in Ida Jean Orlando's *The Dynamic Nurse–Patient Relationship*.[51] One such study was conducted by Rhetaugh G. Dumas and Robert C. Leonard,[52] its aim being to observe the effect of an experimental nursing process on the incidence of vomiting during recovery from anesthesia.

A research team at Rush-Presbyterian—St. Luke's Medical Center and the MEDICUS Systems Corporation have developed a methodology for monitoring quality of nursing care. Emphasis is placed upon an outcome assessment, and the researchers suggest that the relationship between process and outcome may be different for different types of patients. Many factors affect nursing quality, one of which is hospital management control. The quality-monitoring methodology has merit for nursing management in controlling nursing performance at the unit level. Nursing management must know and understand both process and outcomes to make decisions regarding quality of nursing care.[53]

A significant breakthrough has been achieved by the American Nurses' Association, as a result of a contract with the Department of Health, Education, and Welfare in the development of model sets for criteria for screening quality, appropriateness, and necessity of nursing care in settings for which Professional Standard Review Organizations (PSROs) have responsibility. The manual *Guidelines for Review of Nursing Care at the Local Level* describes the development and organization of PSROs, a model for quality assurance in nursing, and explains the process for identifying outcome criteria.[54]

Discussing the difficulty of evaluating nursing, Dorothy M. Smith[55] proposes that practice be measured more indirectly than directly. She thinks measurement of the nursing care of a "patient as a whole" may not be possible. She suggests that measurement of quality nursing might be made on the basis of the "scientific rightness" of the assessment of the patient's nursing problems and the nurse's management of them. Smith proposed that "we need a system—an organized framework wherein we can see plainly and definitely what is to be done and what we must do to accomplish it."[r] She proposed that the nursing problems that professional nurses are called upon to assess and manage daily might form the basis for evaluating quality nursing care. Quality nursing might be measured indirectly by examining the system or organization provided for dealing with these nursing problems. For example, the degree to which communications are systematized might be one of the most important criteria that can be used in assessing quality nursing practice.

The identification of criteria of nursing practice poses many problems. Measurement of quality care will have to be both direct and indirect before a complete assessment of the effects of nursing practice upon patient welfare can be made.

Eleanor C. Lambertsen identifies six criteria for evaluating nursing care related to the plan of nursing care. These are as follows: must be coordinated with the over-all plan of medical care, based on scientific principles, is therapeutically effective, ensures minimum physical and emotional safety and security for the patient, reflects immediate and long-range planning for regaining or maintaining maximum degree of health attainable for the patient, meets the psychosocial needs of the patient, and provides for patient-family participation.[s]

Dorothy Harrison, a nurse and anthropologist, is designing a study that will use electronic devices in measuring patient status which will also evaluate the effect of nursing. She says:

Inasmuch as technology today is advancing at an ever more rapid pace, I believe that nursing as a profession should make use of technological tools to meet its particular needs. Nursing is a discipline that demands not only an understanding of internal physiology and disease processes, but understanding of the whole person in an environment—physical and social. Medicine and most other helping and healing disciplines have tended to see and study separate parts and operations. It is especially important in nursing to see and integrate the whole. In the past, nurses have had to put the pieces that go to make the whole together on a more or less intuitive basis. Ability to do this varies with the particular nurse's alertness, power of observation, knowledge, and skill. An objective analysis and evaluation of this process of integration is needed. It is now possible to make this analysis and evaluation electronically, using electromagnetic field theory. All forms of matter, including living systems, possess constantly interacting electromagnetic properties. Electronics today can be called upon to do things that were heretofore undreamed of, to sense and measure minute electrical activity. I shall therefore attempt to use electronic devices to detect, measure, and study integration of the person, including interaction with some major environmental factors, which will provide nursing with the assessment tools it needs.[t]

Standards for Nursing Practice

Standards should derive from, or be consistent with, an accepted definition of nursing. They should also be sufficiently specific to describe effective practice. Standards may be so inclusive that they describe practice in any setting, or separate standards may be set up for nursing practice in hospitals, homes, schools, industry, penal institutions, and so on. Evolution of standards is on-going—never completed. Definitions of nursing and standards based on them are related to assessing the quality of nursing practice. Definitions and standards appropriate for one era may need revision in the next.

Jean K. McFarlane,[56] engaged in 1970 in a 2-year study of nursing care, comments on the difficulty of establishing criteria (standards) of quality nursing care. She comments that health care professions lack precise goals and the goals of one profession may conflict with the goals of another. Standards for motor skills can be spelled out but the skills of observation, judgment, and applying the results to individuals cannot be spelled out, nor can human relation skills be defined. For these latter it is especially hard to establish criteria of performance.

Grace Fivars and Doris Gosnell,[57] also discussing the problems of evaluation, say it is recognized that in any activity where performance must be evaluated acceptable minimum standards are needed. Establishing standards of performance requires a thorough knowledge of what should be done to complete an assignment and the kinds of behavior it requires.

There seems to be a consensus among nurse educators that a program that prepares nurse practitioners is performance-based if:

1. Competencies (knowledge, skills, behaviors) to be demonstrated by graduates are derived from explicit conceptions of roles stated in measurable terms.
2. Criteria (standards) for assessing competencies make explicit expected levels of mastery under specified conditions.
3. Assessment of the nurse practitioner is based on performance, and evidence of knowledge relevant to planning for, analyzing, interpreting, or evaluating situations or behavior.

Determining Standards of Performance

Having agreed upon a definition of nursing and the scope of nursing functions, the next step would be to identify the components of performance that determine the desired level of proficiency. For example, when a patient's blood pressure is taken, the nurse should be able to complete the activity within a specified period of time, get an accurate reading, and handle the equipment with dexterity. So there are minimum requirements for each performance that, when they occur together, represent adequate performance.

David J. Klaus and his associates[58] say that on developing standards of performance for various nursing behaviors, attention is usually given to absolute (criterion referenced) standards rather to normative standards. By *normative* is meant the performance of many individuals with the same training and experience when it is ordered along a continuum and an arbitrary point along this continuum is selected as the standard of acceptable performance. Most standards are stated in terms of measured performance, or the adequacy of performance in a test situation.

The following are some recent efforts to produce "instruments" for measuring nursing performance:

Charles M. Bidwell and Doris J. Froebe[59] have developed an instrument for evaluating hospital nursing performance for "clinical nurse practitioners" in patient care and administrative "tasks," teaching, and formulation of objectives.

Margaret A. Dunn[60] constructed an instrument to measure the performance of professional nurse practitioners and she reports that it was found to be reliable in describing and evaluating clinical performance. The PETO System[61u] indexes nursing care needs and is a useful management tool for measuring nursing workload and resource planning. It is particularly useful when correlated with a nursing audit. The critical criteria, or seven areas in which evaluations are made, are diet, toileting, vital signs and measurements, respiratory aids, suction, cleanliness, and turning and/or assisted activity. These criteria are derived partly from the work of R. White et al.[62] R. Wilda Routhier[63] developed a tool to evaluate patient care. The tool is a 79-item questionnaire that includes direct and indirect elements of patient care and involves auditing the patient's record. The tool builds upon Irene L. Beland's[64] guide for assessing patients' needs.

Joy E. Gelder[65] describes a *Flow Process Chart* as a simple way of looking at a procedure in a systematic way. The procedure to be analyzed is described in detail. Each step is coded as to whether it is an operation, transportation, storage or waiting, and inspection. Specific questions are asked such as: What is its purpose? Why is it necessary? What should be done? Where should it be done and why? When should it be done and why? Who should do it and how is the best way to do it?

Lawrence L. Weed's[66] *Problem-Oriented Record* system of medical care with its revolutionary computerization provides a logical basis for planning, giving, and evaluating and/or auditing care. It allows health workers (physician, nurse, others) to define and follow clinical problems one-by-one and organize them for solution.

Mabel A. Wandelt and Maria C. Phaneuf[67,68,69] have described three instruments for measuring the quality of nursing care: the *Slater Nursing Competences Rating Scale*, the *Quality Patient Care Scale*, and the *Nursing Audit*. The Slater Scale, with 84 items, measures the nurse's competence in giving care in any setting, over a period of 2 weeks to 1 year. The Quality Patient Care Scale, with 68 items, is derived form the Slater Scale but has a slightly different emphasis. The Nursing Audit, developed by Phaneuf, has 50 items and measures the care received by the patient in his or her own home, a nursing home, or a hospital. It provides a basis for written appraisal of nursing care after discharge of the patient through analysis of patient care records.[v] The Nursing Audit is a useful tool in evaluating the quality of the care provided in any program and setting in which a record is an integral part of providing comprehensive and continuing nursing care.

The Nurse's Role in Research Related to Improvement of Care

Nursing is a health science profession to the extent that its practice is based on science and that its research is practice-oriented. Nurses who participate in research can enrich their own practice and validate, rationalize, and improve their methods. Research challenges nurses to find answers to problems or questions. Research should be a part of every nurse's practice. All practitioners should be able to read and apply findings of research reports and take part in research. Speaking to this point, Dorothy Mereness says:

> Research is not a set of skills which can be added to an individual's educational equipment at will. Rather, it is a way of seeking solutions to problems, a way of thinking and working, a way of collecting data and treating it once it has been collected, a way of making use of the results of a study once these results have been identified—in short, it is a way of life.[w]

As the authors have pointed out, the idea that all who practice nursing should be aware of and participate in research is relatively new. Abdellah and Levine[70] emphasize this in their 1965 publication *Better Patient Care Through Nursing Research*. In 1962, the American Nurses' Association Committee on Research and Studies[71] presented what it called a "Blueprint for Research in Nursing." It is a guide in outline form giving areas in which research is needed. Ten years later, Werley,[72] who directed the Center for Health Research, Wayne State University College of Nursing, comments on the paucity of clinical nursing research but also on some encouraging signs, as, for example, the existence, since the 1950s, of a nursing research department in the Walter Reed Army Institute of Research, the support given by the U.S. Department of Health, Education, and Welfare of clinical nursing research, and its support in universities. Werley identifies 18 reasons for the "paucity" of clinical research. They include "not enough clinical researchers, . . . lack of research role models, . . . instruction often not based on research, . . . students do not gain . . . research awareness, . . . textbooks not based on research-documented content," and "In the last analysis, one might wonder if there is not a lack of meaningful commitment to research on the part of both the profession and the many individuals who profess commitment."[x] There is no doubt that nursing has in the past depended on other disciplines rather than developing its own body of scientific knowledge. Leonard, discussing the development of research in the practice-oriented discipline of nursing, observes that "Nurses are pressed to act, act often, and act swiftly. In the face of the urgent and constant demand for nursing services, a body of nursing practice which incorporates many untested assumptions has become imbedded in hospital policies and textbooks for nursing students. Such principles [assumptions] are likely to be rationalizations for existing practices rather than scientifically based propositions that have been rigorously tested by our best research methods."[y]

While nursing research can be defined as "a systematic, detailed attempt to discover or confirm facts that relate to a . . . problem or problems in the field of nursing . . ." the research is referred to as "clinical" when "the ultimate goal is . . . to improve nursing practice."[z]

Extending the Scope of Nursing Practice[73] is one of the publications that has fostered the development of the expanding role of nursing. Clinical research as a basis for determining the value of an extended role for nurses is the subject of many commentaries.[74-76] *Better Patient Care Through Nursing Research* outlines the major steps in the research process: (1) formulate the problem; (2) review the literature; (3) formulate the framework of theory; (4) formulate hypothesis; (5) define the variables; (6) determine how variables will be quantified; (7) determine the research design; (8) delineate the target population; (9) select and develop methods for collecting data; (10) formulate methods of analyzing the data; (11) determine how results will be interpreted (generalized); and (12) determine methods of communicating results.[aa]

"Clinical research" can be conducted in any clinical setting in which the nurse and patient are together, as, for example, a hospital unit, a nursing home, a school or industrial or penal health service, a clinic, or in a patient's home. The investigator (nurse researcher and/or practitioner) collects data through direct observation of the patient. Phyllis J. Verhonick says, "All too frequently the changes that have been made in nursing practice have been the result of the application of expedient measures rather than systematic investigation."[bb]

It is the responsibility of every nurse to appraise his or her practice and identify ways of improving it. Leonard F. Stevens[77] describes a program at the Veterans Administration Hospital, St. Cloud, Minn., which created a climate that encouraged nurses to evaluate their practices and to make use of studies in doing this more effectively. Research was considered a means of improving nursing practice rather than an end in itself.

Lucille E. Notter[78] comments on the time lag that always exists between research and its implementation despite the increasing opportunities for publication and dissemination of research reports through reviews and source books.

In the 1970s nurse investigators placed increased emphasis upon clinical research. Some excellent examples are provided in the ANA publication, *Research in Nursing: Toward a Science of Health Care*, 1976.

Examples of research in clinical nursing will be found in many chapters of this text. In discussing procedures such as enemata or taking temperatures, studies by nurses are cited; in discussing pain, preparing the patient for surgery, or caring for the dying, numerous studies by nurses are also used as a basis for suggesting methods or ways of helping patients. It is hoped that those who use this text will come to look upon the conduct, use, and interpretation of research as an essential element of nursing practice. Every nurse should at the very least know where to find published research.

The analytical aspects of the nursing literature published in English between 1900 and 1959 are indexed and annotated in the *Nursing Studies Index*.[79] Henderson[80] in 1957 and Abdellah[81] in 1970 published reviews of nursing research, which included clinical studies. Simmons and Henderson in 1964 published *Nursing Research—A Survey and Assessment*.[82] Abdellah with Levine in 1965 published *Better Patient Care Through Nursing Research*[83] which dealt with "how some of the important methodological tools can be applied to problems that are uniquely nursing," giving throughout examples of how these methods have been used and citing hundreds of studies. The bimonthly journal *Nursing Research*, besides publishing full-length reports of major studies, gives abstracts of many others. Abstracts under the heading "Nursing Practice and Related Care" in the May–June 1973 issue outnumber those in any other category. This same trend is noticeable in the *International Journal of Nursing Studies*. It is tempting to mention certain investigations that might be considered "milestones" in the development of clinical nursing research but this is coming to be as difficult as it would be to select outstanding studies in any other health field.

More and more often nurses are working with other health workers on problems of common concern. A good example is the work of the U.S. Department of Health, Education, and Welfare's Center for Disease Control, an agency of the Public Health Service. There, bacteriologists, epidemiologists, nurses, and physicians are studying ways of preventing the spread of infection. An example is the [abortive] nationwide swine flu program directed by the Public Health Service. In some cases nurses studying in this Center are afterwards employed in hospitals as epidemiologists. Most health institutions and agencies realize that practice must change and that it should be under constant surveillance. Nurses are assuming more and more responsibility for this work.

Organization Within Practice Settings that Fosters the Improvement of Care

An analysis of practice settings in which nurses work indicates the need for establishing a formal mechanism for the study of procedures, practices, and method in the care of patients. Figure 17.1 illustrates one organizational approach developed by Henderson that might be used in a hospital.

At Case-Western Reserve University, Jannetta MacPhail directed *An Experiment in Nursing: Planning, Implementing, and Assessing Planned Change*[84] that resulted in an effective approach. A Committee on Nursing Practice Guidelines was established as a counterpart of the Procedures Committee of the Medical Council. The purposes of the Committee on Nursing Practice Guidelines were defined as follows: (1) to review existing policies and procedures, identifying those which pertain to nursing practice, and to recommend the need for policy revisions or the development of policies where none now exist; and (2) to submit policy statements to the Nursing Council for review and preparation of guidelines for the implementation of the policy. This committee had six representatives from medical-surgical nursing, a centralized staff development group faculty appointee, and related clinical specialty representatives.

In any agency, the Research Review Committee usually studies research

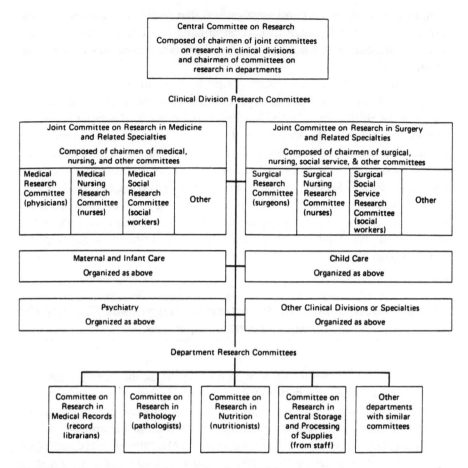

FIGURE 17.1 Suggested organization within a hospital to promote study of method in patient care. (Prepared by Virginia Henderson for meeting of Connecticut League for Nursing, Sept. 29, 1961.)

proposals from all angles but its most important function is to protect human subjects.

In most hospitals the committee on Research in Central Storage and Processing of Supplies, including equipment, is an important one. Representation on this committee must include one or more persons in this field as well as knowledgeable workers in clinical services who can interpret the needs of these services. This committee is responsible for reviewing requests for change in supplies or equipment, getting needed information, and collecting data or testing supplies and equipment and recommending selection. The effectiveness of such committees will depend upon the opportunities they provide for continuing education. This is stressed by Marjorie Cantor[85] and Abdellah.[86]

Ethical Aspects of Clinical Research

Advances made in biomedical science and technology have raised perplexing problems and increased professional and public interest in ethical issues and moral decisions. James Carmody[87] discusses this in a report that includes a bibliography on this subject. The revision of practices based on experiments involving human subjects—the prolongation of life, the survival of malformed neonates, organ transplantation, the control of population—all necessitate ethical decisions. As nursing research moves more and more in the direction of clinical research the legal and ethical aspects of using human subjects for experimentation must be continuously examined. Abdellah discussed this question at some length in a 1967 article.[88]

The most far-reaching study of ethical standards for research with human subjects has been undertaken by the American Psychological Association. It proposes the following ethical principles:

1. It is the personal responsibility of the investigator to make a careful evaluation of the ethical acceptability of each study he plans to undertake, taking into account the following guidelines for research with human beings. To the extent that this appraisal, weighing scientific and humane values, leads the investigator to consider a deviation from any principle, the investigator incurs a correspondingly greater obligation to seek ethical advice and to observe more stringent safeguards to protect the rights of the human research participant.
2. The final responsibility for the establishment and maintenance of acceptable ethical practice in research always remains with the individual investigator. The investigator is also responsible for the ethical treatment of research participants by collaborators, assistants, students and employees, all of whom, however, incur parallel obligations.
3. The investigator should inform the participant of all features of the research that reasonably might be expected to influence willingness to participate. In addition, the investigator should explain all other aspects of the research about which the participant inquires. When full

disclosure is impossible, the investigator incurs increased responsibility to maintain confidentiality, and to protect the welfare and dignity of the research participant.

4. Openness and honesty should characterize the relationship between investigator and research participant. When the methodological requirements of a study necessitate concealment or deception, adequate measures must be taken to ensure the participant's understanding of the scientific grounds for this action and to restore the quality of the relationship with the investigator.

5. The investigator should respect the individual's freedom to choose to participate in research or not and to discontinue participation at any time. The obligation to protect this freedom increases when the investigator is in a position of power with respect to the participant. The decision to limit this freedom increases the investigator's obligation to protect the participant's dignity and welfare.

6. From the beginning of each research investigation, there should be a clear and fair agreement between the investigator and the research participant that defines the responsibilities of each. The investigator has the obligation to honor all promises and commitments included in that agreement.

7. Researchers should protect participants from physical discomfort, harm and danger, and from all forms of mental stress. If the potential for such consequences exists, the investigator should inform the participant of the fact, secure his consent to proceed, and take all possible measures to minimize the distress he may experience.

8. Immediately after the data are collected, the investigator should provide the participant with a full clarification of the nature of the study and remove any misconceptions that may have arisen. Where scientific or humane values justify withholding information, every effort must be made to assure that this has no damaging consequences for the participant.

9. Where research procedures may result in undesirable consequences for the participant, the investigator has the responsibility for employing appropriate measures to detect and remove or correct these consequences, including, where relevant, long-term after-effects.

10. The investigator should keep in confidence all information obtained about research participants. When any known possibility exists that others may obtain access to such information, this possibility, together with the plans for protecting confidentiality, should be explained to

the participants as a part of the procedure for obtaining informed consent.[cc]

The American Hospital Association has recently issued to its member hospitals *A Patient's Bill of Rights* which had consumer participation in its development.[89]

The American Nurses' Association through its Commission on Nursing Research has accepted a commitment to support two sets of human rights. The first is concerned with the rights of qualified nurses to engage in research. The second deals with the human rights of all persons who are recipients of health care services or are participants in research performed by investigators whose research impinges on the patient care provided by nurses.[90]

Every profession has an ethical code that guides its practice. Nursing has been conspicuously vocal about its ethics. A Committee on Ethical Standards was established in the American Nurses' Association in the early 1920s. Tentative codes were presented at intervals, and in 1950, the Association adopted a code. This has undergone major revisions by its present Committee on Ethical, Legal and Professional Standards and has resulted in ten cardinal principles for nurses.[91]

Medical associations have well-defined ethics. The American Medical Association issued a revised "Principles of Medical Ethics" in 1957.[92] While formal recognition by the health professions that patients have rights is important, the critical question is how these "rights" are implemented in daily practice. Edmund D. Pellegrino[93] says what is notably lacking is the critical reassessment of traditional professional roles and functions that will permit the fullest exploitation of new scientific knowledge while protecting the patients' rights.

Experimentation with new procedures, practices, and/or methods should be encouraged. Any changes in procedures or reassignment of tasks that involves two or more types of personnel must be decided by a joint practice committee or a research committee where ethical principles that protect the rights of the patients and workers are operative.

Notes

---

[a]Benjamin A. Kogan, in his work *Health: Man in a Changing Environment* (Harcourt, Brace & World, New York, 1970), says the central and recurring

theme of his book is how people can achieve harmony between their "slowly changing inner environment and their rapidly changing outer environment" (p. IX).

b *Truth*

For what is truth?
Since it is found to be,
Later, no more than sooth-
sayer's early fantasy
So often! But may you
Guard what your conscience tells
Or mind thinks to be true;
For he who conscience sells;
That sale will rue!

Evelyn Princeps

cWilliam Bagley, an educator at Teachers College, Columbia University, discussing standardization in education during the 1920s, used to say that the French Minister of Education claimed that, on looking at his watch during a school day, he could say what every child in every grade of the French schools was doing at that moment. It is small wonder that the first national curriculum in nursing, published by the National League of Nursing Education in 1917, was called *The Standard Curriculum*.

dThe following are examples of studies made by students: (1) the effect of smoking just before measuring body temperature by mouth; (2) the sedative effect of a cold wet sheet pack as compared with a warm wet sheet pack; (3) the optimum temperature for a perineal cleansing solution, an eye or ear irrigation; (4) the amounts of fluid held, or the distention of the colon tolerated, by persons while having a cleansing enema; (5) the fears and discomforts of a person in a body cast; and (6) the safety and comfort factors with different types of lubricants for urinary, nasal, or rectal intubations. A number of such studies were published in nursing journals of this era.

eIn this era, before the development of the sulfa drugs and antibiotics and many of the vaccines, infectious diseases were man's chief enemies. Medical research focused on them very largely and it is not surprising that nursing studies of this period did likewise.

fBecause of the emphasis on education research, Harriet Werley and Fredericka P. Shea describe the Center for Nursing Research at Wayne State University, Detroit, Mich., as "The First Center for Research in Nursing," (*Nurs. Res., 22*:217, [May–June] 1973.)

[g]The history of research in nursing is traced in this report during the period of development [of nursing] 1870–1900; period of expansion 1900–1930; period of stock-taking and upswing in research 1930–

[h]The ANA now has a Commission on Nursing Research and a Council of Nurse Researchers responsible to the Commission, who are nurses with earned doctor's or master's degrees who are engaged in research. (Notter, Lucile E. "The New Council of Nurse Researchers," *Nurs. Res., 21*:293, [July–Aug.] 1972.)

[i]Abdellah, Faye G.: "Surveys Stimulate Community Action," *Nurs. Outlook, 2*:268, (May) 1954.

[j]Abdellah, Faye G.: "Evolution of Nursing as a Profession. Perspective on Manpower Development," *Int. Nurs. Rev., 19*:319, (No. 3) 1972.

[k]Chow, Rita K.: "Research + Primex = Improved Health Services," *Int. Nurs. Rev., 19*:319, (No. 4) 1972. (Primex is a family nurse practitioner or a "primary care extender.")

[l]These methods or techniques are:

1. Opinionnaires or questionnaires answered in writing or verbally by patients, nurses, doctors, and others; accompanied, or unaccompanied by pictures showing persons or situations—comparing what someone thinks the patient needs with what he gets.
2. Analysis of critical incidents showing effective and noneffective, or even destructive, nursing.
3. Interviews, with or without written schedules, "Q-sorts" or pictures, and other descriptive materials, such as case studies.
4. Observation and analysis of patient-nurse (or other) interaction and changes in the behavior or appearance of patients.
5. Clinical tests for changes in physical status such as measurement of blood pressure, body temperature, or gain of weight.
6. Study of patients' records to find evidence of certain services to the patient or of physical changes, psychosocial behavior and the status of patients with relation to independence or rehabilitation.

[m]Monitoring would answer the questions, Were the services medically necessary and of an acceptable professional standard? This would include hospitalization.

[n]This system, usually called "the Weed System," is referred to repeatedly

throughout this text. (See also Weed, Lawrence L.: *Medical Records, Medical Education and Patient Care: The Problem-Oriented Record as a Basic Tool*. Case-Western Reserve University Press, Cleveland, 1969).

[o]*Physician Behavior*—A. Technical management of health and illness, 1. adequacy of diagnosis, 2. adequacy of therapy, 3. parsimony or minimum redundancy in diagnostic and therapeutic procedures, 4. full exploitation of medical technology, 5. full exploitation of professional and functional differentiation; B. Socioeconomic management of health and illness, 1. attention to social and environmental factors, 2. use of larger social units as the units of care wherever appropriate, 3. use of community resources on behalf of the patient, 4. attention to broader community interests; C. Psychological management of health and illness; D. Integrated management of health and illness; E. Continuity and coordination in the management of health and illness. II. *Client-Provider Relationship—A. Some formal attributes of the client-provider relationship; B. Some attributes of the content of the client-provider relationship.*

[p]*Assessment of quality care* was accomplished by three techniques: (1) review of the medical record alone, (2) review of the medical record with the criteria presented in the *Hospital Utilization Review Manual,* and (3) a combination of the medical record, the criterion list, and a case abstract prepared by a nonprofessional. If readers are interested in the specifics they will find a list of criteria for evaluating the care of a patient with pneumonia in the hospital in the monograph by Payne titled *Quality Assurance of Medical Care*, Regional Medical Programs Service, US Department of Health, Education and Welfare.

[q]February 1973, pp. 252–254. Payne is now extending his research to include the development of criteria for ambulatory care.

[r]Smith, Dorothy M.: "Myth and Method in Nursing Practice," *Am. J. Nurs., 64*:68, (Feb.) 1964.

[s]Lambertsen, Eleanor C.: "Evaluating the Quality of Nursing Care," *Hospitals, 39*:61, (Nov.) 1965.

[t]Personal communication.

[u]PETO is an acronym of the surnames of the pediatrics team that developed the system: Marilyn Poland, Nellie English, Nancy Thorton, and Donna Owens, Medical College of Georgia, Augusta.

[v]Quality of care with relation to the following functions is judged:

(1) application and execution of physician's legal orders;
(2) observation of symptoms and reactions;
(3) supervision of the patient;
(4) supervision of those participating in care;
(5) reporting and recording;
(6) application of nursing procedures and techniques;
(7) promotion of health by direction and teaching.

[w]Mereness, Dorothy: "Preparing the Nurse Researcher," *Am. J. Nurs., 64*:78, (Sept.) 1964.

[x]Werley, Harriet H.: "This I Believe—About Clinical Nursing Research," *Nurs. Outlook, 20*:718, (Nov.) 1972.

[y]Leonard, Robert C.: "Developing Research in a Practice-Oriented Discipline," *Am. J. Nurs., 67*:1472, (July) 1967.

[z]Abdellah, Faye G.: "Overview of Nursing Research 1955–1968, part I," *Nurs. Res., 19*:6, (Jan.–Feb.) 1970.

[aa]Abdellah, Faye G., and Levine, Eugene. *Better Patient Care Through Nursing Research*. Macmillan Publishing Co., Inc., New York, 1965, p. 91.

[bb]Verhonick, Phyllis J.: "Clinical Investigations in Nursing," *Nurs. Forum, 10*:81, (Summer) 1971.

[cc]American Psychological Association: "Ethical Standards for Research with Human Subjects," The Association, Draft document (May) 1972.

References

1. Nutting, M. Adelaide: "Florence Nightingale as a Statistician," *Public Health Nurse, 19*:207, (May) 1927.

2. _____. *The Education and Professional Position of Nurses*. U.S. Government Printing Office, Washington, D.C., 1907. (Reissued as *Educational Status of Nursing*, Bull. No. 7 of U.S. Office of Education.)

3. Waters, Ysabella: *Visiting Nursing in the United States*. Charities Publication Committee, [New York], 1909.

4. Galbraith, Lillian M.: "Management Engineering and Nursing," *Am. J. Nurs., 50*:780, (Dec.)1950.

5. American Hospital Association: "Report of Simplification and Standardization Committee," in *Transactions, American Hospital Association Meeting, Detroit*, 1932. The Association, Chicago, 1933.

6. Barnes, Ralph M.: *Motion and Time Study*. 3rd ed. John Wiley & Sons, New York, 1949.

7. Pfefferkorn, Blanche, and Rottman, Marion: *Clinical Education in Nursing*. Macmillan Publishing Co., Inc., New York, 1932.

8. Stewart, Isabel M.: "Possibilities of Standardization in Nursing Technique," *Mod. Hosp., 44*:46, (Oct.) 1919.

9. _____: "An Opportunity to Cooperate in a Plan for Improving Nursing Practice," *Nurs. Ed. Bull.*, n. s. 1:4, 1930.

10. _____: "A Search for More Exact Measures of Reliability and Efficiency in Nursing Procedures," *Nurs. Ed. Bull.*, n. s. 1:4, 1930.

11. Smith, Martha Ruth, and Broadhurst, Jean (eds.): *An Introduction to the Principles of Nursing Care*. J. B. Lippincott Co., Philadelphia, 1937.

12. Simmons, Leo W., and Henderson, Virginia: *Nursing Research—A Survey and Assessment*. Appleton-Century-Crofts, New York, 1964.

13. Henderson, Virginia: "Research in Nursing—When?" (editorial), *Nurs. Res., 4*:99, (Feb.) 1956.

14. Hughes, Everett C., et al.: *Twenty Thousand Nurses Tell Their Story*. J. B. Lippincott Co., Philadelphia, 1958.

15. Kroeger, Louis J., et al.: *Nursing Practice in California Hospitals*. California State Nurses Association, San Francisco, 1953.

16. American Nurses' Association: *Facts About Nursing 74–75*. The Association, Kansas City, Mo., 1976.

17. Canadian Nurses' Association: *Countdown 1973. Canadian Nursing Statistics*. The Association, Ottawa, 1974.

18. American Nurses' Foundation: "Directory of Nurses with Earned Doctoral Degrees," *Nurs. Res., 18*:465, (Sept.–Oct.) 1969.

19. Brown, Esther Lucile: *Nursing for the Future*. Russell Sage Foundation, New York, 1948.

20. National Commission for the Study of Nursing and Nursing Education: *An Abstract for Action*. McGraw-Hill Book Co., New York, 1970.

21. Abdellah, Faye G.: "Overview of Nursing Research, 1955–1968, Part III," *Nurs. Res., 19*:239, (May–June) 1970. (Financial data updated by author Oct. 1976.)

22. Canadian Nurses' Association: *Index of Canadian Nursing Studies*. The Association, Ottawa, 1973.

23. [Finnish] Foundation for Nursing Education: *Sairaanhoidon Vuosikirja X*. The Foundation, Helsinki, 1973.

24. Bayne-Jones, Stanhope: "The Role of the Nurse in Medical Progress," *Am. J. Nurs., 50*:601, (Oct.) 1950.

25. Brown, Amy Francis: *Research in Nursing*. W. B. Saunders Co., Philadelphia, 1958.

26. Meyer, Burton, and Heidgerken, Loretta E.: *Introduction to Research in Nursing*. J. B. Lippincott Co., Philadelphia, 1962.

27. Simmons, Leo W., and Henderson, Virginia: *op. cit.*

28. Skipper, James K., and Leonard, Robert C. (eds.): *Social Interaction and Patient Care*. J. B. Lippincott Co., Philadelphia, 1965.

29. Abdellah, Faye G., and Levine, Eugene: *Better Patient Care through Nursing Research*. Macmillan Publishing Co., Inc., New York, 1965.

30. Fox, David J.: *Fundamentals of Research in Nursing*. Appleton-Century-Crofts, New York, 1966.

31. Wandelt, Mabel T.: *Guide for the Beginning Researcher*. Appleton-Century-Crofts, New York, 1970.

32. Woolridge, Powhatan J., et al.: *Behavioral Science, Social Practice, and the Nursing Profession*. Press of Case-Western Reserve University, Cleveland, 1968.

33. Wald, Florence, and Leonard, Robert: "Toward Development of Nursing Practice Theory," *Nurs.Res., 13*:309, (Fall) 1964.

34. Dublin, Louis I.: "First 1,000 Midwifery Cases of the Frontier Nursing Service in Kentucky,"*Public Health Nurse, 24*:582, (Oct.) 1932.

35. Simmons, Leo W., and Henderson, Virginia: *op. cit.*

36. Abdellah, Faye G., and Levine, Eugene: *Patients and Personnel Speak. A Method of Studying Patient Care in Hospitals*. U.S. Department of Health, Education, and Welfare, Division of Nursing, Washington, D.C., 1957. (USPHS Pub. No. 527.)

37. Sanazaro, Paul J., et al.: "Research and Development in Quality Assurance. The Experimental Medical Care Review Organization Program," *N. Engl. J. Med., 287*:1125, (Nov. 30) 1972.

38. Donabedian Avedis: "Evaluating the Quality of Medical Care," *Milbank Mem. Fund Q., 44*:166, Part 2, 1966.

39. _____: *A Guide to Medical Care Administration*, Vol. II; *Medical Care Appraisal—Quality and Utilization*. American Public Health Association, New York, 1969.

40. _____: *Evaluating the Quality of Medical Care, Program Evaluation in the Health Fields*. (Edited by H. C. Schulberg *et al.*) Behavioral Publications, New York, 1969, p. 186.

41. _____: "Promoting Quality Through Evaluating the Process of Patient Care," *Med. Care, 6*:181, 1968.

42. Williamson, John W.: "Evaluating Quality of Patient Care—A Strategy

Relating to Outcome and Process Assessment," *J.A.M.A., 218*:564, (Oct. 25) 1971.

43. _____, et al.: "Priorities in Patient-Care Research and Continuing Medical Education," *J.A.M.A., 204*:303, (Apr. 22) 1968.

44. Payne, Beverly C.: *Hospital Utilization Review Manual*. University of Michigan Press, Ann Arbor, 1966.

45. Woodham-Smith, Cecil: *Florence Nightingale 1820–1910*. Constable, London, 1950.

46. Hitchcock, Jane E.: "Five Hundred Cases of Pneumonia," *Am. J. Nurs., 3*:169, (Dec.) 1902.

47. Reiter, Frances, and Kakosh, Marguerite E.: *Quality of Nursing Care*. A Report of a Field Study to Establish Criteria 1950–1954, Institute of Research and Studies in Nursing Education, Division of Nursing Education, Teachers College, Columbia University, New York, 1963.

48. Kakosh, Marguerite E.: *Differentiating Characteristics of Professional Nursing Care*. Ed. D. Dissertation, Teachers College, Columbia University, New York, 1954.

49. Aydelotte, Myrtle Kitchell, and Tener, Marie E.: *An Investigation of the Relation Between Nursing Activity and Patient Welfare*. State University of Iowa, Utilization Project, Iowa City, 1960.

50. Nite, Gladys, and Willis, Frank: *The Coronary Patient; Hospital Care and Rehabilitation*. Macmillan Publishing Co., Inc., New York, 1964.

51. Orlando, Ida Jean: *The Dynamic Nurse-Patient Relationship. Function, Process and Principles*. G. P. Putnam's Sons, New York, 1961.

52. Dumas, Rhetaugh G., and Leonard, Robert C.: "The Effect of Nursing on the Incidence of Postoperative Vomiting," *Nurs. Res., 12*:12, (Winter) 1963.

53. Haussman, R. K. Dieter, et al.: *Monitoring Quality of Nursing, Part II. Assessment and Study of Correlates*. U.S. Department of Health, Education, and Welfare, Public Health Service, Bethesda, Md., July 1976 (Pub. No. [HRA] 76–7).

54. American Nurses' Association: *Guidelines for Review of Nursing Care at the Local Level*. The Association, Kansas City, Mo., 1976 (Pub. No. NP-54).

55. Smith, Dorothy M.: "Myth and Method in Nursing Practice," *Am. J. Nurs., 64*:68, (Feb.) 1964.

56. McFarlane, Jean K.: "Study of Nursing Care—The First Two Years of a Research Project," *Int. Nurs. Rev., 17*:102 (No. 2) 1970.

57. Fivars, Grace, and Gosnell, Doris: *Nursing Education: The Problem and the Process*. Macmillan Publishing Co., Inc., New York, 1966, p. 47.

58. Klaus, David J., et al.: *Controlling Experience to Improve Nursing Proficiency*. Background and Study Plan, Report No. 1. American Institutes for Research, Pittsburgh, 1966, p. 40.

59. Bidwell, Charles M., and Froebe, Doris J.: "Development of an Instrument for Evaluating Hospital Nursing Performance," *J. Nurs. Admin., 1*:10, (Sept.–Oct.) 1971.

60. Dunn, Margaret A.: "Development of an Instrument to Measure Nursing Performance," *Nurs. Res., 19*:502, (Nov.–Dec.) 1970.

61. Clark, E. Louise, and Diggs, Walter W.: "The PETO System Offers a New Method of Matching Patient Needs with Available Nursing Care," *Hospitals, 45*:96, (Sept. 16) 1971.

62. White, R., et al.: *Patient Care Classification: Methods and Application*. Johns Hopkins University, Baltimore, 1967.

63. Routhier, R. Wilda: "Tool for Evaluation of Patient Care," *Supervisor Nurse, 3*:15, (Jan.) 1972.

64. Beland, Irene L.: *Clinical Nursing*, 2nd ed. Macmillan Publishing Co., Inc., New York, 1970.

65. Gelder, Joy E.: "The 'Flow Chart' Assists Nursing," *Can. Hosp., 48*:81, (Oct.) 1971.

66. Weed, Lawrence L.: *Medical Records, Medical Education, and Patient Care: The Problem-Oriented Record as a Basic Tool*. Case-Western Reserve University Press, Cleveland, 1969.

67. Wandelt, Mabel A., and Phaneuf, Maria C.: "Three Instruments for Measuring the Quality of Nursing Care," *Hosp. Topics, 150*:20, (Aug.) 1972.

68. Phaneuf, Maria C.: "Quality of Care: Problems of Measurement Part I—How One Public Health Nursing Agency Is Using the Nursing Audit," *Am. J. Public Health, 59*:1827, (Oct.) 1969.

69. _____: *The Nursing Audit, Profile for Excellence*. Appleton-Century-Crofts, New York, 1972.

70. Abdellah, Faye G., and Levine, Eugene: *Better Patient Care Through Nursing Research*. Macmillan Publishing Co., Inc., New York, 1965.

71. American Nurses' Association: "ANA Blueprint for Research in Nursing," *Am. J. Nurs., 62*:69, (Aug.) 1962.

72. Werley, Harriet H.: "This I Believe . . . About clinical Nursing Research," *Nurs. Outlook, 20*:718, (Nov.) 1972.

73. U.S. Department of Health, Education, and Welfare: *Extending the Scope of Nursing Practice*. A Report of the Secretary's Committee to Study

Extended Roles for Nurses. US Government Printing Office, Washington, D.C., (Nov.) 1971.

74. Diers, Donna: "Application of Research to Nursing Practice," *Image*, 5:7 (No. 2) 1972.

75. Notter, Lucille E.: "The Vital Significance of Clinical Nursing Research," *Cardio-Vasc. Nurs., 8*:19, (Sept.–Oct.) 1972.

76. Verhonick, Phyllis J. "Clinical Investigations in Nursing," *Nurs. Forum, 10*:81, (Summer) 1971.

77. Stevens, Leonard F.: "Look at Your Own Practice," *Am. J. Nurs., 65*:106, (June) 1965.

78. Notter, Lucille E.: "The Editor's Report—January 1973," *Nurs. Res., 22*:3, (Jan.–Feb.) 1973.

79. Henderson, Virginia (ed.): *Nursing Studies Index. An Annotated Guide to Reported Studies, Research Methods, and Historical and Biographical Materials in Periodicals, Books, and Pamphlets Published in English* (1900–1959). J. B. Lippincott Co., Philadelphia, 1964–1972, 4 vols.

80. Henderson, Virginia: "An Overview of Nursing Research," *Nurs. Res., 6*:61, (Oct.) 1957.

81. Abdellah, Faye G.: "Overview of Nursing Research, 1955–1968," Parts I, II, III. *Nurs. Res., 19*:6, (Jan.–Feb.) 1970; *19*:151, (Mar.–Apr.) 1970; *19*:239, (May–June) 1970.

82. Simmons, Leo W., and Henderson, Virginia: *op. cit.*

83. Abdellah, Faye G., and Levine, Eugene: *Better Patient Care Through Nursing Research*. Macmillan Publishing Co., Inc., New York, 1965.

84. MacPhail, Jannetta: *An Experiment in Nursing: Planning, Implementing, and Assessing Planned Change*. Case-Western Reserve University, Frances Payne Bolton School of Nursing, Cleveland, 1972, p. 8.

85. Cantor, Marjorie: "Standard 5—Education for Quality Care," *J. Nurs. Admin., 3*:49, (Jan.–Feb.) 1973.

86. Abdellah, Faye G., et al.: *New Directions in Patient-Centered Nursing*. Macmillan Publishing Co., Inc., New York, 1973.

87. Carmody, James: *Ethical Issues in Health Services. A Report and Annotated Bibliography*. U.S. Department of Health, Education, and Welfare, National Center for Health Services Research and Development, Report HSRD #70-32, (Nov.) 1970.

88. Abdellah, Faye G. "Approaches to Protecting the Rights of Human Subjects," *Nurs. Res., 16*:316, (Fall) 1967.

89. American Hospital Association: *A Patient's Bill of Rights*. The Association, Chicago, 1972.

90. American Nurses' Association: *Human Rights Guidelines for Nurses in Clinical and Other Research*. The Association, Kansas City, Mo., 1975 (Pub. No. D–46).

91. American Nurses' Association: "Code for Nurses," *Am. J. Nurs.,* 68:2581, (Dec.) 1968.

92. American Medical Association: "Principles of Medical Ethics," *J.A.M.A., 164*:1484, (July 27) 1957.

93. Pellegrino, Edmund D.: "Ethical Implications in Changing Practice," *Am. J. Nurs., 64*:110, (Sept.) 1964.

Chapter 18

On the Role of
Research in Nursing

Cordial greetings to colleagues gathered in Edinburgh to report on and discuss research related to our education, our practice and its management. I wish I were with you, but I look forward to reading the report on this historic meeting of more than 900 nurses from 24 countries.

Being in my ninetieth year I inevitably see events in the light of history. It pleases me, for instance, to know that Edinburgh is the site of this conference since it was here, I believe, that nursing education established its first connection with a university. While the present-day method of investigation we call "research" is used to solve problems everywhere—in industry as well as professional services—the discipline this approach demands is rarely acquired outside the university.

We must be grateful to nurses and their supporters in every country who have helped to make the resources of higher education available to those who practice nursing. At the same time we should realize that this alone will not insure an ability to use the scientific method of investigation effectively nor will it endow us with the habit of an analytical approach to practice which is the hallmark of scientists.

In all modesty we must acknowledge that Florence Nightingale, who never went to college, did more with her statistical studies to affect the care of hospitalized patients and the conditions under which British soldiers lived in their barracks than any nurse of today has accomplished for comparable groups of citizens through implementation of his or her recommendations based on research.

Miss Nightingale, sometimes called "the first medical statistician," could persuade the British Government to change conditions in hospitals and conditions affecting the health of military personnel because her studies showed convincingly that existing ones were harmful. Until nurses of today employ research to materially affect the *practice* of nursing and other health services it will remain, what I believe it is now, very largely an academic exercise that enhances our self-esteem and our position in academia but has relatively little effect on human welfare.

Having helped many graduate nurses studying at Teachers College in New York City to supplant their loyal adherence to nursing methods taught in their basic programs with the questioning spirit of scientific inquiry, I have looked forward to seeing nurses (the most numerous of health workers in mots countries) affect radical changes in health services worldwide in homes, hospitals, industries, schools and prisons, or correctional institutions.

When nurses' sensitivity to human needs (their intuition) is joined with the ability to find and use expert opinion, with the ability to find reported research and apply it to their practice, and when they themselves use the scientific method of investigation, there is no limit to the influence they might have on health care worldwide.

Unfortunately the art of nursing (intuition as a source of knowledge and the value of experience) is distrusted and too few nurses have the skills necessary and are given the time to find reported research conducted by other health disciplines. And alas, the studies conducted by nurses (the reports of which I happen to have read) are rarely focused on prevention or cure of disease, alleviation of discomfort caused by disease, coping with handicaps or the promotion of a peaceful death when death is inevitable. And the report of studies I read are more often than not so limited in scope that they fail to provide convincing evidence on which to base a change in practice.

For reasons too numerous and complicated to consider here, nurses conducting research have had more help and encouragement from social scientists than from the physical and biological scientists and physicians. "The nursing process" (in my opinion nothing more than the universal problem-solving process) has established a false dichotomy between the objectives and methods of nurses and others, and a dichotomy between the objectives of patients–clients and health workers. In other words, it has narrowed rather than broadened our concept of "nursing research."

If research focused on health is to further human welfare, I think it must enhance the ability and opportunity for health care providers to collaborate rather than compete and, most especially, to work with the public in reaching common goals.

Toward these ends—in conferences such as this—the following questions might be discussed:

- Should the curricula for all health care providers give students of the various disciplines opportunities to work together in studying their common and overlapping functions?
- Should students of these various disciplines have an opportunity to conduct joint research on common problems?
- Should students and practitioners have, or make, an opportunity to work with informed citizens or groups in the community concerned with health problems?

To illustrate the use and importance of a collaborative approach, I suggest that only with this approach can the optimum value of personal, medical, or health, records be realized by the public and health care providers.

Recognizing importance of self-help and the necessity of sudden change in their habitats military personnel (in the United States) are given copies of their medical records: in Japan the elderly who must (if unemployed) receive health care in their homes are given by the government a record in which entries are made by caregivers, and certain groups here and elsewhere are considering the use of microchips to make it easy to own, transport and store health records.

Since nurses are being asked to accept major responsibility for providing primary care they could very appropriately assume leadership, but of necessity work with others, in (1) identifying the essential elements of a health record, (2) freeing it from all forms of jargon, and (3) making copies available to subjects of the record, or their guardians, as a fundamental tool in health education and the promotion of self-help. In its most useful form this research would demand interdisciplinary and international collaboration. And I can think of no other development that might more profoundly affect the nature and quality of health service.

PART IV

Nursing in Society

Introduction

$\mathbf{M}$iss Virginia Henderson is a citizen of the world. Since 1950 she has traveled extensively at the invitation of professional nurse leaders and governments to consult about nursing practice, research, and education. Several years ago, aware of her age, I asked her to visit the Nursing staff at University Hospitals of Cleveland, if she were still traveling. She wrote to say the dates we selected could be sandwiched between trips she was to make to Pakistan and the United Kingdom. The Aga Khan invited her to participate in the opening of the new nursing school in Karachi and the British nurses were to listen to her presentation on nursing in a technological era.

Canadian nurses were the first of many to award Miss Henderson an honorary degree, and the Royal College of Nursing of the United Kingdom made her an honorary fellow. Numerous awards and honorary degrees have been given her and are among her papers at the Mugar Library, Boston University. Many awards have been made by nursing organizations in countries around the world and others are from institutions where she has consulted. The first university nursing education center in France was opened in 1992 and Miss Henderson was the featured educational consultant.

Miss Henderson has used her extensive travel to inform her opinions about health care. She is an advocate of a tax-supported health care service like America's educational system, and opposes the use of industrial techniques and profit motives for improving this essential human service. She speaks authoritatively about the effectiveness and efficiency of the national health services she has visited in Europe, Japan, and Canada, and particularly the satisfaction and peace of mind the citizens of these countries have with their health services.

One theme evident in Miss Henderson's writing is her use of language that contains no jargon. She writes to communicate to anyone who seeks to understand nursing. No special indoctrination is required to understand her (and our) work. In fact, in the Preface to the 6th edition of *Principles and Practice of Nursing*, Virginia Henderson describes the book as being useful "to those who want to guard their own or their family's health or take care of a sick relative or friend." Like Nightingale's publication of *Notes on Nursing*, Miss Henderson makes nursing available to anyone who can read.

Recently, Miss Henderson has campaigned for patients' rights and responsibilities for their own health records. As it is, the records are intended for health professionals to communicate with each other, and not with patients. Miss Henderson sees the records as an excellent tool to use to involve patients in their own care, particularly to educate them about their illness. She supported the efforts undertaken by a Blue Cross agency that was experimenting with computerized records being affixed to a membership card so they were always with the patient.

Miss Virginia Henderson was as unfailing in her beliefs in the skills of nurses as her mentor Miss Annie Goodrich was when she wrote *The Social and Ethical Significance of Nursing*.

References

Goodrich, A. W. (1973, facsimile). *The social and ethical significance of nursing: A series of addresses*. New Haven: Yale University School of Nursing.

Henderson, V., & Nite, G. (1978). *Principles and practice of nursing* (6th edition). New York: Macmillan.

Nightingale, F. (1859). *Notes on nursing: What it is and what it is not*. London: Harrison.

Chapter 19

Nursing as an Aspect of Health Care

The Goal of All Health Care

What is nursing and what is the function of the nurse? These are questions with which society should be concerned; but those who practice, administer, teach, study, conduct research on, or legislate for nursing *must* answer these questions since consciously or unconsciously they operate under some concept of nursing and the function of the nurse. If the concept is clear and valid, it can guide them to consistent and constructive action; if it is confused and uninformed, it can lead to inconsistent, ineffective, or even harmful action. These questions could be asked and statements made about any health occupation and its members. In the last analysis, all health workers are trying to promote the health and happiness of the individual and the preservation of the species. Each category of health worker must try to define its role in this joint effort.

All organisms behave instinctively to preserve their lives. For some, this instinctive, protective behavior is sufficient, and such organisms (the simpler forms of life) are independent of their parents throughout their separate existence; complex organisms (the higher forms of life) require parental protection and teaching. Generally speaking, the more complex the organism, the longer the period of dependency on adults.[1]

As a species develops communal life, or a society, all members, not only parents, may protect, teach, and nurture the young and protect the sick and helpless; or special members of the community may be assigned these functions. Studies of insect and animal life, as well as studies of human life, show such divisions of labor, or specialized helping functions. Communities of ants, for example, are said to have "nurses" and "sanitarians," the latter disposing of dead bodies. Bees have comparable specialists within the hive.[2,3]

Human societies allow the young shorter or longer periods of dependence on parents, nurses, and teachers according to the particular culture. Even today, in different parts of the world, the dependence of the young man lasts only through puberty or well into adulthood. The dependency of children, the very old, and the sick has been such a threat to the survival of some peoples, particularly nomads, that infanticide and euthanasia were practiced.[a]

In some cultures, the *care* of the young, the sick, and the infirm has been the responsibility of all women rather than designated members; the treatment of disease, or *cure*, has usually been assigned to designated men, sometimes priests, sometimes "medicine men." The "cures" of the latter supplemented the "care" given the sick by women.

As societies increase in size and organization, these basic functions of caring for (nurturing or nursing), teaching about, and curing disease (doctoring) are again subdivided. The assignment of their component functions to groups of men or women depends to a large extent on the status of males and females in the society, and on differences in their education and roles. If there is no agreement among the major categories of workers and their subdivisions as to who does what, there is chaos. If nurses, teachers, or doctors (or any of their subdivisions) get too numerous or too powerful in a society, or develop practices inimical to the welfare of the population, they may make the society as a whole unduly dependent on them or they may pervert the instinctive behavior that preserves the individual and protects the species. If the different categories or subdivisions of workers have ill-defined functions and are competitive, they may develop along the lines of self-interest rather than in ways that will further the common good. It is for these reasons, among others, that the functions of nurses, teachers, and doctors, and the subdivisions of these essential health workers must be considered *interdependently* and their roles in society continually studied in relationship to each other rather than as separate entities. Common goals for health workers, a certain amount of common knowledge, and cooperative relationships are essential to effective health care. This is particularly true for nurses and doctors, who are the oldest and largest groups of specialized health workers in most societies.

There are many indications today that health workers, especially nurses and doctors, are realizing the necessity of cooperation and that they are trying to identify the commonalities in their practice and the particular roles of each in health care. In order to understand the difficulties they face in changing their roles and relationships, it is necessary to know something about the history of medicine and the history of nursing. A thorough study of each is rewarding, and full-length works are included among the suggested readings at the end of this chapter. The following historical sketch does nothing more than give some of the significant differences in the origins and concepts of nurses and doctors.

Medicine and Nursing. Their Origins, the Public's Image of Doctors and Nurses, their Preparation and Cultural Influences

Any study of medicine and nursing involves a study of cultural settings. Henry E. Sigerist makes the following statement:

> Medical theories always represent one aspect of the general civilization of a period. . . .
> If we attempt to see the theories of medicine as products of their time . . . then we understand the religious character of Babylonian medicine. We understand why the Greek physicians interpreted the phenomena of health and disease in philosophic terms.[b]

Fielding Garrison explains the omniscience of the "medicine man":

> Primitive medicine is inseparable from primitive modes of religious belief. . . . the diagnosis and treatment of disease, . . . was only one phase of a set of mystic processes designed to promote human well-being, such as averting the wrath of angered gods or evil spirits, fire-making, making rain, purifying streams or habitations, fertilizing soil, improving sexual potency or fecundity, preventing or removing blight of crops and epidemic diseases. These powers, originally united in one person, were he god, hero, king, sorcerer, priest, prophet, or physician, formed the savage's generic concept of "making medicine". . . .[c]

Primitive healers still function among North and South American Indians and have their equivalents in other tribal societies on every continent today. Physicians practicing modern Western medicine in such cultures may collaborate with the indigenous "healers."[d] Prevention of disease in primitive systems is thought to depend on placating the omnipresent spirits. If this belief is disregarded, the "scientific" treatment may be ineffective. Anthropologists note that individuals in primitive societies who believe they are doomed to die may respond negatively to a scientific regimen that would under other circumstances be lifesaving.

Egyptians are said to have refined primitive medicine and, in observing the dead body, which they prepared elaborately for entry into the next world, derived explanations for many illnesses. Babylonian medicine, as has been noted, was essentially religious, with metaphysical "cures." Ancient Chinese medicine was influenced by Confucian philosophy which taught that Yang—the masculine element—and Yin—the feminine—are balanced in health. This principle still influences Chinese health care and may be the Eastern counterpart of the Western concept of balance in the negatively and positively charged elements of the fluid-electrolyte system of the body, accepted as essential to health. Traditional Eastern and modern Western medicine are practiced side by side in China today. Research in both ancient and modern practice is encouraged in the People's Republic of China.[4]

V. Djukanovic and E. P. Mach, reporting a joint UNICEF-WHO study under the title *Alternate Approaches to Meeting Basic Health Needs in Developing Countries* (WHO, Geneva, 1975), suggest the extent to which primitive concepts persist and are combined in currently effective health programs on various continents.

Sigerist dates "the new epoch" of medicine from the Indo-European peoples. He says, "the parallelism in the development of Greek and Indian medicine is striking, both in chronology and in content." He believes that "we glorify the Greeks" and disregard other ancient medical systems except as precursors of Greek medicine and this approach to history is "utterly naive and viciously wrong." A thorough study, he thinks, shows that "Western and Indian medicine were closely related and equally effective not only in antiquity but also in the Middle Ages."[e] It is interesting that one of the effective UNICEF-WHO health programs is based on the 3000-year-old Ayurvedic medicine of India, which, according to those reporting the study, is used by most peoples living in India and neighboring countries. They say that "as an integral part of Indian culture it cannot be ignored."[f] Indian physicians (400,000 of them) are trained to use this ancient system which includes a psychosomatic approach to health in preventive and curative aspects. Medical research in India, as in China, is focused on indigenous as well as Western medicine.

As Sigerist notes, most historians say that "Western medicine" is derived from Greek medicine, because both are based on critical analysis of observation. Hippocrates is called "the father of medicine," and most medical students of today take the Hippocratic Oath at graduation. The Greeks saw humans as differentiated from the rest of nature by their capacity for thought or reason; they recognized that emotions affected the body and believed that man had a "soul." Being healthy was a Greek virtue. Vern and Bonnie Bullough[5] say that the rudiments of health were common knowledge, and self-care rather than constant recourse to health workers characterized the Greek citizen.[g] Relatively little is known about nursing in Greece, as distinct from medicine. Physicians had trained helpers and some say they were nurses. Edwin B. and Myra E. Levine[6] suggest that Hippocrates is "father" to both medicine and nursing.

The Greeks emphasized exercise, rest, and diet rather than medication. Their health spas were also temples where there were statues of the gods of medicine and health—Asclepius (or Aesculapius, Roman spelling)[h] and his daughters Hygeia, the goddess of health, and Panakeia, the goddess of healing.

Edgar Jackson[7] says that Aesculapius was thought to restore disordered function, while Hygeia symbolized the quality of wholeness, or health. Some see this distinction as typified today by the work of doctors on one hand and nurses on the other. Mack Lipkin says:

> Hygeia, the guardian of health, symbolized that blessed state achieved by living a sane life in a good environment. Her sister was reputed to heal by her great knowledge of drugs and manipulations. As [R. J.] Dubos [*Mirage of Health*, Harper & Row, New York, 1959, p. 182] points out, ever since there has been an oscillation between the two points of view of medicine. . . . Since the teachings of Hygeia require self-discipline, they are commonly ignored. The help of the healer, Panakeia, is sought more often.[i]

Fielding H. Garrison credits the Romans with advancing surgery "including obstetrics and ophthalmology." He says it "reached a stage of perfection which it was not to reach again before the time of Ambroise Paré (sixteenth century)."[j]

According to Edmund D. Pellegrino, "Many of the Roman ideas of disease were corruptions of the Greek."[k] One of their methods of treatment depended on "keeping the pores of the skin open." The Roman baths were a combination of clubhouse and spa. The "baths" or "watering places," so numerous in many countries throughout the nineteenth and early part of the twentieth centuries, had these characteristics also. The people of Japan today put great emphasis on communal bathing, and the Scandinavian sauna is popular around the world. But hydrotherapy as such is not typical of the present age.

Judao-Christian thought dominated the Western world following the decline of the Roman Empire and throughout the Middle Ages, the latter sometimes being called "The Age of Faith."[1] Its monotheistic philosophy emphasized the worth and uniqueness of the individual, the unity of body and soul, or the total personality. Christians were, to some extent, resigned to suffering in this world but stressed heaven as the reward of a well-spent life. One road to heaven was succoring the sick and helpless. Nursing became a Christian virtue and hospitals and hospices flourished in the Middle Ages. Some of the best-known men and women of the early Christian centuries were made famous, or even raised to sainthood, by a selfless devotion to the sick, the poor, and the unfortunate. Highborn persons often joined religious orders that owned and operated hospitals or hospices, or they cared for the sick and helpless at home. Groups whose chief work was nursing were formed all over the known Western world. While some were secular, many were religious. During the Crusades, military chivalric nursing orders were founded, and it was not unmanly to belong to them, although the members of these orders treated as well as nursed the sick, or combined medicine and nursing.[8] Some hospitals and hospices established in the Middle Ages and a number of nursing orders founded then are still functioning today. Lucie Young Kelly identified the latter in a 1975 publication.[9]

Arabian medicine, practiced during the Middle Ages within the Moslem Empire, was based on translations of the Greeks and was enhanced by rigorous study of chemistry, physiology. and pharmacy. Arabian physicians developed a rational system of medical care and were respected members of society. The Mohammedan religion embraced the teachings of some of the major contemporary religions, so Moslem learning was broad rather than narrow. A strict hygienic regimen was part of religious practice. Arabic-Hebraic medicine was the most enlightened of any during the Middle Ages, and it kept alive some of the advances made by the Greeks. However, because dissection of the human body was prohibited by the Mohammedan religion, misconceptions of anatomy and physiology persisted.

During the Renaissance, there was an intense interest in learning, rediscovery of the classics, and the study of man. This period was marked by geographic exploration and by the development of libraries and universities.

Schools of medicine, theology, philosophy, and law were included in the Renaissance universities, although there were medical schools in the universities at Boulogne, Montpellier, and Paris during the Middle Ages.[10]

While Renaissance medicine was based largely on translations of Greek texts, dissection of the human body and experimentation were introduced, and this led to important changes in thought and practice. Pellegrino makes the following observation:

> Modern man was born sometime in the Renaissance at that indefinite but crucial point when his thought turned from a primary interest in philosophy and theology to the investigation of himself and his world with the tools of experimentation and mathematics.[m]

While medicine from the Middle Ages onward has had a place in the university, the preparation of physicians and surgeons and their social status have varied. As late as the nineteenth century, many of them learned the medical arts through an apprenticeship. Hospitals controlled some medical schools and others might be operated for profit. Vernon W. Lippard[11] says that the British system was dominated by the hospital schools of London. He maintains that the medical school in the United States had its roots not only in the British system but also in the German system centered in universities. As a whole, medical education in the United States rated below that in Europe at the time of the Flexner Report (1910).[12] Not until after this report on American medicine were proprietary medical schools and correspondence courses eliminated in the United States. Today, American medical schools are within universities and doctors have a uniform, rigorous, and costly preparation. At present, medicine is more scientific and technical than humanistic.

This trend toward the development of a medical technology from a science is not new. Hans Peter Dreitzel says:

> This conception of medicine as a science developed during the Enlightenment. It was Paracelsus, who, still in the Middle Ages, first effectively rejected theological and magical conceptions of illness and opened the way to the modern development of medicine.[n]

Medical historians attribute to René Descartes, French philosopher of the seventeenth century (sometimes called "the Age of Reason"), a trend toward a mechanistic view of man and life, for, instead of seeing the human body and soul as one, Descartes thought the soul pure spirit and the body pure matter. Cartesian thought was widely discussed and had a profound effect on many aspects of life in France and elsewhere.° Pellegrino says that, while Descartes finally admitted his defeat, he tried to develop a theory of medicine "based on infallible demonstrations." Pellegrino attributes reintroduction of the notion of disease as a total disturbance to Immanuel Kant, German philosopher of the eighteenth century and his followers, who emphasized "transcendental, subjective, imaginative systems." This encouraged study of psychology and psychiatry.

In an article titled "Educating the Humanist Physician," Pellegrino calls this "an ancient ideal reconsidered." He makes the following observation:

> In the growing litany of criticism to which our profession is increasingly exposed, there is one that in many ways is more painful than all the rest. It is the assertion that physicians are no longer humanists and that medicine is no longer a learned profession. Our technical proficiency is extolled, but in its application we are said to be insensitive to human values. We are, in short, presumed to be wanting as educated men and as responsive human beings.[p]

Actually, medicine based on the scientific method of investigation, or "modern medicine," is historically still young. Except for psychiatry, it is largely an application of the physical and biologic sciences.

The microscope, developed by Anton van Leeuwenhoek (1632–1723), made it possible to study the structure and function of the cell. Claude Bernard's[13] nineteenth-century concept of keeping the lymph around the cell (relatively) constant, or in physiologic balance, revolutionized the practice of medicine. Now the scanning electron microscope has ushered in a new era in the study of microbiology, histology, and cell physiology. Lennart Nilsson and Jan Lindberg make the following comparison between the capabilities of the ordinary microscope and the scanning electron microscope:

> The common laboratory microscope uses light rays to illuminate an object. Anything smaller than the wavelength of visible light, i.e., smaller than half a thousandth of a millimeter, is beyond the capacity of the light microscope and cannot be reproduced. This limitation does not apply to the scanning electron microscope, which uses a beam of electrons instead of visible light. Magnetic fields are used to direct and focus the beam so that it behaves like a ray of light. The "camera" of the electron microscope picks up the activity of the electron beam as it scans the preparation to be

studied and produces a picture on a screen in somewhat the manner of a television camera.

The definition in depth of the scanning electron microscope is up to five hundred times greater than that of the light microscope. For this reason, this type of microscope is used to study and photograph surface structures. Its magnifying power varies between 20,000 and 60,000.[q]

It is hard to imagine the full effect that use of electronic photography will have on study of cell structure and function and ultimately on public understanding of health and disease; and there are other recent technologic developments that may greatly alter health care. Bioelectric medicine, the collaboration of engineers and physicians, is radically changing diagnostic procedures; the laser beam may drastically alter surgery; and modern methods of communicating make health discoveries common knowledge. Nilsson's and Lindberg's book, *Behold Man*,[14] Lewis Thomas's *The Lives of a Cell*,[15] and the film "The Incredible Machine" (the last shown first on public television in 1975) can give even a child a clearer picture of the microscopic structure of tissues and of some body functions than great scientists had in earlier decades.

While contemporary medicine is largely a technical application of physiology, this cannot be said of modern psychiatry, which is based largely on psychology, anthropology, and sociology. With the exception of psychiatry, modern medicine is criticized for being too dependent on technology. The *art of medicine*, as opposed to the *science of medicine*, has its roots in human values. Modern medicine is believed by some critics to overemphasize its science and underrate its art.[r] Contemporary medicine is even thought by some critics to do more harm than good. Ivan Illich develops this theory under the title *Medical Nemesis. The Expropriation of Health* (Pantheon Books, New York, 1976) and Rich J. Carlson under the title *The End of Medicine* (John Wiley & Sons, New York, 1975). They consider the people of many countries exploited by industrialized health care which, unevenly distributed but universally sought, is making people unrealistic in their expectation of escaping pain and incapable of self-care. Its spiraling cost is believed by many to put a disproportionate burden on society. While a full explanation of the aggrandizement of medical science as opposed to its art would be presumptuous at this point, some reasons are clear to the most superficial student. Through technical research, the causes of many diseases have been identified and the development of cures and preventive methods established; anesthesia has been developed; and, through animal experimentation, surgery has progressed to the point where surgeons daily perform lifesaving operations that would, until this century, have been thought impossible. Surgery was, until this age, quite rightly feared and distrusted, as was the surgeon. Only in this century has the surgeon in Europe enjoyed the same social acceptance as the physician. The technical accomplishments of this era have fostered pride in medical "progress" rather than self-criticism.[s]

Organized medicine in many countries, most particularly the United States, has opposed rather than supported attempts to distribute health care equably—attempts to make it as universally available as education. Tax-supported education has been rooted in value systems and dominated by social science; tax-supported health care is often referred to as the largest, or next to the largest, "industry"; it is technologic and dominated by the physical and biologic sciences.

While nursing has been greatly influenced by and in some instances is inseparable from medicine, its history—its development in most cultures—is different. The fact that physicians where usually men and nurses were usually women may partially explain the difference. Vern and Bonnie Bullough's study, *The Subordinate Sex—A History of Attitudes Towards Women*[16] and Jo Ann Ashley's work, *Hospitals, Paternalism, and the Role of the Nurse*[16a] show some of the ways in which attitudes toward women have affected nursing and medicine. Margaret Mead,[17] an anthropologist, frequently observed that most cultures tend to assume that the woman's share of the work is easier and less intellectually demanding than the man's. It is only in this century that nursing has been accepted in any country as a university discipline, whereas medicine has had a place in universities since the latter began.[t] Nursing as an art is as old as the art of medicine; nursing as a science is much younger than medicine as a science. The humanistic element in nursing still dominates the scientific.

It is hard to identify the beginning of the science of nursing. If enough was known about the early training programs, it might be seen that some nurses were introduced to the science of the time and place, but Anne L. Austin,[18] whose *History of Nursing Source Book* is a compilation of excerpts from writings on nurses and nursing from ancient to modern times, dates the "profession of nursing" from the Nightingale era. The existence of nursing science may even now be questioned by some, but there are courses of study in nursing science here and in Europe.[19–21]

Like medicine, nursing can be traced to primitive cultures, and in some form has existed in all cultures. The art of nursing has flowered in religious communities throughout the centuries and in some secular and military orders. Like medicine, it has been influenced by dominant philosophies. Since nursing has usually been seen as woman's work, woman's status has affected nursing's status, just as man's status has affected medicine's status. Even today, a doctor is usually referred to as "he," a nurse as "she."

In some societies, however, there is no sharp distinction between medicine and nursing, between doctors and nurses. Margaret Read, discussing traditional systems of care in sickness and the role of the traditional practitioners, says:

> Health personnel and anthropologists have distinguished several kinds of healer. First, there are the women, whose skills in the use of home remedies, widespread across the world, are shared by countless others. Women's techniques include such practices as the use of purgatives and emetics, poulticing, inducing sweating by various processes, and all the traditional birth practices.[u]

In a 1957 study of Navaho Indians cited by Read, among 73 diagnosticians, 43 were men and 30 were women. In countries such as India, where women led sheltered lives, men performed the functions of nurses outside the home, most particularly the functions that necessitated touching the bodies of adult males.

Differentiation of function between doctors and nurses, between the practice of medicine and nursing, is especially difficult in military services. The barber surgeons of the Middle Ages, attached to European armies, both treated and cared for the sick and injured.[22] Schools for Russian feldshers, military and civil, that have existed since the eighteenth century, today offer 3- to 4-year programs that combine medicine and nursing, as the latter are conceived in the United States. Today's feldshers are taught by doctors and nurses. The recently established schools for physician's assistants in the United States are following the feldsher pattern to some extent.[23,24]

To understand "modern nursing," the nurse's function and status, it should be stressed that nursing schools did not (like medical schools) originate in the universities. While there were apprenticeship training programs for nurses in a variety of settings in many countries, the independent Nightingale School of Nursing (with St. Thomas's Hospital in London used as its practice field) is generally considered the first true school of nursing. Established under the influence of Florence Nightingale, it reflected her philosophy. She was deeply religious and committed to the service of her fellow man. She thought the life of a nurse "the happiest of any." Like the Greeks, she trusted in cleanliness, fresh air. good food, rest, sleep, and (with less emphasis) exercise as support for nature's curative forces. She seems to have feared the physician's interference with nature and to have believed both physicians and nurses ignorant about the fundamentals of health. She decried their overriding interest in disease and their relative indifference to helping people achieve good health.[25] Mrs. Cecil Woodham-Smith,[26] whose biography of Florence Nightingale is one of the more definitive, concluded that her work in nursing was the greatest of all her contributions to society. She said Miss Nightingale saw nursing as helping people to live; she saw the body and soul as inseparable; she looked upon the patient as a member of a family and a community and upon nursing as an expression of the nurse's citizenship and religion. Florence Nightingale was a competent mathematician and statistician. She was one of the first to use health statistics as leverage in effecting health legislation for England and other parts of the British Empire. In this age, Miss Nightingale might have been called a sociologist and economist as well as a statistician.

Women who have shaped nursing since the Nightingale era have, like her, tended to emphasize the psychosocial aspects of nursing—to see nursing as significant in changing the social order. Ethel Bedford Fenwick in England and Lillian Wald, Lavinia Dock, and Annie W. Goodrich in the United States are examples of those who believed nursing to be a complex and creative social service growing out of the needs of contemporary society. Miss Goodrich entitled her collective works *The Social and Ethical Significance of Nursing.*[27] These women worked in the Women's Suffrage movement. Lillian Wald persuaded President Theodore Roosevelt to create the U.S. Children's Bureau, which, among other functions, controlled child labor.[28] Public health nurses (community nurses) have always considered the family rather than the individual as the patient, or client, and have responded to a wide range of social needs.[v] In recent years, psychiatric nurses have developed the psychosocial aspects of care to a high degree. Most nurses in many countries give at least lip service to the concept of family-centered health care.

While institutional nursing is often impersonal and may seem to be dominated by technological medicine, nursing as a whole has remained a service derived from the universal human needs of the very young, the helpless, and the sick. Certain branches of nursing have concentrated on health teaching, on promotion of health, and on prevention of disease.

The points made in the preceding historical review are the following:

Health care is an integral part of every culture or is affected by the philosophy and the social values of the culture. Looking at health care worldwide, all stages of its development can be found today, from the primitive to so-called "modern medicine." Both Occidental, or "Western medicine," and Oriental, or Eastern medicine, are derived from many cultures. Primitive and ancient practices may survive intact, they may be blended with newer methods, or they may subtly influence practice and the public image of the health worker. "Modern" Western medicine, while not even today free from the occult or from mysticism, derives from classic (Greek) medicine (according to Sigerist, from the Indo-Grecian culture), and has been, in certain countries, a university discipline since the Middle Ages. Western medicine in this age is based largely on the application of the physical sciences and is influenced to a high degree by institutional technology. Eastern medicine puts more emphasis on the totality of man and on the metaphysical aspects of treatment.

Nursing as a profession dates from the latter half of the nineteenth century, but generic nursing has existed in every culture. The founder of modern nursing and subsequent leaders have conceived of "professional" nursing as a social service with revolutionary capabilities. While influenced by its association with domestic service, with religious and military groups, and more recently with institutional technology, nursing remains essentially a nurturing, family-centered service. Nursing has based much of its practice on the application of the biologic sciences of physiology and bacteriology but, to a greater extent than medicine, on the social sciences—on psychology, human development, sociology, and economics. Nursing research is most often derived from the social sciences. While the following may be an oversimplification, it would seem that Western medicine has been focused on disease control and research in the physical and biologic sciences; nursing on meeting the human needs of the very young, the old, the sick, and the helpless, drawing on the psychosocial sciences in an effort to improve the lot of mankind. Nursing has been, more than has medicine, a substitute for self-care.

All health care in every culture is affected by the dominant religions or ethics, especially as they relate to the protection of the very young, the old, the sick, and the helpless. The World Health Organization has taken the position that health care is a universal right. Most nations are trying to achieve this goal. New categories of health workers have been created, and functions and responsibilities among established categories of health workers have been redistributed. The current emphasis in medicine on primary care and family practice and in nursing on physical assessment and clinical research suggests a trend toward overlapping functions, common goals and shared responsibility.

As both medicine and nursing emphasize prevention, and as doctors and nurses recognize the importance of self-help by the client or patient, the interdependence of physicians and nurses with health educators will be as apparent as the interdependence of physicians and nurses. Each society must answer the following questions: What should all citizens know about health? When should they learn it? Who should teach it? Where should it be taught?

Medicine, Nursing, Health Education, and Social Service

Assuming that promotion of health and prevention of disease are more important to human welfare and less costly to society than the cure of disease (both are generally conceded), it would seem that there is no limit to what the average citizen might profitably know about health promotion and disease prevention. However, people should not only know how to be healthy and avoid disease, but they *must want to be healthy*. Health must be valued—a sought after ideal or goal. Healthy habits must be acquired, and the earlier in life the better, for unhealthy habits are hard to break. The single most important condition in promoting health is that the individual *wants to be healthy.*

Knowledge of health is constantly unfolding, so, if the general public is to profit by the growing body of knowledge, people must continue to learn throughout the life span, and acquire the ability to change habitual behavior in applying new knowledge. The preceding statements suggest that there should be no fence around knowledge on which to base health practice, that acquiring this knowledge is a lifetime quest.

It is not easy to outline how to inculcate health values, goals, and ideals. Few persons of any schools of thought doubt that family, clan, tribal, or societal influences contribute toward the development of values, goals, and ideals. In childhood, individuals are most likely to adopt the values of parents; in adolescence, they accept the values of their age group or of adult role models; and later, they are more susceptible to the values of the social class to which they belong. Only in maturity are people relatively free to create a highly individualized pattern of behavior. These statements suggest that health motivation is a widely shared responsibility and that actions contributing to it pervade all aspects of life.

Promotion of health and prevention of disease are indeed everybody's business, as many have said. Mark Van Doren,[29] studying liberal education in 1943, concluded that health was one of its goals, that good health is characteristic of the "liberally" educated. Those who agree with him must see doctors and nurses and all other health workers as sharing with educators of all age groups the responsibility for teaching health promotion and disease prevention Carlson[30] and others suggest that a health dollar spent on education is more effective than one spent on medical care.

The word doctor comes from *docere*, meaning to teach, and some persons see teaching as the principal service the physician performs. John B. Dillon,[31] a physician, decries the overemphasis on research and technologic medicine and on specialization. Speaking of the reform in medical education stemming from Abraham Flexner's study, he says that Flexner considered prevention of disease through education of the public the physician's most important function and that he deeply regretted what happened to medical education in this century.

With the tendency toward specialization in American medicine and with the increasing importance attached to medical research, physicians have had less and less time to know their patients and to teach them, even in the unstudied manner of the family practitioner.[32,w] The inadequacy of the health care system, especially as it relates to disease prevention, is widely discussed. Most developed countries have organized or reorganized health care in recent decades, stressing its preventive aspects and giving the recipients of care more influence. James O. and Donna M. Hepner,[33] calling for reorganization of health care in the United States, refer to "the new consumerism."

Different countries provide health services for all citizens; for example, the system in the People's Republic of China, where military, industrial, and rural workers are trained to teach health, give preventive and remedial care, and to collaborate with more thoroughly trained professional nurses, doctors, and others, distributing the task of health education among a wide variety of workers; also the Russian network of health services, designed to bring preventive and remedial services to all citizens; and the nationalized health service of Great Britain. In Britain, one or more general medical practitioners, working with one or more district nurses, a health visitor, and a health officer, constitutes one of the building units for the national health service. These workers are available to every citizen of the area they serve, and they offer health education and preventive and remedial services.

In all these and other countries that have nearly eliminated a private fee-for-service system of medical care and established a tax-supported health service, preventive and curative services are available to all, and health teaching is an integral part of the service. In such national plans, the physician shares the responsibility for health teaching with other workers.

In the United States, some segments of the population have tax-supported health care that is preventive as well as remedial. There is a general trend toward universal health insurance, or prepaid preventive and remedial care. While the United States is almost, if not the only, developed country that does not have a national health program comparable to that of the British Isles or the (provincial) programs in Canada, in the USSR, mainland China, or the Scandinavian countries, it is generally believed that some plan of national health insurance will be adopted in the near future. When this happens, teaching people to be healthy and to avoid disease will be essential on economic as well as humane grounds.

The extent to which health workers have collaborated and should collaborate with teachers interested in health education in primary and secondary education is hard to assess. Many eminent health educators in the schools have been physicians; joint commissions, composed of members of national health organizations and national educational organizations, have provided guidelines for practice; physicians, nurses, and other health workers employed in school health and college health systems have tried, and are trying, to answer the questions, Who teaches what about health? To whom, and where?[x]

There has been a tendency in the past for physicians to think "a little knowledge [of medicine] is a dangerous thing"; a tendency to guard medical secrets, to expect patients to trust physicians to prescribe the right drug, the proper treatment. Nurses have been taught to refer to physicians any questions from patients on diagnosis, prognosis, or therapy. These beliefs and practices, limiting what was taught patients and who taught it, are now challenged. Books and journals about all major diseases written for the general public are available, as are films, television programs, and multisensory media of all sorts. Widely distributed "bills" listing the "rights of patients" include their right to be informed. Patients can and do bring suit against practitioners who treat them without explaining the purpose and the risks of treatment. It is no longer feasible for physicians, or any other therapists, to avoid educating patients, and with the kind of information now available to the general public, teaching must be increasingly sophisticated. Knowledge needed by a newspaper science editor to write a good article on open heart surgery, nuclear medicine, or treatment of leprosy may equal or exceed that of the average physician; the same statement might be made about producers of films and other multisensory teaching aids in the field of health. While the practice of medicine increases in complexity, the mysterious elements are disappearing, and the public is almost demanding that the sources of information be available to everybody.

Medical libraries have been traditionally open to physicians only. Gradually, they were opened to nurses and other health workers. Now, in the United States, medical libraries that accept funds from public sources must be open to the public.[y] Libraries in universities, once called "medical," are now called "health science libraries or information centers," and they serve the entire university community. Many persons believe all "medical" libraries (national, provincial, state, or local community) should be renamed to more accurately describe the scope of the contents and to invite the broadest possible usage.

There is an implication in what has been said so far that health may be promoted, disease prevented, cured, or controlled, if there are health workers and others to teach patients and their families and to give supportive care and remedial treatment. While these are the services stressed in this book, none is effective if patients or clients lack an adequate diet, shelter, and the other necessities of healthful living.[z] Many religious orders giving health care have provided a variety of social services; hospitals and other institutions employ social workers to help patients and their families with socioeconomic problems and in some countries, in certain eras, nurses, particularly those in community nursing, were prepared for both nursing and social work. Family physicians were once, in a more personal culture, also friends and often helped a family alter living conditions so that recovery from disease was possible. The advice of the family physician was sought on many social problems. With the development of district, public health, or community nursing, families have had the same sort of help from nurses in coping with social problems, and some private duty nurses have played the same role.

In the United States, the interdependence of the various aspects is recognized in the title of a single department within the federal government—the Department of Health, Education, and Welfare. In states and local communities, there may not be this structural unity but joint committees or commissions and planning boards may attempt coordination of services. While physicians, dentists, nurses, social workers, clinical psychologists, health educators, and other health workers must concentrate their energies on performance of their respective functions, their efforts may be relatively ineffective if they work in isolation and are unconcerned with other aspects of health care. Critics of health care available in the United States see a lack of planning, inadequate coordination, overlapping functions among workers, and unfulfilled needs of the people. Critics also say that health care imposes an unsupportable burden on most families. Contemporary articles on health care suggest a rapidly changing scene with terms such as ferment, crisis, chaos, transition, conflicting roles, emerging concepts, issues, new directions, and a new era appearing in titles of books and articles.[34–42]

The importance of flexibility is stressed so that in each age, in each place, health needs of people may be served most effectively with resources available. No plan that sacrifices the welfare of the receivers of care to those who give it or the other way around will be tolerated by a society indefinitely.[aa]

It may seem that, for a book about nursing, undue attention has been paid so far to the practice of medicine and the practice of teaching. The next topic to be discussed is the definition of nursing and the function of the nurse. Before discussing this subject, it seems important to emphasize nursing's close relationship to medicine particularly; to point out that the functions of doctors and nurses have differed from one era to another, have often overlapped, and in some cases have been combined; and to stress that nursing, as a profession, is much younger and less established than medicine. The public image of the nurse has been less prestigious than that of the physician, but not in all eras less sympathetic.

It has been suggested in the preceding pages that teaching is inherent in both medicine and nursing, that promoting health and preventing disease is largely a matter of teaching, and that even remedial medicine depends for its efficacy upon the informed self-help of patients and their families. The functions, roles, and responsibilities of health workers and health educators are described as interdependent; coordinated planning is essential if the goal of an effective health service for all citizens is to be reached. Every community, state, and nation is trying to establish its health goals, assess its resources, and develop the services essential to the realization of its health objectives. This process of cooperative planning is much more established and more effective in some countries than in others. It can drastically change the functions and relationships of health workers with patients, and with each other.[43–47]

Regardless of the rapidly changing scene, it is helpful to review efforts in the past to define nursing and to also give the *working definition of nursing* on which the content of this book is based. The following definition, as expressed in a booklet, *ICN Basic Principles of Nursing*,[bb] has been accepted by the International Council of Nurses as its working definition of nursing. The heart of this definition, which will be discussed in more detail later, is as follows:

> Nursing is primarily assisting individuals (sick or well) with those activities contributing to health, or its recovery (or to a peaceful death) that they perform unaided when they have the necessary strength, will, or knowledge; nursing also helps individuals carry out prescribed therapy and to be independent of assistance as soon as possible.

Health care should be considered as a whole, even though working definitions of the roles of each class of practitioners are useful, in fact, necessary. Health workers must be generalists as well as specialists. Nursing can never be defined for all time and for all ages and without reference to the roles and numbers of physicians and medical technicians, dentists and dental hygienists, social workers, pharmacists, physical therapists, health educators, sanitarians, clinical psychologists, and others. In every age, every community, and every health agency, an attempt should be made to understand and cope with the over-all problem of providing health care. The services needed and the numbers and competences of available workers should determine what each does. The resulting plan may demand a willingness on the part of all those concerned to forget traditional roles to some extent, to abrogate privileges, and to share functions and responsibilities.[cc]

Defining Nursing and the Function of the Nurse

Some Definitions of Nursing and Nurses by Individuals from the Nightingale Era to the Present

Nurses, physicians, and others have been defining nursing for many years. Florence Nightingale seems to have looked upon both physicians and nurses (if they functioned effectively) as nature's colleagues. In the conclusion of her small volume, *Notes on Nursing, What It Is and What It Is Not,* she makes the following statement:

It is often thought that medicine is the curative process. It is no such thing: medicine is the surgery of functions, as surgery proper is that of limbs and organs. Neither can do anything but remove obstructions; neither can cure; nature alone cures. Surgery removes the bullet out of the limb, which is an obstruction to cure, but nature heals the wound. So it is with medicine: the function of an organ becomes obstructed; medicine, so far as we know, assists nature to remove the obstruction, but does nothing more. *And what nursing has to do in either case, is to put the patient in the best condition for nature to act upon him.*[dd] [italics ours]

Nightingale thought all disease "at some period or other of its course, . . . a reparative process, not necessarily accompanied with suffering. . . ."[ee] The writer has heard nurses of this era say that they thought the Nightingale definition of 1860 the most helpful. In any event, the Nightingale philosophy dominated nursing well into the twentieth century. She is regarded as a genius by nurses and nonnurses alike, and her concept of the body as self-healing is generally accepted today.

With the evolution of medical science, development and proliferation of medical and nursing schools, and enactment of medical and nursing legislation, definitions of medicine and nursing that would clearly differentiate the practice of doctors and nurses were needed, although each was referred to as an art rather than a science until recently. W. S. Thayer, an eminent physician, referred in 1919 to medicine as an art, and said, "it is difficult to overstate the contribution of the trained nurse." He spoke of the nurse's function as "wholly complementary' [to medicine] and said that without the nurse "the proper practice of the art of therapy is inconceivable."[ff]

Sir William Osler, speaking to nurses, commented on the "art of nursing" and its roots in prehistoric practices. He said:

Nursing as an art to be cultivated, as a profession to be followed, is modern: nursing as a practice originated in the dim past, when some mother among the cave-dwellers cooled the forehead of her sick child with water from the brook, or first yielded to the prompting to leave a well-covered bone and a handful of meal by the side of a wounded man left in the hurried flight before an enemy.[gg]

In 1934, writing about the nature of nursing, Effie J. Taylor accepted the idea that it was "adapting prescribed therapy and preventive treatment to the specific physical and psychic needs of the individual." However, she said "The real depths of nursing can only be made known through ideals, love, sympathy, knowledge. and culture, expressed through the practice of artistic procedures and relationships."[hh]

In 1946, Annie W. Goodrich published the following statement that stressed the nurse as an activator of medical and social sciences. She suggested the range of service but seemed to accept the idea that the nurse was "directed" by a "qualified" instructor. In the following paragraph, the reader is left wondering who gave this direction:

> Nursing is that expression of social activities that seeks under qualified instruction and direction to interpret through action the findings of the medical and social sciences in relation to bodily ills, their care, cure and prevention, including all factors, personal and environmental, that bear upon the achievement of the desired objective, a healthy citizenry.[ii]

Following World War II, there was a demand for a reevaluation of the nurse's function. J. C. Meakins, a Canadian physician, joined the chorus with an article entitled "Nursing Must Be Defined."[48]

In 1947, Esther Lucile Brown, who was conducting a nationwide investigation of nursing in the United States, asked a nationally selected committee of nurses to produce a statement on the "probable nature of nursing in the latter half of this century." She cited it as follows in her report, *Nursing for the Future*:

> . . . the professional nurse will be one who recognizes and understands the fundamental [health] needs of a person, sick or well, and who knows how these needs can best be met. She will possess a body of scientific nursing knowledge which is based upon and keeps pace with general scientific advancement, and she will be able to apply this knowledge in meeting the nursing needs of a person and a community. She must possess that kind of discriminative judgment which will enable her to recognize those activities which fall within the area of professional nursing and those activities which have been identified with the fields of other professional or nonprofessional groups.[jj]

While this statement suggests a vital role for nursing, it fails to specify the difference between nursing and other health services. The phrases "health needs," "nursing needs," and "how these needs can best be met" must be explained if the statement is to help readers who are trying to differentiate between the practice of nursing and other medical arts and sciences.

During the late 1940s, an advanced course in medical-surgical nursing at Teachers College, Columbia University, in New York City, was organized around common nursing problems (for example, adapting care to age needs and to preoperative and postoperative states or the communicability of the patient's disease) rather than around diseases of body systems, which was at that time the common pattern. In the fifth edition of *The Principles and Practice of Nursing*, Part V was entitled "Common Problems in Nursing Practice," and an explanation was given of this problem-solving approach.[kk] In 1951, R. Louise McManus, in a study emanating from Teachers College, Columbia University, offered the following definition of nursing function:

> . . . the unique function of the professional nurse may be . . . : (1) the identification or diagnosis of the nursing problem and the recognition of its interrelated aspects, (2) deciding upon a course of nursing actions to be followed for the solution of the problem, in light of immediate and long-term objectives of nursing, with regard to prevention of illness, direct care, rehabilitation, and promotion of highest standards of health possible for the individual.[ll]

In 1960, Faye G. Abdellah and her associates published *Patient-Centered Approaches to Nursing*,[49] which presented 21 problems as a foundation on which to build a nursing program; in 1970, Mae M. Johnson and Mary Lou C. Davis presented a text on method entitled *Problem Solving in Nursing Practice*.[50] Parenthetically, since 1970, Lawrence L. Weed has promoted the "problem-oriented" approach to medical practice, including medical records. Many nurses have participated in this movement and adapted their records accordingly. While the problem approach has been gaining acceptance by teachers of nursing and the importance of nursing research has been recognized, the hunt for a satisfying definition of nursing goes on.

Between 1953 and 1955, the writer visited 27 states interviewing nurses, student nurses, physicians, social scientists, and others to find out what studies of nursing and nurses had been made in these states and what studies were thought needed. In answer to the second question, the usual response was "Investigations to more clearly establish the function of the nurse."[51]

In 1961, Ida Jean Orlando, in connection with a USPHS-funded "project" on integrating mental health with other aspects of the basic curriculum, published *The Dynamic Nurse–Patient Relationship*. In discussing the "task of the professional nurse," she differentiated between *nursing* [a cold] and *doctoring* [a cold]. The latter, she thought, implied using "the products of medical science—pills, inhalers and the like." She made the following statement:

> The *purpose of nursing is to supply the help a patient requires in order for his needs to be met.* The nurse achieves her purpose by initiating a *process* [italics ours] which ascertains the patient's immediate need and helps to meet the need directly or indirectly. She meets it directly when the patient is unable to meet his own need; indirectly when she helps him obtain the services of a person, agency, or resource by which his need can be met.
>
> The nurse, in achieving her purpose contributes simultaneously to the mental and physical health of her patient. This is so because in helping him she affects for the better his sense of adequacy or wellbeing. These may be small changes but they are helpful at the moment and may have cumulative value. Nursing in its professional character does not add to the distress of the patient. Instead the nurse assumes the professional responsibility of seeking out and obviating impediments to the patient's mental and physical comfort. In order for the nurse to develop and maintain the professional character of her work she must know and be able to validate how her actions and reactions help or do not help the patient or know and be able to validate that the patient does not require her help at a given time.[mm]

Orlando's description of nursing as a *process* has had wide acceptance. Her insistence that nurses ask patients to confirm or correct their (the nurses') perceptions of patients' needs has also had wide acceptance as part of the "nursing process." Validating the effect of nursing is also accepted as part of the process.[nn]

Margaret M. Lamb, who was at the time chairman of the General Nursing Council for Scotland, asked in 1970 "Nursing Is What?" and answered the question in part by saying that:

> The nurse exists . . . to nourish or cherish the patient. . . . The bulk of nursing is physical care. . . . I submit that nursing yesterday, today and tomorrow is caring for people and that unless it is built on an ideal of service to others it is built on shifting sand. . . .[oo]

M. L. Badouaille,[52] a New Zealand nurse, explained in 1973 why she thought nursing was "different" from other health services. If time and space allowed citations of books and articles from around the world, it would be apparent that there is a universal and continuing effort to define nursing.

Most recently, definitions of nursing have tended to stress the nurse's interest in health promotion, in contrast with the cure of disease. Rozella M. Schlotfeldt in 1972 wrote as follows:

> My purpose here is to set forth a straightforward and unambiguous conceptualization of nursing in terms of the profession's goal and the phenomena with which nurses must be concerned if they are to fulfill their social responsibilities. Simply stated, *the goal of nursing as a field of professional endeavor is to help people attain, retain, and regain health.* The phenomena with which nurses are concerned are man's health-seeking and coping behaviors as he strives to attain health. Nurses are independent, professional practitioners whose field of work is health care.[pp]

Marjorie Ramphal, as president, addressing the ANA's Congress on Nursing Practice, made this statement in her summary:

> The goal of nursing is to help the patient, as needed, in pursuit of his goal of behavioral integrity. Behavioral integrity means that the patient's interrelated behavioral patterns directed toward fulfilling major needs result and are likely to continue to result in biological, psychological and social health.[qq]

In a pamphlet published in 1976 by the National League for Nursing, Shirley Chater, a nurse educator, gave the following definition of nursing as compared with medical practice:

> Nursing is a process through which *care* is provided to individuals, families, or community groups *primarily* around circumstances and situations that arise from health-related problems. Medical practice, on the other hand, is primarily cause- and cure-oriented. It is important in the above definition to stress the word *primarily*, for settings, numbers, and other circumstances can change the degree of overlapping functions between the nursing and medical professions. For instance, in remote areas nurses often come closer to practicing medicine than nursing. Similarly, a physician may sit beside his patient in the recovery room caring for the subtle circumstances that arise during the postoperative course, practicing something more akin to nursing than to medicine.[rr]

There is a consensus that nursing function, like all other aspects of health service, should derive from the needs of the patients, or clients. Janet M.

Kraegel and her associates,[53] studying the appropriate use of nurses at St. Mary's Hospital, Milwaukee, Wisconsin (under a USPHS grant), identified 22 "patient needs" and classified them as physical, socio-psychological, and environmental. They showed how the structure and organization of a patient care unit could be organized around these needs.

While the call for a definition of nursing has been loud and clear, some persons think too much time and energy have been devoted to a question that answers itself. For example, Frances Storlie, an American nurse, writing in 1970, expressed the following opinion: "Nursing need never be defined. . . . The danger of definition is loss of mystery, loss of aura, and diminishing beauty. The substance of nursing will resist being reduced to so-called facts no matter how precise the research."[55]

The foregoing definitions of nursing by individuals that have been cited are just a few of those that might be included. Definitions used in official and legal documents, discussed in the following pages, may have, in the last analysis, more effect on nursing practice than the opinions of individuals, although they too must be arrived at by a consensus of individuals.

Some Definitions of Nursing and Nurses by Organizations

Organizations have found it necessary to define nursing for many reasons. Internationally, nationally, and by state and province, nurses have sought cooperation based on a definition of the nature of nursing, on an ethical code, on legislation, and on the scope of practice, or on nursing curricula.

The International Council of Nurses has based its membership on the assumption that in each country represented in the Council there was an association of "trained nurses" whose constitution and by-laws were "in harmony with those of the Council."[tt] The Council stands for self-government by nurses in their associations. At first it was assumed that "a trained nurse" meant the same thing worldwide, but it was soon apparent that this was not so. With the development of *nurse registration* in the United States, the international effort to define nursing can be traced in Daisy Caroline Bridges' *A History of the International Council of Nurses, 1899–1964,*[54] in its official journal, the *International Nursing Review* and in reports of ICN Congresses.

The following definition of "a nurse" was adopted by the ICN's Council of Nurse Representatives in 1975.

A nurse is a person who has completed a programme of basic nursing education and is qualified and authorized in her/his country to practice nursing. Basic nursing education is a formally recognised programme of study which provides a broad and sound foundation for the practice of nursing and for post-basic education which develops specific competency. At the first level, the educational programme prepares the nurse, through study of behavioral, life and nursing sciences and clinical experience, for effective practice and direction of nursing care, and for the leadership role. The first-level nurse [professional nurse] is responsible for planning, providing and evaluating nursing care in all settings for the promotion of health, prevention of illness, care of the sick and rehabilitation; and functions as a member of the health team. In countries with more than one level of nursing personnel, the second-level programme prepares the nurse, through study of nursing theory and clinical practice, to give nursing care in co-operation with and under the supervision of a first-level nurse.[uu]

Efforts within the ICN to keep the definition of a nurse sufficiently explicit to have meaning and sufficiently general to make it possible for countries with different patterns of nurse education to be members of the Council have persisted.

In 1973, the Council of National Representatives (CUR) of the ICN approved the following statements on the "professional nurse" and the "auxiliary nurse" to be forwarded to the International Labor Organization in hopes that it would use them in its next edition of the *International Standard Classification of Occupations*:

Workers in this unit group [professional nurses] assist individuals, families, groups and communities in the promotion and preservation of health as well as contributing to recovery and rehabilitation in illness.

They participate in the development and implementation of the therapeutic and educational plans of the health team.

Their functions include: (1) carrying out the therapeutic programme, including personal services concerned with hygiene and comfort as they cover the range of basic human needs; (2) creating and maintaining a physical and psychological environment, conducive to health improvement, convalescence, recovery, or the achievement of a dignified death; (3) enlisting the interest of the patient and his family in seeking the conditions necessary to attain recovery, rehabilitation and optimal self-maintenance; (4) counseling people, sick and well, in measures promoting physical, mental and social well-being; (5) instituting measures of, and encouraging the pursuit of, disease prevention; (6) developing goals for nursing activities and coordinating them with those of all other members of the health team in order to achieve the broadest health care benefits for those involved; (7) participating in the teaching of nursing and other health personnel; (8) assisting in the administration of the delivery of health care in institutional or community settings.

[Professional nurses] have successfully completed a recognized nursing education programme qualifying them to be registered or licensed as a nurse by the appropriate authority.

. . . the professional nurse, specialized [is] one who provides specialized nursing in a particular branch of nursing practice: consultation, administration, teaching or research, applied to nursing; has recognized preparation in the field of specialization.

Auxiliary nurses . . . provide care which does not require the training and theoretical knowledge of a professional nurse. They work in an organized health service which provides guidance and supervision.[vv]

The passage of a Nurse Practice Act in each state began when laws were enacted by New Jersey, New York, North Carolina, and Virginia. Such acts incorporate statements on the function of the nurse, or the nature and scope of nursing practice. The ANA, through its Council of State Boards, has defined nursing and constructed model Nurse Practice Acts. In 1937, the following definition of nursing, published by the ANA, is reflected even today in Nurse Practice Acts:

A blend of intellectual attainment, attitudes and mental skills based upon the principles of scientific medicine acquired by means of a prescribed course in a school of nursing affiliated with a hospital, recognized by the state and practiced in conjunction with curative and preventive medicine by an individual licensed to do so by the state.[ww]

Other definitions, such as that in the 1937 *A Curriculum Guide for Schools of Nursing,*[55] said that nursing was, in effect, helping people to keep well, or regain their health when ill. Although these definitions were, in a sense, official definitions, there is considerable evidence that they were neither specific nor broad enough to satisfy everyone.

During the 1950s, the American Nurses' Association spent $400,000 studying the functions of the nurse. Twenty-one separate studies in 17 states were reported by Everett C. Hughes and his associates in *Twenty Thousand Nurses Tell Their Story.*[56] While this exhaustive nationwide study threw light on what nurses were doing (one study identified more than 400 activities) and what nurses themselves and the public then thought of the nurse, it failed to define nursing to everybody's satisfaction. People have continued to ask what is unique about nursing and what is the function of the nurse.

In 1967, the National Commission for the study of Nursing and Nursing Education, organized by the American Nurses' Association and the National League for Nursing, began its work under grants from the Mellon (then Avalon) and Kellogg Foundations and an anonymous donor. It continued its work under continued support from these and additional sources. In its first major publication, *An Abstract for Action,* Jerome P. Lysaught reviewed the development of nursing in America and noted the relationship of nursing and medical care. He seemed to think that the development of "nursing science" is "retarded," that "nursing has many miles to go before it can reach full professional status."[xx] While recognizing that nursing had a unique role, no one definition seems to be favored in the Commission's report. Recommendations in this report and the subsequent papers published as a volume under the title *Action in Nursing: Progress in Professional Purpose*[57] (1974) emphasize throughout the importance of the nurse's role, on unity of purpose among nurses, on essential steps in becoming a full-blown profession, on the necessity of assuming the responsibilities of a profession but, at the same time, cooperating with other categories of health workers.

Not only in the Commission's report but in many critiques of health care, there is increasing recognition of overlapping roles of nurses, physicians, and others (discussed later in more detail) and of the importance of legislation that permits overlapping roles. In 1972, a Joint Commission on Practice with representatives of the ANA and the AMA was appointed. It is funded by the two associations and the W. K. Kellogg Foundation. A study of Nurse Practice Acts and Medical Practice Acts was initiated by the Joint Commission. In the report *Statutory Regulation of the Scope of Nursing Practice—A Critical Survey,*"[58] Virginia Hall, an attorney, seemed to conclude that nurses were then practicing medicine, as so defined, as well as nursing, as so defined, and that they must continue to do so if the needs of the public are to be met. In any event, Hall instanced and commented on the varying definitions in Nurse Practice Acts and suggested that instead of modifying existing Nurse Practice Acts, an over-all solution might be to exempt professional nurses from the prohibition against the practice of medicine in Medical Practice Acts.

It is safe to say that in no other era has there been such wide disagreement on the definition of nursing and the function of the nurse.[yy]

The effort to differentiate between the practice of nursing and other health practices and to differentiate between nursing research and other health-related research has led to a study of nursing "theory" and nursing "concepts." The following is a brief review of some efforts along these lines. Nursing conferences in past decades tended to focus on function, and later on research. In recent years they were more apt to deal with theory and concepts. Curricula are planned to reflect a particular philosophy on, or concept of, nursing.

Philosophies, Concepts, Theories, and Systems Underlying Definitions of Nursing and the Function of the Nurse

All health services are influenced by prevailing philosophies or cultural values, by political environments in which they exist. Nursing, like all other health services, is affected by attitudes toward sex, age, color, race, religious beliefs, physical fitness, intellectual ability, creative ability, educational achievement, self-expression, self-discipline, equality of opportunity, respect for authority, and respect for life—human and nonhuman. To be specific, a culture that values the young more than the old is likely to provide better health care for infants and children than for the aged and dying; a society committed to equal opportunity is more likely to make health service universally available than one that is not; a people who look for reward in an afterlife may put less emphasis on health care than one that looks for its respect on this earth; and a culture committed to protecting animal and insect life has a different system of health care (including diet) from one that makes the welfare of other forms of life dependent on what that particular culture believes best for humans.

Some nurse educators, nurse researchers, and others have emphasized the importance of identifying goals or stating the philosophy underlying nursing. Mildred A. E. Newton's study, *Florence Nightingale's Philosophy of Life and Education* (Ed.D. dissertation, Stanford University, Palo Alto, Calif., 1949), showed the extent to which her values affected nursing for many years; the *Curriculum Guide*,[59] prepared under the sponsorship of the National League of Nursing Education in 1937, stressed educational philosophy; its proposed curriculum was dominated by the concept of adaptation as an educational goal. In 1962, Sister Madeleine Clémence Vaillot[60] discussed existentialism as a philosophy of commitment and its meaning for her in nursing.[zz] Other examples might be given to show that throughout its history nursing has identified its philosophic base. There is, however, considerable evidence that the *insistence* on identifying philosophy, concepts, theories, or systems in which nursing operates is new. Of 1464 master's theses and papers written between 1930 and 1955, there were only a few that dealt with philosophic, political, cultural, or ethnic questions.[61] Martha M. Brown,[62] a nurse reporting a study in 1969 on "nurses, patients, and social systems," makes the categorical statement that, conceptually, nursing is a "primitive discipline." The profession is, perhaps, overly sensitive to such criticism. In any event, faculties of schools of nursing seeking accreditation know they had better state the philosophy or the concept of nursing on which they base their curricula, and research proposals must often embody a philosophic statement, a concept or theory of nursing. National regional conferences focus on such topics, as do journal articles and full-length books.[63-78]

Theory comes from the Greek *theōria*, a beholding, spectacle, contemplation, speculation. Webster's gives six meanings other than these, but the following is the sense in which it is used here:

> The general or abstract principles of any body of facts real or assumed; pure, as distinguished from applied, science or art: as, the *theory* of music or of medicine.

Ernest Nagle[79] calls a theory "an intellectual tool." Using it in this sense, the following questions must be asked: Has nursing, as distinct from other branches of health practice, "a body of facts real or assumed?" Is research in nursing from which such a body of facts would be derived, different in content and method from research in health education, in psychology, chemistry, physics, physiology, pathology, microbiology? Medicine, interpreted as diagnosis and therapy—whose research might be assumed to most closely resemble nursing research—not only borrows from all these sciences but collaborates in its research with scientists in these fields. This idea of borrowing from other fields seems to be rejected by some nurses. Gean Mathwig says:

> . . . I endorse the philosophy that by definition of a profession, the theoretical knowledge of a profession evolves from that profession. . . .
> . . . the theoretical core of nursing knowledge evolves not from administration, anthropology, biology, psychology, sociology, nor any other discipline, but rather from the field of nursing per se.[A]

Florence Wald, a nurse, and Robert Leonard, a sociologist,[80] described the development of "nursing practice theory" as distinct from the theory of practice in any other health field.

M. Isabel Harris accepted the definition of theory as a "more or less plausible or scientific acceptable principle to explain phenomena." She saw it as "a conceptual structure built for a purpose"[B] which, in nursing, was practice. She traced the development of nursing theory from Florence Nightingale in whose writings she thought theory *implicit*; she thought *explicit* theory recent.

Rosemary Ellis discussed the characteristics of a significant theory and said it was "one that enlightens us about the patient and what happens to him."[C] She said *studies of nurses* might or might not contribute to the development of significant theories for nursing, and she proposed that practitioners were the theorists in nursing.

Imogene M. King reviewed the literature, "synthesized ideas," and concluded that "the essential characteristics of nursing were those properties that had persisted in spite of environmental changes." She said, "If nursing is a science, then the body of knowledge taught, learned, and used by professional nurses is characterized by certainty, structure and generalizations."[D] (She thought these the characteristics of science.)

King presented a series of diagrams to clarify her concepts of how nurses work with individuals, groups, and social systems to help individuals and groups "attain, maintain, and restore health." In the following definition of nursing, King seems to synthesize the positions of Virginia Henderson, Ida Orlando, Hildegard Peplau, and Martha E. Rogers:

> Nursing is a process of action, reaction, interaction and transaction whereby nurses assist individuals of any age and socioeconomic group to meet their basic needs in performing activities of daily living and to cope with health and illness at some particular point in the life cycle.[E]

Margaret A. Newman made the following statement about nursing theory, implying that the borrowing phase is over:

> Nursing theory has evolved through several phases: borrowing theory from other disciplines; analyzing nursing practice situations to seek conceptual relationships; and developing a conceptual framework.[F]

Dorothy E. Johnson took another position in a paper entitled "Theory in Nursing: Borrowed and Unique." She said:

It is extremely hazardous to attempt to differentiate between borrowed and unique theory in nursing. It is hazardous first of all because the man-made, more or less arbitrary division between the sciences is neither firm nor constant. It appears there is an essential unit in knowledge, corresponding to a unity in nature, which defies established boundaries, and continuously presses for the larger, more cohesive view. Moreover, knowledge does not innately "belong" to any field of science. It is not exactly happenstance that a given bit of knowledge is discovered by one discipline rather than another, but the fact of discovery does not confer the right of ownership. Viewed in this light borrowed and unique have no real permanence, nor any real meaning.[G]

(Johnson's position on theory in nursing seems eminently reasonable to the writer and it is one with which she concurs.)

It seems to be useful to many persons to express concepts of nursing schematically—as systems. For instance, Martha Rogers[81] used the coiled spring to express the concept of continuing change, continuing interaction between the nurse and the client. College courses are built around the idea of systems analysis, and almost any activity can be diagrammed as either a closed or open system.[82,83] Ludwig Avon Bertalanffy made the following distinction between open and closed systems:

From the physical point of view, the characteristic state of the living organism is that of an open system. A system is closed if no material enters or leaves it; it is open if there is import and export and, therefore, change of the components. Living systems are open systems, maintaining themselves in exchange of materials with environment, and in continuous building up and breaking down of their components.[H]

Reference has been made to King's diagrammatic exposition of nursing theory as a system. Kraegel and her associates reported a study at St. Mary's Hospital, Milwaukee, Wisconsin, in which the management of patient care was revised to meet basic human needs. The plan was described and diagrammed as a system."[84,85]

The following are some of the *concepts* of the registered nurse that have been discussed during this century:

The professional registered nurse is (1) nature's helper in restoring the body to health; (2) a mother substitute—the professional mother; (3) the physician's assistant in caring for the ill and preventing disease; (4) the physician's complement—the physician concentrating on *cure*, the nurse on *care*; (5) a substitute for the physician; (6) a coordinator of the services of all health workers; (7) a manipulator of the environment and a trainer and director of personnel with less preparation than that of the professional nurse; (8) a health educator; (9) someone who, through the nursing process, enables the client or patient to make the best use of health resources; (10) someone who applies "nursing science" for the betterment of mankind; (11) someone who "intervenes" in the client's or patient's behalf in a crisis or time of need; (12) the patient's and family's helper in meeting their health needs[86-100]

These concepts are not mutually exclusive. Many persons would combine two or more in giving their idea of a nurse. In the United States, Canada, and some other countries, all nurses are, at least theoretically, health educators as well as caregivers. In England, a health visitor is a community nurse who is primarily a health educator, while a district nurse is primarily a caregiver. Many persons recognize the overlapping functions of professional nurses and physicians and admit that nurses, especially public health nurses, have always been substitutes for the physician in situations where the latter's services were unavailable.

Throughout this chapter, the concept of a physician as a healer or a worker interested in cure of disease has been stressed, as has been the concept of the nurse as a caretaker or as a worker more interested than the physician in promoting health. However, if health workers listen to current criticism of medical care or health care, or if they note the growth of the self-help movement, the concept of what constitutes "good" health care might change radically, and with it, the concept of the way nurses and physicians function.[101-107] At present, their respective functions are overlapping, confused, and sometimes in conflict with those of other health workers.

The Overlapping and Collaborative Roles of Nurses, Physicians, and Other Health Workers

Some people see nurses and physicians as having separate and distinct functions; others see both as responding to the health needs of individuals in every situation according to the worker's particular competence and according to competences of the health manpower available. While the latter view has always influenced health care, there seems to be more discussion of the relationship of nursing and medicine now than in the past, and since the demand for health service is mounting, the question is increasingly critical.

The prevailing point of view is that health care should be universally available. In most people's minds this entails periodic visits to (or from) health workers from conception to the grave. Illich[108] thinks that this concept makes "patients" of well people throughout life and prevents development of "normal" or desirable self-reliance. Others might concur in this opinion, but the trend toward spending more and more of the gross national product (GNP) on health has not been reversed nor has the trend toward developing more and more categories of workers. Physicians seem to be increasingly willing for nurses and others to assume a greater share of responsibility for health assessment, for supervision of "well" children and the chronically ill, and for almost total care of the aged. While some physicians seem to want to claim that they "supervise" nurses in all these roles, others believe this is neither practical nor desirable and are willing for nurses to be legally, and in every other way, accountable for their practice even though it encompasses functions that are generally considered the domain of medicine.

The question of the overlapping roles of doctors, physician's assistants, feldshers, nurses, and other health workers is apparent in the discussions at two recent conferences with an international focus. One was in England, the report of which is entitled *The Greater Medical Profession,*[109] and the other was in the United States, the report of which is *Intermediate-Level Health Practitioners.*[110] The overlapping functions of private medical practitioners, health officers, nurses (district nurses, health visitors, and nurse-midwives), and social workers is seen in the British publication *The Health Team in Action*[111]—a series of essays based on a BBC television program. Overlapping functions are apparent in many British publications, a few of which are listed among the references for this chapter.[112-116]

In Canada, nurses, physicians, and others are studying the function of the nurse. Under the sponsorship of the Department of National Health and Welfare, a study has been in progress on the function of the nurse since 1971. Doctors, nurses, and others are making task analyses in six universities of nursing practice, particularly that in Northern outposts. The resulting documents clearly show the extent to which nurses carry out diagnostic and therapeutic procedures that traditionally lie within the province of medicine. (The Canadian study is discussed in more detail under the next subhead—"The Nurse as Therapist (The Extended Role)."[117-123]

In the People's Republic of China, health care has undergone radical revision. There "barefoot" and "Red Guard doctors" (workers with far less preparation than registered nurses in the United States or feldshers in Russia) are in factories, rural communes, and elsewhere assuming responsibility for diagnosing and treating minor diseases and ailments. Many observers report the health program (which involves continuing education of all workers) strikingly effective in many respects.[124-126]Almost as striking are the accomplishments in Russia, although the system is quite different from that in the People's Republic of China. Feldshers and midwives in the health services of the USSR function in many situations as would physicians if they were present. Nurses in Russia seem to have less autonomy and are more likely to work with physicians who play the major role in determining what they are taught and how they function.[127-129]

While the accomplishments of Red Guard and barefoot "doctors" in the People's Republic of China and those of feldshers in the USSR as "physician extenders" seem striking, there is evidence from many quarters that health progress can be achieved under many systems when health is the goal of the people, when the people are involved, and when environmental conditions essential to health are understood and there is a common effort to bring them about. The report of a joint study by UNICEF and WHO describes programs in Bangladesh, Cuba, India, Niger, Nigeria, People's Republic of China, Tanzania, Venezuela, and Yugoslavia. Most of them are characterized by combining native (often ancient) systems of medicine with contemporary Western medicine, emphasizing health education and the development of self-reliance. Representatives of the community, usually chosen by the people, are prepared to give primary care; a community council is involved in making and implementing a plan for improved living conditions and developing self-reliance in health and other aspects of social welfare. The point is made in the report that "Organizing the delivery of health care so that part of it 'belongs' to those it is designed to serve has enormous advantages."[1] The primary caregivers are known to and trusted by the people they serve. They share the lot of the people and often toil with them in farming or other manual labor.

In summary, if health care is studied internationally, it is clear that not only do doctors' and nurses' roles overlap but that the roles of both are filled by a wide variety of workers. Nevertheless, the extended (or expanded) role of the nurse is the most widely discussed topic in nursing meetings and in nursing journals. The following is an attempt to suggest the nature and range of the discussion, especially in the United States and Canada.

The Nurse as Therapist (The Extended Role)

While the term "extended" or "expanded" role is new, some people maintain that the "trained" nurse of the Nightingale era often functioned in this capacity as it is now described and that some doctors then treated nurses as collaborators rather than as "hand-maidens" as is so often implied by critics of the doctor–nurse relationship. Private duty nurses, caring for patients in their homes, undoubtedly worked in partnership with physicians. It is interesting to find in a 1902 directory of trained nurses in four major cities of the Eastern seaboard an article by a doctor on the ideal nurse and another on what doctors "owe trained nurses."[130] A 1923 directory lists, in one small pamphlet, the nurses and physicians of New Haven County, Connecticut.[131]

The extended role involves assessing clients' health status, diagnosing, and prescribing treatment or giving primary care, which means admitting clients or patients to the health care system. Barbara G. Schutt,[132] in 1972, reviewed the history of "primary care nursing" and concluded that nurses have always been "in the primary care business but haven't cared to talk about it." She noted the following terms used for nurses giving primary care in 1972: pediatric nurse practitioner[j]; pediatric nurse associate; family nurse practitioner (PRIMEX); clinical associate (of the family physician); adult health practitioner; medical nurse practitioner; nurse midwife; nurse practitioner. To these might now be added psychiatric nurse practitioner, geriatric nurse practitioner, school nurse practitioner, and industrial nurse practitioner. "Clinical specialist" and "nurse clinician" are other terms used to denote postbasic preparation that prepares the worker for the extended role.[K]

Schutt studied the Frontier Nursing Service in Kentucky, noting that its staff had been giving primary health care for 40 years.[133] As evidence of this, the nurse-midwifery service there delivered its first 1000 babies with only one death,[134] which is a demonstration of excellent primary maternal and newborn care. Although the Frontier Nursing Service operates under *Medical Directives* (7th ed., the Service, Wendover, KY, 1975), which can be interpreted as delegation of authority from medical advisers or consultants, it is clear that its staff nurses have, since the inception of the Service, been functioning independently in giving primary care.[L]

It bears repeating that the functions of all health workers vary from place to place and from one decade to another. Their functions depend on the public's concept of health, what it expects from trained workers, the numbers and varieties of workers available, and the services they are prepared to give. No category of workers can be considered in isolation. The report of a 1976 international conference on nursing contains the following statements:

> . . . the legal and professional problems inherent in the changing role of nursing have recently been . . . the subject of close study in collaboration with other health disciplines at the policy level.
>
> The part played by nurses has expanded . . . professional nurses have been taking over some of the duties traditionally reserved for the doctor.
>
> . . . summary definitions [of nursing] seem inadequate since nurses are increasingly called upon to do work which puts them in danger of being accused of practicing medicine.[M]

Laws regulating practice affect function, but when they are in conflict with human needs, people tend to disregard them. The fact that almost everybody accepts the United Nations dictum that health care is a universal human right is forcing people to accept professional nurses as givers of primary care.[N] As noted, national prepaid health insurance is the rule rather than the exception in developed countries, and some developing countries have adopted it. Even in most countries that have no national health insurance, all citizens assume that health care is a right.

If the peoples of this earth are to receive health care as a basic human right, a wide variety of systems is necessary, since the kinds and numbers of health workers vary from country to country. Physicians and "trained" nurses are almost nonexistent in some parts of the world. It is reported, for instance, that in Tanzania there was in 1972 one physician for every 28,000 of the population "with a correspondingly low ratio of other health professionals and auxiliaries." In rural India, the ratio of physicians may fall lower than one to 11,000, while it may be as high as 1:1200 in cities.[135] In the United States, Canada, Great Britain, Scandinavia, and other economically favored parts of the world, the ratio of physicians to the population in cities may be as high as one physician to every 500 of the population and one to 1000 in some rural areas, and in the USSR, the ratio is reported to be about one physician to every 370 inhabitants.[136] In economically favored countries, the supply of nurses has increased rapidly; the ratio of registered nurses may range from 1:250 to 1:400. At the turn of the century, it is variously reported that the ratio of physicians to the population equalled or exceeded the ratio of "trained nurses" in the United States; in 1976, the ratio of registered nurses *far exceeded* that of physicians and the ratio of auxiliary nursing personnel to the population exceeded that of registered nurses.

While the worldwide goal of one professional nurse to 5000 inhabitants and one health auxiliary for every 1000 inhabitants has not been reached, the ratio of professional nurses exceeds the ratio of physicians on every continent except Asia.[137,138] It seems obvious that the system of meeting the health needs must vary from country to country and even from decade to decade and that in this era nurses are almost forced to give primary care.

Nursing journals from all over the world carry articles on the extended role of the nurse. In June, 1972, the International Council of Nurses released the following statement on the "developing role of the nurse":

> In the light of scientific and social change and the goals of social and health policy to extend health services to the total population, nursing and other health professions are faced with the need to adapt and expand their roles. In planning to meet health needs it is imperative that nurses and physicians collaborate to promote the development and optimum utilization of both professions. A variety of practices may evolve in different settings including the creation of new categories of health workers. Although this may require nurses to delegate some of their traditional activities and undertake new responsibilities, the core of their practice and their title should remain distinctly nursing and education programmes should be geared to prepare them for their duly recognized role.[o]

In 1970, the American Medical Association's Committee on Nursing published a position statement supporting increased numbers of nurses, expansion of role, preparation of nursing at "all levels," increased involvement of nurses in direct medical care of patients, and collaboration of medicine and nursing.[139] The Canadian Nurses' Association and the Canadian Medical Association issued a joint statement on the interdependent role of nursing and medicine and agreed upon an experimental approach in developing an extended role for the nurse.[140,141] While physicians in the United States have also developed physician's assistants as "extenders" of medical care, physicians in Canada have not done so.

Since the Canadian experience is more contained and easier to follow, it might be described before that in the United States. Canadians seem to have realized for years that many nurses, but particularly those in the medical services of the North, were practicing a combination of nursing and medicine. Articles in nursing journals for decades reported the broad scope of the community nurse's practice in northern outposts. Nurses serving Indians and Eskimos may be the only professionals in health stations for months, and while they may be able to consult physicians by telephone, it has been impracticable for nurses to consult them every time they had to decide whether and how to treat a sick patient or whether to have the patient flown to an appropriate hospital.

Ruth E. May, describing the Canadian experience of a university nursing school and medical school collaborating in preparation of graduate students for outpost nursing, said it had its roots in a 1964 investigation of the Royal Commission on Health Services. This involved visits by a medical educator to the Canadian Arctic and other remote areas.[142] A resulting program at Dalhousie University Medical School, Halifax, Nova Scotia, is the prototype of those established later in other universities.

A study made by a Committee on Clinical Training of Nurses for Medical Services in the North, appointed by the Department of National Health and Welfare, was reported by its chairman, Dorothy J. Kergin, in 1970.[143] As a result of the findings of this committee, clinical courses of study for graduate nurses were begun in the Universities of Alberta, McGill, Manitoba, Ontario, Toronto, Sherbrooke, and Western Ontario to improve the competence of nurses in isolated nursing stations in the North.[144] With the exception of the course at Ontario University, they were funded by the Medical Services Branch of the Department of National Health and Welfare and it was stipulated that the universities were obligated to evaluate the effectiveness of the courses. This led to a "task analysis" of nursing in these stations, or the skills the Kergin report indicated were needed. A list of these skills clearly showed that nurses were functioning within the traditional scope of medicine as well as in the traditional scope of nursing.[145]

In 1971, the Department of National Health and Welfare called a conference to discuss assistance to the physician, which was attended by invited physicians, nurses, and consumers. The conference decided to expand the role of the nurse rather than develop a new category of worker (a physician's assistant of the feldsher type).[146] In 1973, the Canadian Nurses' Association and the Canadian Medical Association issued a joint statement endorsing this decision.[147]

At each of the universities mentioned above, a "validating panel" consisting of a nurse, a physician, and a content specialist determined whether a course objective (a skill) was necessary for a "clinically trained nurse." The hundreds of "objectives" (procedures) identified are reported in a 600-page document with the following 30 chapter headings: History and Physical Examination; Laboratory Procedures; X-ray Procedures; Pharmacology; Fluids and Electrolytes; Nutrition; Growth and Development; Obstetrics and the Newborn; Gynecology; Ophthalmology; Otorhinolaryngology; Dentistry;

Respiratory System; Cardiovascular System; Gastro-intestinal System; Genitourinary System; Central Nervous System; Musculoskeletal System; Dermatology; Haematology; Deficiency and Metabolic Disorders; Endocrine System; Psychiatry; Communicable Diseases and Immunization; Immunology and Allergies; Burns; Accidents; Surgical Procedures; Adult Flowsheets; Pediatric Flowsheets.[P]

From the evidence just cited, it is clear that a broad scope of nursing practice is recognized in Canada and it would seem that doctors and nurses accept an overlapping function. Because the health programs of each province are different, generalizations may be challenged. It is not possible to review the recent legislation affecting the legal scope of nursing practice throughout Canada. It is interesting, however, that the unified health legislation of Quebec, which in 1973 promulgated the Professional Code (S.Q. 1973, ch. 43), brought 38 "professional corporations" under an umbrella act. Nicole Du Mouchel and Odile LaRose reported that 21 professions had exclusive right to practice "as well as reserved title" and 17 had reserved title only. Nursing is one of the 21 exclusive professions, each of which is governed by a special act. The Nurses Act (S.Q. 1973, ch. 48) defines the practice of the profession as follows:

> Every act the object of which is to identify the health needs of persons, contribute to methods of diagnosis, provide and control the nursing care required for the promotion of health, prevention of illness, treatment and rehabilitation, and to provide care according to a medical prescription constitutes the profession of nursing.
>
> A nurse may in practicing the profession inform the population on health problems.[Q]

From this definition, the Order of Nurses of Quebec has developed the philosophy, objectives, and functions of nurses in maternal, infant, preschool, school, adult, and aged health services which were published in 1974 under the title *Community Health Nursing*. It is perhaps significant that the Centre within the [International] Organization for Economic Cooperation and Development (OECD), Paris, got a "Group of Experts" to study the "Ontario Experience" in educating health professions "in the context of the health care system." The 1975 report of this study (financed by the Josiah Macy, Jr. Foundation) suggests complete acceptance of an extended role for the nurse.[148]

While the preceding discussion of primary care by nurses in Canada is obviously simplistic and incomplete, it does suggest that physicians and nurses are collaborating effectively in planning and implementing plans.

In the United States, recognition of the ability of nurses to give primary care seems to have come from a number of centers during the 1960s. In 1964, Pellegrino, in "Nursing and Medicine; Ethical Implications in Changing Practice," urged "joint discussion" in the readjustment of functions.[149] Since this time, in his work at several medical centers, he has promoted reexamination of the functions of health personnel. During a 1972 conference on interdisciplinary education in the health professions, Pellegrino made the following observation:

> A major deterrent to our efforts to fashion health care that is efficient, effective, comprehensive, and personalized is our lack of a design for the synergistic interrelationship of all who can contribute to the patient's well-being. We face, in the next decade, a national challenge to redeploy the functions of health professions in new ways, extending the roles of some, perhaps eliminating others, but more closely meshing the functions of each than ever before.[R]

Barbara Bates, another physician, who was associated with Pellegrino in the Department of Medicine at the University of Kentucky Medical Center, began her study there of the working relationships of physicians and nurses which she has, with nursing participation, continued at the University of Rochester. In 1970. Bates wrote:

> Medicine and nursing have common goals: the preservation and restoration of health. Yet their roles in achieving these objectives are not identical and may be visualized as two overlapping circles, each with its own content but sharing a common ground. The primary [chief] role of medicine comprises diagnosis and treatment—the "cure" process described by Schulman, Mauksch and others. In contrast, the primary [chief] role of nursing lies in the care process, expressive in nature, and consisting of caring, helping, comforting and guiding. Neither role is an exclusive domain. Both professions feel responsible for trying to meet patients' psychologic needs. Furthermore, as technology advances, a steadily enlarging area of overlapping roles is made up of tasks instrumental to diagnosis and treatment, delegated by doctor to nurse.[S]

Few would question the statement by Bates that neither role is an exclusive domain; however, some would question the premise that nurses can

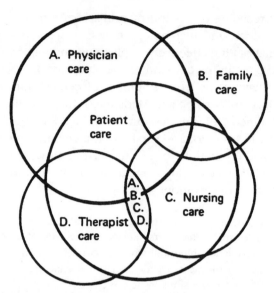

FIGURE 19.1 Diagram showing overlapping of (A) physician care, (B) family care, (C) nursing care, and (D) therapist care. (Adapted from National Commission for the Study of Nursing and Nursing Education: *An Abstract for Action.* Jerome P. Lysaught, director. McGraw-Hill Book Co., New York, 1970, p. 39.)

only perform a diagnostic or treatment "task" if it is delegated by a doctor. Can the doctors, then, only perform "caring, helping, comforting and guiding" tasks if delegated by a nurse?[T] Bates and others have shown the overlapping functions of health workers with overlapping circles (see Fig. 19.1). It may be useful to stress here that, according to the kind of help people need and according to the persons available to give this help, the physician, the nurse, the social worker, the physical therapist, the prosthesis maker, the vocational counselor, or others may be the most valuable or major helper. In 1966, the writer tried to show with a series of "pie graphs" (see Fig. 19.2) the fallacy of assuming that any one health worker was always the dominant member, or the appropriate "captain," of the team.

Sir George Godber, discussing "The Greater Medical Profession," in 1975 commented on "the undoubted decline in understanding between the medical and nursing professions, as the right of the latter to share in decision making is too little realised. . . . I am a doctor and I believe that the medical role in health care is central, but coordinating rather than domi-

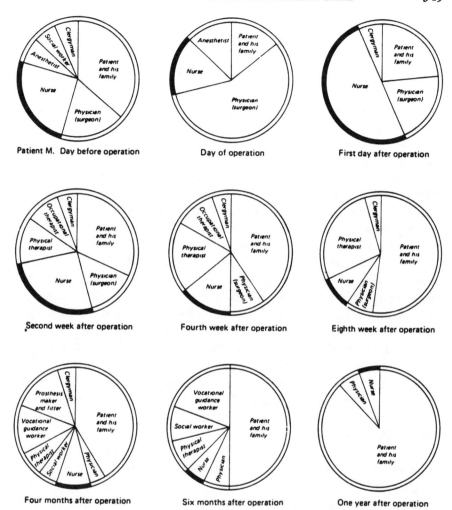

FIGURE 19.2 Diagrams that show the changing dominance in the roles of patients and their families, physicians, nurses, and other health workers during the various phases of illness and rehabilitation. (Adapted from Henderson, Virginia: *The Nature of Nursing*. Macmillan Publishing Co., Inc., New York, 1966.)

nant. Some of the other professional contributions can be, at times, more important and they are quite distinct from that which the physician can make."[U]

While the health care available in medical centers within the United States tends to establish a standard of care (possibly because most health workers are trained in these centers), many nurses in recent decades have reminded their colleagues and the public that in remote and sparsely populated areas they, like the Canadian nurses, are forced to substitute for all other health workers, including physicians.

Any study of the extended role of the nurse takes into account nurse-midwifery (already mentioned in connection with the Frontier Nursing Service) and the care of infants and children by pediatric nurses.

Henry Silver, a physician, in association with Loretta Ford, a nurse, is credited with having inaugurated at the University of Colorado in 1965 the first Pediatric Nurse Practitioner Program.[150] Nurses with baccalaureate degrees who were given special preparation saw well infants and children and treated minor illnesses and conditions in consultation with physicians. This program received so much attention that *Time Magazine* ran a feature article in 1966 entitled "Where Doctors Don't Reach" (*88*:71, July 22).

In 1969, Silver, collaborating with the School of Nursing, University of Colorado, established the Child Health Associate Program which enabled graduates to "practice pediatrics under close physician supervision" as defined under a new Colorado law. These child health associates came into the program with 2 years of college and had 3 years of professional studies that included a 1-year internship.[151,152]

Many programs similar to those in Colorado have been instituted and assessments made of graduates. A few reports of each are listed at the end of this chapter.[153-166]

The Maternal and Child Health Service, Health Services Administration, U.S. Department of Health, Education, and Welfare, has funded a 3-year study by the American Nurses' Association to develop research methods for evaluating the impact of pediatric nurse practitioner (PNP) programs and their graduates on the health care of children.[167]

The nurse-midwife was probably the first nurse accepted as giving primary care in the United States; the pediatric nurse practitioner and the child health associate were perhaps the next to be accepted. However, some psychiatric nurses have functioned as therapists for decades. In the review of nursing research reported by Leo W. Simmons and Virginia Henderson in 1964,[168] more studies of nursing in psychiatry were reported than in any other clinical field and parallel upgrading of their preparation and practice was noted. For decades. some psychiatric nurse specialists have been giving primary care in private practice, in clinics, and in hospitals.[169-172]

While the extended role of the pediatric nurse was being developed at the University of Colorado, C. E. Lewis, a physician, and Barbara Resnick, a nurse, developed a primary role for the nurse in a medical ambulatory service at the University of Kansas. This experience was reported in journals and as a final report in 1968 to the U.S. Public Health Service, the funding agency.[173-176] Barbara R. Noonan[177] has reported on 8 years in a medical nurse clinic at the Massachusetts General Hospital in Boston and on her changing role as she assumed a caseload of her own.

In the decade of the 1970s, the primary care role of the nurse has been developed in almost every clinical setting—maternal and child care, medical nursing, and psychiatry and in most of the occupational settings discussed in Chapter 3—hospitals, clinics, nursing homes, offices, industries. schools, private homes. In 1973, Mary H. Browning and Edith P. Lewis compiled articles on the expanded role of the nurse in a volume which was published by the American Journal of Nursing Company.[178] While most articles indicate that patients, nurses, and physicians respond positively to an extended role for the nurse, change in human relationships is not easy, and nurses in this role describe many of the difficulties they encounter. Robert Galton, a physician, and his associates make the following comment:

> The movement toward a physician-nurse team care of patients with complementary roles has not developed as quickly as was originally projected. Both patients and physicians are loathe to have anything interfere with the traditional relationship. Physicians have expressed anxiety about losing their patients to nurses.[V]

Throughout the 1960s and 1970s, the US Department of Health, Education, and Welfare has sponsored studies of the extended role. The Secretary's Committee to Study Extended Roles for Nurses published a report in 1971. The Committee was composed of 11 physicians and 10 nurses, and the staff director was Faye G. Abdellah. The report stated that "health care should reflect patient needs rather than professional prerogatives, and those who provide health care should work as a team whenever the needs of the patient and his family warrant. . . . Nursing practice . . . may be compartmentalized under . . . primary care, acute care, and long-term care." Primary care, as used in the report, was defined as "(a) a person's first contact in any given episode of illness with the health care system that leads to a decision of what must be done to help resolve his problem; and (b) the responsibility for the continuum of care, i.e., maintenance of health, evaluation and management of symptoms, and appropriate referrals."[w] This report carried weight and, perhaps more than any other publication in the United States, established the extended role as an accomplished fact. By 1975, there were 74 "nurse practitioner" programs in 34 states that awarded a B.S. degree and/or certificate and 53 programs in 34 states that awarded a master's degree.[179]

The conclusions and recommendations of the Secretary's Committee are very much in line with those in the report of the National Commission for the Study of Nursing and Nursing Education.[180] The American Nurses' Association took a similar stand on the extended role and collaborated with the National Commission in activating its recommendations. The ANA's ongoing Joint Practice Commission with the American Medical Association to study the functions of nurses and physicians and their overlapping functions is a model for state and local commissions of this sort.[181]

The development of the *physician's assistant* by the medical profession in the United States and their role as primary care providers must be considered in even a brief discussion of the nurse's extended role. Just as feldshers were developed in Russia during the seventeenth century to nurse (and treat) sick and wounded soldiers and sailors, medical technicians were developed in most countries to nurse (and treat) military personnel or to "extend" the services of physicians and professional nurses. Patrick B. Storey prepared a report on USSR feldshers for the National Institutes of Health in 1972.[182] The contribution of Russian feldshers to health care is described in greater detail in a pamphlet prepared by the Ministry of Health of the USSR for, and distributed by, the World Health Organization in 1974. By 1956, there were almost 300,000 employed feldshers. In the 1970s, they belong to categories such as feldsher-generalist, midwife, sanitarian, laboratory technician, and dental assistant or dental mechanic. The formal feldsher training programs began in the seventeenth century, some for physician's assistants in civil life and some for military feldshers. the latter being longer and more rigorous programs. They now have 8 years of primary education and the feldsher curriculum is about 4 years in length. Students are taught by physical, biologic, and social scientists, physicians, nurses, and others.[183] Generally speaking, feldshers function more independently in the USSR than registered nurses do in the United States.[184] Feldsher programs are said to prepare graduates to give medical care in the absence of the physician. In the USSR, both feldshers and nurses are classified as "middle-level medical personnel"; both are taught by physicians (who administer the schools), and both, if they show special ability, may later study medicine without having to pass an entrance examination to medical school.[185]

In World War I, but more particularly in World War II, a wide variety of medical aides were developed in the United States military forces, with preparation that ranged from weeks to months or even years. Some medical technicians remained in military service to function in this capacity; others went into schools of nursing in civil life; others were interested in becoming assistants to physicians rather than becoming nurses. Physicians in the United States who had found them helpful in military service and other physicians who were impressed with the work of feldshers in Russia promoted the creation of physician's assistants. Eugene A. Stead, a physician of Duke University, Durham, North Carolina is credited with leadership in initiating such programs. With K. G. Andreoli, he reported the progress of the Duke program in 1967.[186] In 1968, Thelma Ingles, a nurse who had worked with Stead, also described the program which welcomed nurses as applicants.[187]

In 1970, Ernest B. Howard, vice-president of the American Medical Association, speculated that 100,000 nurses who could be "quickly trained" to expand physicians' abilities to serve patients could relieve the physician shortage, including the resumption of house calls.[188] This unilateral action excited a negative response from organized nursing and tended to discourage recruitment of nurses into the physician's assistant programs that had by 1974, 48 AMA accredited programs.[189] The programs may be called physician's assistant, physician's associate, or MEDIC or MEDEX programs—the latter being programs for military personnel with medical experience. They are under the direction of medical schools, community colleges, public or private universities, or hospitals. About 1000 graduates are now produced annually, the total by September, 1975, was estimated as 3000—the ratio of male to females being 7:3. Thirty-six states had, by the end of 1975, legislation sanctioning physician's assistants or MEDEX.[X,190] There is considerable disagreement on the extent to which the functions of nurses and physician's assistants overlap and on the professional relationship of nurses and physician's assistants. A great variety of opinion exists.[191-194] While their numbers are few, physician's assistants are organized and have an official publication (*The P.A. Journal—A Journal for New Health Practitioners*). At present, their numbers, the length of training, their role in health care, and their relationship to nursing are quite different from those of feldshers in Russia. Alfred M. Sadler and his associates, discussing the independence and dependence of health workers and the expanding roles of physician's assistants, speak of the "legally dependent and flexible status" of physicians' assistants in contrast to the status of nurses who are "striving for an independent function."[195] Whatever the difference, it is as necessary for nurses in the United States to have effective working relationships with physicians' assistants as it is for nurses in the USSR to have effective working relationships with feldshers.

Whether or not there is one body of knowledge on health and disease or whether it can be parceled out as psychology, physiology, health education, medicine, dentistry, pharmacy, nursing, nutrition, and so on, is debatable. The fragmentation of health care and the elaboration of health workers goes on and on. And within each category of health worker, as, for instance, medicine and nursing, specialization results in further fragmentation of health care.

Some physicians still seem to think that everyone entering the health care system should see an internist, a diagnostician, a family health physician, or a primary care physician. Texts such as Mark Lipkin's *The Care of Patients, Concepts and Tactics,*[196] addressed to medical students, barely mentions nurses (or physician's assistants), and Robert E. Rakel, a physician writing on "Primary Care—Whose Responsibility?"[197] seems to say that the answer lies in training a sufficient number of primary care physicians. Admitting the value of thorough training and seasoned clinical judgment, this goal is unattainable in even the most economically favored countries even if their complements of doctors were equally distributed.

In 1972, the National Joint Practice Commission of the American Nurses' Association and the American Medical Association was initiated with equal numbers of physician and nurse practitioners. Shirley A. Smoyak has described its origin and purpose.[198] At its 1974 conference, *Building for the Future,* such subjects were discussed as the roles of physicians' assistants and expanded roles of nurses, interdisciplinary education, and legal aspects of joint practice.[199] The Commission is studying medical and nursing practice acts[200] and has published a bibliography with abstracts on joint practice.[201]

Private foundations are sponsoring studies of primary care and roles of physicians, nurses, physicians' assistants, and others. Two conferences funded by the Josiah Macy, Jr. Foundation were reported under the titles *The Greater Medical Profession*, 1973 (held in England) and *The Intermediate-Level Health Practitioners*, 1974 (held in the United States). The Josiah

Macy, Jr. Foundation funded a study by the Secretary-General of the [International] Organization for Economic Cooperation and Development, reported in 1975 under the title *New Directions in Education for Changing Health Care Systems.* The Foundation also financed the Center for Educational Research and Innovation (CERI).[Y] Support for the development of physicians' assistants has come from a number of foundations—the Carnegie Corporation, the Commonwealth Fund, the Rockefeller Foundation, and the Robert Wood Johnson Foundation, as well as from the U.S. Department of Health, Education, and Welfare.

In all these conferences and publications, the unequal distribution of health manpower is stressed, as are the wasteful use of expensively prepared workers in some places, the insupportable cost of health care, the overuse of resources in some countries, with consequent fostering of dependence, and the effectiveness of community involvement and indigenous health workers who understand the people's problems and who have their trust.

There can be little doubt that the role of the physician is changing, as is that of the nurse. In a WHO conference on health economics, it is noted that one way of "containing costs" is to "ensure that the degree of technical complexity involved [in the workers' preparation] is appropriate for the task to be performed."[Z] Because their education is the most lengthy and costly, doctors are advised to turn over to other health workers any tasks the latter can safely perform. This principle, and the fact that there are not enough physicians to give the care the peoples of the world believe to be their right, is forcing physicians in every country to relinquish many of their traditional functions. A collaborative role for physicians and nurses is essential if the goal of providing a universal health service is to be reached.[AA]

In the writer's opinion, every health institution would profit by the creation of *an interdisciplinary committee on practice to assess the needs of the clientele to be served and the available health manpower, and the allocation of functions and responsibilities among the available workers.* All categories of clinical health professionals should retain some direct service to the client or patient, for without this human interaction, the service loses its chief reward and the opportunity for the worker to sense the patient's problem, the kinds of research needed, and possible changes that might be made to improve the service.

Albert Schweitzer, who left successful musical and theological careers to be a medical missionary, said he wanted to be able:

. . . to work without having to talk. For years I have been giving myself out in words and it was with joy that I had followed the calling of theological teacher and preacher. But this new form of activity [the practice of medicine] I couldn't represent to myself as being talking about the religion of love but only as an actual putting it into practice.[BB]

He quotes Goethe's *Faust*, "In the beginning was the Deed." Nursing is a service primarily of deeds. Annie W. Goodrich used to say there was no such thing as a "menial act," but that a person could have a menial attitude toward any kind of work. Esther A. Werminghaus in her biographical sketch of Annie W. Goodrich says:

Gradually a new symbol is emerging. . . . Miss Goodrich has referred to her as "the complete nurse." A few schools can produce a good many complete nurses, but it is Miss Goodrich's unfaltering contention that all nurses must be complete nurses before we can expect to realize the great social potentialities of professional nursing.[CC]

An Operational Definition of Nursing Used in This Book[DD]

Admitting the importance of theory, of identifying values and goals, and of unifying these into a system which might also be called a philosophy, the writer believes it still necessary to have a specific operational definition of nursing. And because so many health workers would claim the over-all goals for nursing that have been cited, it is helpful to define nursing so that it is differentiated from health education, the practice of medicine, clinical psychology, or social service. In fact, it is necessary, even in an age of rapid change, as long as students in these fields are educated in different programs and their respective practice is regulated by separate laws and regulations.

Under any health care system, each category of worker should be recognized as having a peculiar or *unique* function, no matter how many functions they have in common with others. Certainly the members of each vocational group should be more competent in performing some activities than are the workers in any other vocation. So the questions must be asked: What *is nursing* that is not also medicine, physical therapy, social work, etc.?; and What is *the unique function of the nurse?* The writer assumes responsibility for the following analysis but cannot take full credit for it since association with hundreds of nurses and others interested in nursing has contributed to clarification of these concepts—right or wrong. They are presented in the hope that they may help others, whether they agree or disagree, to develop a working concept of the place of nursing in society.

Nursing is primarily helping people (sick or well) in the performance of those activities contributing to health, or its recovery (or to a peaceful death) that they would perform unaided if they had the necessary strength, will, or knowledge. It is likewise the unique contribution of nursing to help people to be independent of such assistance as soon as possible. Nursing has a part in other activities that contribute to the accomplishment of what Goodrich refers to as "a healthy citizenry," just as medicine, whose unique function is diagnosing disease and prescribing therapy, may be engaged cooperatively in all activities concerned with health in its fullest meaning. From the preceding definition of nursing, the definition of the *unique* function of nurses follows: *To help people, sick or well, in the performance of those activities contributing to health or its recovery (or to a peaceful death) that they would perform unaided if they had the necessary strength, will, or knowledge. It is likewise the function of nurses to help people gain independence as rapidly as possible.* This part of their work nurses initiate and control; of this they are masters. In addition (or as part of this defined function if it is broadly interpreted), nurses help patients carry out therapeutic plans as initiated by physicians. Nurses also, as members of a cooperative health team, help its other members, as they in turn may help nurses to plan and carry out with patients and their families the total program of care. No member of the team should make such heavy demands on other members that they are unable to perform their special or unique function. Nor should any member of the team be diverted by nonmedical activities such as cleaning. clerking, and filing, as long as their unique task must be neglected. All members of the team should consider the person (patient) served as the central figure, and should realize that primarily they are all *assisting him or her.* If patients do not understand, accept, and participate in planning the program of care, the effort of the health team is largely wasted. The sooner people recognize the nature of their health problems, the reasons they are ill, the rationale of treatment, the sooner they can care for themselves—even carry out their own treatments—the better off they are.

This concept of the nurse as a substitute for what patients lack to make them "complete," "whole," or "independent," be it the lack of physical strength, will, or knowledge, may seem limited to some who read this.[EE] The more one thinks about it, however, the more complex is the nurse's function, as so defined. Think how rarely one sees independence, completeness, or wholeness of mind and body! To what extent good health is a matter of heredity, to what extent it is acquired, is controversial, but it is generally admitted that intelligence and education, by and large, tend to parallel health status. If, then, most people find "good health" a difficult goal to reach, how much more difficult it is for health workers to help others reach it. Nurses must, in a sense, get "inside the skin" of each patient in order to know what help he or she needs from them. *The nurse is temporarily the consciousness of the unconscious, the love of life of the suicidal, the leg of the amputee, the eyes of the newly blind, a means of locomotion for the newborn, knowledge and confidence for the young mother, a voice for those too weak to speak,* and so on.

It is this necessity for estimating the individual's need for momentary or hourly care, support, encouragement, and health guidance that makes nursing a service of the highest order. Many of the activities involved are simple until their adjustment to the particular demands of the client or patient makes them complex. In health, for example, breathing is effortless; but the nurse who places a patient in position for proper chest expansion following a rib resection, or who operates a respirator, performs a complex function. Eating is also effortless with appetite; but when that is lacking, it becomes a problem. To brush the teeth in health seems easy to most persons (actually few know enough about mouth hygiene); but to thoroughly clean the mouth of an unconscious patient is so difficult and dangerous that few skilled nurses accomplish it effectively and safely.

Perhaps enough has been said to indicate that the primary responsibility of the nurse is that of helping people with their daily patterns of living, or with the following activities that they ordinarily perform without assistance: breathing, eating; eliminating, resting, sleeping and moving, cleaning the body and keeping it warm and properly clothed. Nurses also help provide for those activities that make life more than a vegetative process. namely, social intercourse, learning, occupations that are recreational and those that are productive in some way. In other words nurses help people maintain or create health regimens that, were they strong, knowing, and filled with the love of life, they would carry out unaided. It is this intimate, demanding, and yet inexpressibly rewarding service that nurses are best prepared to render. And because nurses are the most numerous of all health workers in most countries, and nursing service in most institutions is the only 24-hour service, nursing is the only service organized to give this most essential help.

In addition to this unique function of nurses, they help patients identify and express their health needs: they help them find and use the health resources of the community and carry out such treatments prescribed by therapists, or physicians, as they cannot perform unaided. And in the absence of physicians and other licensed therapists, nurses may function in these capacities. While nurses are not primarily therapists, as defined in this book, nursing may include therapy, since everybody, in the absence of a physician, must of necessity treat himself or herself.

Notes

[a]Eike-Henner Kluge's *The Practice of Death* is a treatise on the extent to which past and present-day cultures practice abortion, infanticide, suicide, and genocide. (Yale University Press, New Haven, Conn., 1975.)

[b]Sigerist, Henry E.: *A History of Medicine*. Volume 1. *Primitive and Archaic Medicine*. Oxford University Press, New York, 1951, p. 11.

[c]Garrison, Fielding H.: *An Introduction to the History of Medicine,* 4th ed. W. B. Saunders Co., Philadelphia, 1960, p. 20.

[d]Mike Samuels, a physician, calls the body "a three million year old healer." In his book, *The Well Body Book,* written with Hal Bennett for the public and designed to help people stay healthy, Samuels gives credit to Rolling Thunder (an American Indian) "who taught me healing." (Random House/Bookworks, New York, 1973, p. vi.) A nurse, R. S. Bryan, writes about "My Friends the Witchdoctors," *Nurs. Times, 68*:1220, (Sept. 28) 1972.

[e]Sigerist, Henry E.: *op. cit.,* p. 3.

[f]Djukanovic, V., and Mach, E. P. (eds.): *op. cit.,* p. 3.

[g]Self-help is thought by many to be our best hope today. Keith E. Sehnert titles an article "Miracle Drugs and Lifesaving Machines May Make Headlines But It's the Individual Who Is the Cornerstone of a Sound Medical System," (*Fam. Health,* 7:41, [Nov.1 1975).

[h]Beatrice J. Kalisch, in an article titled "Of Half Gods and Mortals: Aesculapian Authority," suggests that this influence persists, leading some wag to say that "M.D. stands for Minor Diety." (*Nurs. Outlook, 23*:22, [Jan.] 1975).

[i]Lipkin, Mack: *The Care of Patients: Concepts and Tactics*. Oxford University Press, New York, 1974, p. 55.

[j]Garrison, Fielding H.: *op. cit.,* p. 108. (The erroneous concept that obstetrics is a branch of surgery is deeply rooted in the literature.)

[k]Pellegrino, Edmund D.: "Medicine, History, and the Idea of Man," *Ann. Am. Acad. Pol. Sci., 346*:9, (Mar.) 1953.

[l]Dates given by authorities for the Middle Ages and the European Renaissance vary. They range roughly from 400 to 1500 for the former and 1300 to 1700 for the latter.

[m]Pellegrino, Edmund D.: *op. cit.*

[n]Dreitzel, Hans Peter (ed.): *The Social Organization of Health*. Recent Sociology No. 3. Macmillan Publishing Co., Inc., New York, 1971, p. vii.

[o]Descartes' writings were the subject of conversation in the fashionable as well as the intellectual world. There are many references to such conversations in Madame de Sévigne's letters to her daughter from the court of France in Paris. (de Sévigne, Marie de Rabutin-Chantal: *The Letters of Madame de Sévigne*. Carnavelet Ed. W. T. Morrell and Co., London, 1928.)

[p]Pellegrino, Edmund D.: "Educating the Humanist Physician," *J.A.M.A., 227*:1288, (Mar. 18) 1974.

[q]Nilsson, Lennart: *Behold Man—A Photographic Journey Inside the Body*. In collaboration with Jan Lindberg. Little, Brown & Co., Boston, 1974, p. 248.

[r]See, for example, Jan Howard and Anselm Strauss, *Humanizing Health Care* (John Wiley & Sons, New York, 1975) and articles such as that of John P. Geyman, "On Depersonalization in Medicine," (*J. Fam. Practice, 3*:239, [June] 1976).

[s]Many critics of health care point out that even though technically excellent care is available in a country, it will not affect the health indices materially until a political system is developed that makes necessary care available to all citizens and that provides them with adequate food and a healthful environment. Health is said to be a social problem and the organization of health care a political task. Roger Hurley maintains that a failure to provide a satisfactory organization should be attributed to a society (in this case American) rather than to its medical profession. (Hurley, Roger: "Health Crisis of the Poor," in Dreitzel, Hans Peter [ed.]: *The Social Organization of Health*. Macmillan Publishing Co., Inc., New York, 1971, p. 113 [Recent Sociology No. 3].)

[t]Even in Sweden where nursing is generally thought to have flourished, its schools are under the National Board of Education, while medical schools are under the office of the chancellor of the Swedish universities. Responsibility for training physical therapists, in contrast, comes under both. (Teng-

stam, Anders: *Patterns of Health Care and Education in Sweden,* Centre for Educational Research and Innovation [CERI], Organisation for Economic Co-operation and Development, Paris, France, 1975, p. 27.)

ᵘRead, Margaret: *Culture, Health and Disease. Social and Cultural Influences on Health Programs in Developing Countries.* J. B. Lippincott Co., Philadelphia, 1966, p. 16.

ᵛSome of the developing countries are giving health care high priority and nurses are playing a significant role in planning and giving health care. F. O. Okedigi discusses the "Economics of Health Care Delivery" in "Nigeria's Second National Plan 1970–1974" in its "Sociological Perspective" (*Niger Nurse,* 5:31, [Apr.–June] 1973).

ʷThe reader should not assume that there is any intention to belittle the importance of research in the field of health. It is only when the cause of disease is established that the best preventive program can be designed; it is only possible to teach the optimum diet when controlled experiments demonstrate its essentials.

ˣIn 1973, the first international conference on "education in the health sciences" was held. Such meetings should encourage the development of common objectives and help to remove interdisciplinary barriers. ("A 'First'—An International Conference on Education in the Health Sciences" [News], *Int. Nurs. Rev., 20*:71, [May–June] 1973.)

ʸSome medical centers and hospitals set up patients' libraries as separate from the library that serves the health workers. (See Collen, F. Bobbie, and Soghikian, Krikor: "A Health Library for Patients," *Health Services Reports, 29*:236, [May–June] 1974.) While librarians especially prepared to help the general public seem to me to promise better service, the writer believes that the entire range of the literature should be available to patients or potential patients. The health occupations should have no "trade secrets," no "private" source of information. It is the mark of professionals to share their knowledge and to make those they serve independent of them. Lucie Young Kelly, writing about "the patient's right to know" and the laws enforcing this right, expresses the opinion that "this movement may have a much more dramatic impact on health care than any series of exotic scientific discoveries." (*Nurs. Outlook, 24*:26, [Jan.] 1976.)

ᶻIt must be recognized that the provision of health care is an economic, a political, issue. Victor R. Fuchs, an economist, expresses this in the title of a 1974 publication, *Who Shall Live? Health, Economics, and Social Choice,* Basic Books, Inc., New York, 1974.

ᵃᵃEverett Hughes, a sociologist, compared health care to the task a group of workers faces who must get a load of faggots up a mountain—every one of them. To accomplish this, he said that if any worker dropped a faggot another worker must pick it up. In like manner, if physicians or nurses or dietitians drop any of the tasks they have traditionally performed, some other worker must pick them up. His point was that no one health group should feel free to define its function or change its established role until it is assured that related groups are willing to change their roles so that the health care goals can still be reached. (Hughes, Everett, *et al.: Twenty Thousand Nurses Tell Their Story*, J. B. Lippincott Co., Philadelphia, 1958.)

ᵇᵇThis booklet, written in 1960 and revised in 1969, which is now distributed by national nursing organizations and by the ICN, has been translated into 27 languages.

ᶜᶜDiscussing the proposed 1970 revision of the British National Health Service, the Ministry of Health spokesman said, "The establishment of an integrated Health Service will make it necessary to consider how far particular specialised training programmes are still appropriate, whether existing personnel can with further training undertake wider functions, and *whether new forms of generic training need to be developed.*" (Ministry of Health: *The National Health Service—the Administrative Structure of the Medical and Related Services in England and Wales*, H. M. Stationery Office, London, 1968, Section 106.)

ᵈᵈNightingale, Florence: *Notes on Nursing, What It Is and What It Is Not.* (Republication of First American edition published by D. Appleton & Co., 1860.) Dover Publications, Inc., New York, 1969, p. 133.

ᵉᵉNightingale. Florence: *op. cit.*, p. 7.

ᶠᶠThayer W. S.: "Nursing and the Art of Medicine," *Am. J. Nurs., 20*:187, (Dec.) 1919.

ᵍᵍOsler, Sir William: *Aequanimitas and Other Addresses,* Blakiston Co., Philadelphia, 1925, p. 163.

ʰʰTaylor, Effie J.: "Of What Is the Nature of Nursing?" *Am. J. Nurs., 34*:476, (May) 1934.

ⁱⁱGoodrich, Annie A.: *A Definition of Nursing* (privately printed, 1946); also in the "Report of the Biennial," *Am. J. Nurs., 46*:741, (Nov.) 1946.

ʲʲBrown, Esther Lucile: *Nursing for the Future.* Russell Sage Foundation, New York, 1948, p. 73.

ᵏᵏAttention was called in this discussion to the work of William R. Houston, who, in *The Art of Treatment* (Macmillan, 1936), advocated the organization of medical courses around the principal method of therapy (the medical problem) rather than around diseases of body systems.

llMcManus, R. Louise: "Assumptions of Functions of Nursing." in *Regional Planning for Nursing and Nursing Education*. Teachers College, Columbia University, New York. 1951. p. 54.

mmOrlando, Ida Jean: *The Dynamic Nurse–Patient Relationship*. G. P. Putnam's Sons, New York, 1961, pp. 8, 9.

nnIn 1972, Orlando elaborated on her concept of the nursing process and reported an evaluative study entitled *The Discipline and Teaching of Nursing Process* (G. P. Putnam's Sons, New York).

ooLamb, Margaret M.: "Nursing Is What?" *Int. Nurs. Rev., 17*:373 (No. 4) 1970.

ppSchlotfeldt, Rozella M.: "This I Believe . . . Nursing Is Health Care," *Nurs. Outlook, 30*:245, (Apr.) 1972.

qqRamphal, Marjorie: "Further Thoughts re Scope [of Nursing]." Paper addressed to Congress on Nursing Practice, Pleasantville, N.Y., Jan. 21, 1972, p. 16 (mimeographed).

rrChater, Shirley: *Operation Update: The Search for Rhyme and Reason*. National League for Nursing, New York, 1976, pp. 5, 6.

ssStorlie, Frances: "Nursing Need Never Be Defined." *Int. Nurs. Rev., 17*:255, (No. 3) 1970.

ttBridges, Daisy Caroline: *A History of the International Council of Nurses, 1899–1964. The First Sixty-Five Years*. Pitman Medical Publishing Co., Ltd. London, 1967, p. 234.

uuInternational Labour Office: *Employment and Conditions of Work and Life of Nursing Personnel*. Report VII (2), International Labour Conference, 61st Session, 1976. The Office, Geneva, 1976, p. 84. (Response of the ICN to questionnaire from the ILO.) See also "ICN Adopts Definition of 'a Nurse,'" *Int. Nurs. Rev., 22*:163 (Nov.-Dec.) 1975.

vv"CNR Approves Definition for International Standard Classification of Occupations" (news), *Int. Nurs. Rev., 20*:153, (No. 5) 1973. (The proposed definition was prepared by the ICN Professional Services Committee.)

ww"Professional Nursing Defined" (editorial), *Am. J. Nurs., 37*:518, (May) 1937.

xxNational Commission for the Study of Nursing and Nursing Education: *An Abstract for Action*. (Jerome P. Lysaught, Director.) McGraw-Hill Book Co., New York, 1970, p. 44.

[yy]Although the discussion here focuses on the United States, uncertainty about the scope of nursing practice, or the function of the nurse, is worldwide. A Finnish publication puts the problem in the same terms that might be used here: "The objectives of social policy and health policy determine the needs which nurses have to meet. At the present time nurses are uncertain what needs are their particular responsibility, due to poor definition of the field of responsibility, quality of education, etc." (Vainio, Aune: "A Review of the Activities of the Development Seminar on Nursing Care/Health Science," *Sairaanhoidon Vuosikirja [Helsinki], 11*:53, 1974.)

[zz]Sister Madeleine quotes Rollo May as saying all science needs a philosophical base—and she agrees.

[A]Mathwig, Gean: "Nursing Science—The Theoretical Core of Nursing Knowledge," *Image, 4*:20, (No. 1) 1971.

[B]Harris, M. Isabel: "Theory Building in Nursing. A Review of the Literature," *Image, 4*:6, (No. 1) 1972.

[C]Ellis, Rosemary: "The Practitioner as Theorist," *Am. J. Nurs., 69*:1434, (July) 1969.

[D]King, Imogene M.: *Toward a Theory for Nursing: General Concepts of Human Behavior*. John Wiley & Sons, New York, 1971, pp. IX, 15.

[E]King, Imogene M.: *op. cit.*, p. 25.

[F]Newman, Margaret A.: "Nursing's Theoretical Evolution," *Nurs. Outlook, 20*:449, (July) 1972.

[G]Johnson, Dorothy E.: "Theory in Nursing: Borrowed and Unique," *Nurs. Res., 17*:206, (May–June) 1968.

[H]Von Bertalanffy, Ludwig: "The Theory of Open Systems in Physics and Biology," in Emery, F. E. (ed.): *Systems Thinking*. Penguin Books, Ltd., Harmondsworth, Eng., 1969, p. 70.

[I]Djukanovic, V., and Mach, E. P. (eds.): *Alternative Approaches to Meeting Basic Health Needs in Developing Countries. A Joint UNICEF-WHO Study*. World Health Organization, Geneva, 1975, p. 16.

[J]Some patients call them "the lady pediatrician."

[K]In the opinion of the writer, such titles should not suggest that it is the exception for nurses to be in practice, to be involved in clinical nursing, or to be concerned with the family, or even functioning as a physician's associate, since all of these conditions should be the rule rather than the exception. Titles should rather indicate the clinical field (as maternal and child health, psychiatry, surgery, or medicine) and the length and depth of the nurse's preparation. For example, a "surgical nurse specialist" should mean that the nurse has studied surgical nursing in a postbasic program. Eventually, as nursing education is upgraded, this should imply the completion of a graduate program in a university. In some institutions. nurses are numbered or lettered as Nurse 1, Nurse 2, or Nurse 3, or Nurse A, Nurse B, or Nurse C to designate different levels of competence or different functions. This has the disadvantage of requiring interpretation.

[L]For the first time in 1975, the Frontier Nursing Service had a physician as a director.

[M]International Labour Office: *Employment and Conditions of Work and Life of Nursing Personnel.* International Labour Conference, 61st Session, 1976, Report Vll (1). The Office, Geneva, 1976, pp. 12, 16, 24.

[N]United Nations: *Universal Declaration of Human Rights.* "It is a fundamental human right for every person to have a standard of living adequate for the health and well-being of himself and his family including food, clothing, housing and medical care and necessary social services."

[O]International Council of Nurses: News Release. Statement on the Developing Role of the Nurse. No. 9-73, June 1972.

[P]Hazlett, C. B.: "Task Analysis of the Clinically Trained Nurse (C.T.N.)," *Nurs. Clin. North Am., 10*:699, (Dec.) 1975.

[Q]Du Mouchel, Nicole, and LaRose, Odile: "Community Health Nursing in Quebec," *10*:721, (Dec.) 1975.

[R]Pellegrino, Edmund D.: "lnterdisciplinary Education in the Health Professions: Assumptions, Definitions, and Some Notes on Teams." Reprinted from *Report of a Conference: Educating for the Health Team.* National Academy of Sciences, Institute of Medicine, Washington, D.C., October 1972.

[S]Bates, Barbara: "Doctor and Nurse: Changing Roles and Relations," *N. Engl. J. Med., 283*:129, (July 16) 1970.

[T]It can hardly be denied that every adult and many children "diagnose" and treat aches and pains, injuries, and dysfunction of all sorts daily. More nonprescription than prescription drugs are sold in most countries. Why should not nurses advise people on self-help when they are the only, or the most informed, persons available?

[U]Godber, Sir Georee: "Ira V. Hiscock Lecture, 1975. The Greater Medical Profession," *Yale J. Biol. Med., 49*:137, 1976.

[V]Galton, Robert, *et al.*: "Observations on the Participation of Nurses and Physicians in Chronic Care," *Bull. N.Y. Acad. Med., 49*:112, (Feb.) 1973.

^WU.S. Department of Health, Education, and Welfare: *A Report of the Secretary's Committee to Study Extended Roles for Nurses.* U.S. Government Printing Office, Washington, D.C., 1971, pp. 2, 4, 8.

^XPrograms that prepare nurses to give primary care are called PRIMEX programs.

^YThe World Health Organization has designated the Center for Educational Development, University of Illinois College of Medicine, as a "WHO Collaborating Institute in Medical Education." In 1973, it published a collection of papers under the title *Development of Educational Programmes for the Health Professions*[202] which suggests an international trend toward interdisciplinary education and collaborative practice.

^ZWorld Health Organization: *Health Economics.* Report on a WHO Interregional Seminar. The Organization, Geneva, 1975, p. 16 (Public Health Papers No. 64)

^{AA}Many studies of nurses in extended roles and of physician's assistants have been reported. E. D. Cohen *et al.* prepared a bibliography of such reports in 1974. (*An Evaluation of Policy Related Research on New and Expanded Roles of Health Workers: Annotated Bibliography.* Yale University School of Medicine, Office of Regional Activities and Continuing Education, New Haven, Conn.)

^{BB}Schweitzer, Albert: *Out of My Life and Thought.* (Translated by C. T. Campion.) Henry Holt & Co., New York, 1933, p. 114.

^{CC}Werminghaus, Esther A.: *Annie W. Goodrich; Her Journey to Yale.* Macmillan Publishing Co., Inc., New York, 1950, p. 7.

^{DD}Eileen Pearlman Becknell and Dorothy M. Smith in *System of Nursing Practice, A Clinical Nursing Assessment Tool* (F. A. Davis Co., Philadelphia, 1975) use this definition and show how it can be implemented in a problem-oriented system of care and problem-oriented record.

^{EE}Dorothea Orem and her associates subscribe to this concept of nursing but they call this lack of knowledge, will, or strength the client's "health deficit." They think it is the nurse's function to make up this deficit.

References

1. Frazer, James George: *The Golden Bough.* Macmillan Publishing Co., Inc., New York, 1926.

2. Topoff, Howard F. "The Social Behavior of Army Ants," *Sci. Am.,* *227*:71, (Nov.) 1972.

3. Wilson, Edward O.: "Animal Communication," *Sci. Am., 227*:53, (Sept.) 1972.

4. Sidel, Victor W., and Sidel, Ruth: *Serve the People. Observations on Medicine in the People's Republic of China.* Beacon Press, Boston, 1973.

5. Bullough, Vern, and Bullough, Bonnie: *Emergence of Modern Nursing.* Macmillan Publishing Co., Inc., New York, 1969.

6. Levine, Edwin B., and Levine, Myra E.: "Hippocrates, Father of Nursing, Too?" *Am. J. Nurs., 65*:86, (Dec.) 1965.

7. Jackson, Edgar: *The Pastor and His People.* Channel Press, Manhasset, N.Y., 1963.

8. Hume, Edgar Erskine: *Medical Work of the Knights Hospitalers of Saint John of Jerusalem.* Johns Hopkins Press, Baltimore, 1940.

9. Kelly, Lucie Young: *Dimensions of Professional Nursing.* 3rd ed. Macmillan Publishing Co., Inc., New York, 1975, p. 21.

10. Hastings, Randall: *The Universities of Europe in the Middle Ages.* Clarendon Press, Oxford, 1895.

11. Lippard, Vernon W.: *A Half-Century of American Medical Education 1920–1970.* Josiah Macy, Jr. Foundation, New York, 1974, p. 3.

12. Flexner, Abraham: *Medical Education in the United States and Canada. A Report to the Carnegie Foundation for the Advancement of Teaching.* The Foundation, New York, 1910.

13. Bernard, Claude: *Introduction to the Study of Experimental Medicine.* (Translated by Henry C. Greene.) Macmillan Publishing Co., New York, 1927.

14. Nilsson, Lennart: *Behold Man—A Photographic Journey Inside the Body.* In collaboration with Jan Lindberg. Little, Brown & Co., Boston, 1974.

15. Thomas, Lewis: *The Lives of a Cell. Notes of a Biology Watcher.* Viking Press, New York, 1974.

16. Bullough, Vern, and Bullough, Bonnie: *The Subordinate Sex—A History of Attitudes Towards Women.* University of Illinois Press, Urbana, 1973.

16a. Ashley, Jo Ann: *Hospitals, Paternalism, and the Role of the Nurse.* Teachers College Press, New York, 1976.

17. Mead, Margaret: *Male and Female.* William Morrow & Co., New York, 1949.

18. Austin, Anne L.: *History of Nursing Source Book.* G. P. Putnam's Sons, New York, 1957, p. 257.

19. National League for Nursing: *Extending the Boundaries of Nursing*

Education—The Preparation and Role of the Nurse Scientist. Papers and summary from second conference of Council of Baccalaureate and Higher Degree Programs, Cleveland, Mar., 1968. The League, New York, 1968 (Pub. No. 15–342).

20. National League for Nursing: *Doctoral Programs in Nursing/Nurse Scientist Graduate Training Grants Program—1973.* The League, New York, 1973 (Pub. No. 15–1558).

21. Eriksson, Katie: "Sairaanhoidon Kehittäminen Oppiaineena," (An Approach—How to Develop Nursing Science.) *Sairaanhoidon Vuosikirja XI*:9 (Helsinki) 1974.

22. Henderson, Virginia: "Barber Surgeons of France in the Sixteenth Century." Teachers College, Columbia University, New York, 1931 (unpublished study).

23. World Health Organization: *The Training and Utilization of Feldshers in the USSR.* A Review Prepared by the Ministry of Health of the USSR for the World Health Organization. The Organization, Geneva, 1974, pp. 9, 18.

24. Sadler, Alfred M., et al.: *The Physician's Assistant Today and Tomorrow. Issues confronting New Health Practitioners,* 2nd ed. Ballinger Publishing Co., Cambridge, Mass., 175.

25. Nightingale, Florence: *Notes on Nursing.* Dover Publications, New York, 1969. (Republication of first American edition, 1860.)

26. Woodham-Smith, Mrs. Cecil: *Florence Nightingale, 1820–1910.* Constable & Co., Ltd., London, 1950.

27. Goodrich, Annie W.: *The Social and Ethical Significance of Nursing.* Macmillan Publishing Co., Inc., New York, 1932.

28. "The National Children's Bureau" (editorial), *Am. J. Nurs., 9*:389, (Mar.) 1909.

29. Van Doren, Mark: *Liberal Education.* Henry Holt, New York, 1943.

30. Carlson, Rick J.: *The End of Medicine.* John Wiley & Sons, New York, 1975.

31. Dillon, John B.: "How Did it Happen?" *Calif. Med. 113*:86, (Aug.) 1970.

32. Carnegie Commission on Higher Education: *Higher Education and the Nation's Health—Policies for Medical and Dental Education.* McGraw-Hill Book Co., New York, 1970.

33. Hepner, James O., and Hepner, Donna M.: *The Health Strategy Game. A Challenge for Reorganization and Management.* C. V. Mosby Co., St. Louis, 1973.

34. "Nursing in the Decade Ahead," *Am. J. Nurs., 70*:2115, (Oct.) 1970.

35. Brodt, Dagmar E.: "Excellence or Obsolescence: The Choice for Nursing," *Nurs. Forum, 9*:19 (No. 1) 1970.

36. Christman, Luther: "What the Future Holds for Nursing," *Nurs. Forum, 9*:12, (No. 1) 1970.

37. Somers, Anne R.: *Health Care in Transition: Directions for the Future.* Hospital Research and Educational Trust, Chicago, 1971.

38. National League for Nursing: *Crisis in Nursing—Changing Roles.* Papers presented at 1973 NLN Biennial Convention. The League, New York, 1973 (Pub. No. 20–1503).

39. Roe, Anne, and Sherwood, Mary: *Nursing in the Seventies.* John Wiley & Sons, New York, 1973.

40. Taffe, P.: "Nursing Today—A Profession—A Vocation—A Job?" *Aust. Nurses J., 2*:31, (Oct.) 1973.

41. Dyson, R.: "Changes in Professional Roles—Implications for the Future," *Can. J. Psychiatr. Nursing,* (Jan.–Feb.) 1973.

42. National League for Nursing: *Current Issues in Nursing Education.* Papers presented at 11th Conference of Council of Baccalaureate and Higher Degree Programs, Kansas City, Mo., Nov. 1973. The League, New York, 1974.

43. Bowman, Rosemary Amason, and Culpepper, Rebecca Clark: "National Health Insurance: Some of the Issues," *Am. J. Nurs., 75*:2017, (Nov.) 1975.

44. Gartner, A.: "Health Systems and New Careers," *Health Serv. Res., 88*:124, (Feb.) 1973.

45. National League for Nursing: *Goals for a National Health Insurance Program.* The League, New York, 1974.

46. Brousssean, B. L.: "The Transfer of Functions Between Health Professions," *Can. Hosp., 49*:44, (Sept.) 1972.

47. Wagner, D. L.: "Issues in the Provision of Health Care for All," *Am. J. Public Health, 63*:481, (June) 1973.

48. Meakins, J. C.: "Nursing Must Be Defined," *Am. J. Nurs., 48*:622, (Oct.)1948.

49. Abdellah, Faye G., et al.; *Patient-Centered Approaches to Nursing.* Macmillan Publishing Co., Inc., New York, 1960.

50. Johnson, Mae M., and Davis, Mary Lou C.: *Problem Solving in Nursing Practice,* 2nd ed. William C. Brown, Dubuque, Iowa, 1975.

51. Simmons, Leo W., and Henderson, Virginia :*Nursing Research. A Survey and Assessment.* Appleton-Century-Crofts, New York, 1964, p. 33.

52. Badouaille, M. L.: "Why Nursing Is Different," *N.Z. Nurs. J.,* 66:29, (July) 1973.

53. Kraegel, Janet M., et al.: *Patient Care Systems.* J. B. Lippincott Co., Philadelphia, 1974.

54. Bridges, Daisy Caroline: *A History of the International Council of Nurses, 1899–1964. The First Sixty-Five Years.* Pitman Medical Publishing Co., Ltd., London, 1967.

55. National League of Nursing Education, Committee on Curriculum: *A Curriculum Guide for Schools of Nursing.* The League, New York, 1937, p. 20.

56. Hughes, Everett C., et al.: *Twenty Thousand Nurses Tell Their Story.* J. B. Lippincott Co., Philadelphia, 1958.

57. Lysaught, Jerome P. (ed.): *Action in Nursing: Progress in Professional Purpose.* (A collection of 33 articles and pamphlets related to work of National Commission for the Study of Nursing and Nursing Education.) Mc-Graw-Hill Book Co., New York, 1974.

58. Hall, Virginia: *Statutory Regulation of the Scope of Nursing Practice—A Critical Survey.* National Joint Practice Commission, Chicago, 1975.

59. National League of Nursing Education, Committee on Curriculum: *op. cit.*

60. Vaillot, Sister Madeleine Clemence: *Commitment to Nursing. A Philosophical Investigation.* J. B. Lippincott Co., Philadelphia, 1962, p. 27.

61. Simmons, Leo W., and Henderson, Virginia: *op. cit.,* p. 119.

62. Brown, Martha M.: *Nurses, Patients and Social systems. The Effect of Skilled Nursing Intervention upon Institutionalized Older Patients.* University of Missouri Press, Columbia, 1969, p. 96 (University of Missouri Studies Vol. XLVI).

63. Fielo, Sandra B.: *A Summary of Integrated Nursing Theory,* 2nd ed. McGraw-Hill Book Co., New York, 1975.

64. Harris, M. Isabel: "Theory Building in Nursing. A Review of the Literature," *Image,* 4:6, (No. 1) 1972.

65. Jacox, Ada: "Theory Construction in Nursing: An Overview,"*Nurs. Res., 23*:4, (Jan.–Feb.) 1974.

66. Johnson, Dorothy E.: "Theory in Nursing: Borrowed and Unique?" *Nurs. Res., 17*:206, (May–June) 1968.

67. King, Imogene M.: *Toward a Theory for Nursing.* John Wiley & Sons, New York, 1971.

68. Ketefian, Shake (ed.): *Translation of Theory into Nursing Practice*

and Education with a Bibliography on Change. Proceedings of 7th Annual Clinical Sessions, New York, Apr. 27, 1974. New York University, Division of Nurse Education, New York, 1974.

69. Kintzel, Kay Corman (ed.): *Advanced Concepts in Clinical Nursing.* J. B. Lippincott Co., Philadelphia, 1971.

70. Mathwig, Gean: "Nursing Science—The Theoretical Core of Nursing Knowledge," *Image, 4*:20, (No. 1) 1971.

71. Mitchell, Pamelia (ed.): *Concepts Basic to Nursing.* McGraw-Hill Book Co., New York, 1973.

72. Murphy, Juanita F.: *Theoretical Issues in Professional Nursing.* Appleton-Century-Crofts, New York, 1971.

73. Murray, Ruth, and Zeniner, Judith: *Nursing Concepts for Health Promotion.* Prentice-Hall, Inc., Englewood Cliffs, N.J., 1975.

74. Newman, Margaret A.: "Nursing's Theoretical Evolution," *Nurs. Outlook, 20*:449, (July) 1972.

75. Nursing Development Conference Group: *Concept Formalization in Nursing Process and Product,* Little, Brown & Co., Boston, 1973.

76. Riehl, J. P., and Roy, Sister Callista: *Conceptual Models for Nursing Practice.* Appleton-Century-Crofts, New York, 1974.

77. Rogers, Martha E.: *An Introduction to the Theoretical Basis of Nursing.* F. A. Davis Co., Philadelphia, 1970.

78. Strauss, Anselm: "The Structure and Ideology of American Nursing: An Interpretation," in David, Fred (ed.): *The Nursing Profession: Five Sociological Essays.* John Wiley & Sons, New York, 1966.

79. Nagle, Ernest: *The Structure of Science.* Harcourt, Brace & World, New York, 1961, p. 106.

80. Wald, Florence, and Leonard, Robert: "Toward Development of Nursing Practice Theory," *Nurs. Res., 13*:309, (Fall) 1964.

81. Rogers, Martha E.: *op. cit.*

82. Santayana, George: "The Process of Nursing as an Open System," In Kintzel, Kay Corman (ed.): *Advanced Concepts in Clinical Nursing.* J. B. Lippincott Co., Philadelphia, 1971.

83. Von Bertalanffy, Ludwig: *General Systems Theory.* George Brazillier, New York, 1968.

84. Kraegel, Janet M.: "A System of Patient Care Based on Patient Needs," *Am. J. Nurs., 72*:257, (Apr.)1972.

85. Kraegel, Janet M., et al.: *Patient Care Systems.* J. B. Lippincott Co., Philadelphia, 1974.

86. Bowar-Ferres, Susan: "Loeb Center and Its Philosophy of Nursing," *Am. J. Nurs., 78*:810, (May) 1975.

87. University of Kansas Medical Center, Department of Nursing Education. McGraw-Hill Book Co., New York, 1974.

88. Giblin, Elizabeth S.: "Symposium on Assessment as Part of the Nursing Process," *Nurs. Clin. North Am., 6*:113, (Mar.) 1971.

89. Henderson, Virginia: "Is the Role of the Nurse Changing?" *Weathervane, 27*:12, (Oct.) 1968.

90. Jamann, JoAnn Shafer: "Providing for the Maintenance of Health," in Kintzel, Kay Corman (ed.): *Advanced Concepts in Clinical Nursing.* J. B. Lippincott Co., Philadelphia, 1971, p. 14.

91. Marriner, Ann: *The Nursing Process: A Scientific Approach to Nursing Care.* C. V. Mosby Co., St. Louis, 1975.

92. Mauksch, Hans O.: "The Nurse: Coordinator of Patient Care," in Skipper, James K., Jr., and Leonard, Robert C.: *Social Interaction and Patient Care.* J. B. Lippincott Co., Philadelphia, 1965.

93. Nightingale, Florence: *op. cit.*

94. Orlando, Ida Jean: *The Dynamic Nurse–Patient Relationship.* G. P. Putnam's Sons, New York, 1961.

95. Rogers, Martha E.: *op. cit.*

96. Sand, René: "The Nurse—Sentinel of Health," *Aust. Nurses, J., 52*:80, (Apr.) 1954.

97. Schulman, S.: "Basic Functional Roles in Nursing: Mother Surrogate and Healer," in Jaco, E. G. (ed.): *Patients, Physicians and Illness: Sourcebook on Behavioral Science and Medicine.* Free Press, Glencoe, Ill., 1958.

98. Sobol, Evelyn G., and Robischon, Paulette: *Family Nursing: A Study Guide.* C. V. Mosby Co., St. Louis, 1975.

99. Sutterley, Doris Cook, and Donnelly, Gloria Ferraro: *Perspectives in Human Development—Nursing Throughout the Life Cycle.* J. B. Lippincott Co., Philadelphia, 1973.

100. Woolley, F. Ross, et al.: *Problem-Oriented Nursing.* Springer Publishing Co., New York, 1974.

101. Dubos, René: *Mirage of Health.* Doubleday & Co., Garden City, N.Y., 1959.

102. Cochrane, A. L.: *Effectiveness and Efficiency: Random Reflections on Health Services.* Nuffield Provincial Hospitals Trust, London, 1972.

103. Illich, Ivan: *Medical Nemesis:The Expropriation of Health.* McGlelland & Stewart, London, 1975.

104. Malleson, Andrew: *Need Your Doctor Be So Useless?* George Allen & Unwin, London, 1973.

105. Meador, Clifton: "The Art and Science of Non-Disease,"*N. Engl. J. Med., 272*:92, (Jan. 14) 1965.

106. Shey, Herbert H.: "Iatrogenic Anxiety," *Psychiatr. Q., 45*:343, (No. 1) 1971.

107. Vayda, Eugene: "A Comparison of Surgical Rates in Canada and in England and Wales," *N. Engl. J. Med., 289*:1224, (Dec. 6) 1973.

108. Illich, Ivan: *op. cit.*

109. Royal Society of Medicine, and Josiah Macy, Jr. Foundation: *The Greater Medical Profession.* The Foundation, New York, 1973.

110. Josiah Macy, Jr. Foundation: *Macy Conference on Intermediate-Level Health Personnel in the Delivery of Direct Health Services. Intermediate-Level Health Practitioners.* The Foundation, New York, 1973.

111. Bloomfield, Ron, and Follis, Peggy (eds.): *The Health Team in Action.* BBC Publications, London, 1974.

112. Anderson, J. A. D., et al.: "Attachment of Community Nurses to General Practices: A Follow-up Study," *Br. Med J., 4*:103, (Oct. 10) 1970.

113. Anderson, Evelyn R.: *The Role of the Nurse.* Royal College of Nursing, London, 1973.

114. "Reorganization—1974 or 1984? Where the Nurses Will Stand," *Br. Med. J., 2*:603, (June 9) 1973.

115. Moore, M. F., et al.: "First Contact Decisions in General Practice. A Comparison Between a Nurse and Three General Practitioners," *Lancet, 1*:817, (Apr. 14) 1973.

116. Wilson, Barnett J.: "A Description of the Working environment and Work of the Unit Nursing Officer," *Int. J. Nurs. Studies, 10*:185, (Aug.) 1973.

117. Apitzer, W. O., et al.: "Nurse Practitioners in Primary Care. 3. Southern Ontario Randomized Trial," *Can. Med. Assoc. J., 108*:1005, (Apr. 21) 1973.

118. Canada. Department of National Health and Welfare, Committee on Clinical Training of Nurses for Medical Services in the North: *Report.* (Chairman, D. Kergin.) The Department, Ottawa, 1970.

119. Canadian Nurses' Association: *Joint CMA/CNA/CHA Conference, Health Action, Sept. 23–24, 1972.* Canadian Nurses' Association, Ottawa, 1972.

120. Carpenter, Helen: "The Canadian Scene," *Int. Nurs., Rev., 21*:43, (Mar.–Apr.) 1974.

121. DeMarsh, Kathleen G.: "Red Cross Outpost Nursing in New Brunswick," *Can. Nurs.*, 69:24, (June) 1973.

122. Hazlett, C. B.: "Task Analysis of the Clinically Trained Nurse," *Nurs. Clin. North Am.*, 10:699, (Dec.) 1975.

123. Jones, Phyllis E.: "A Program in Continuing Education for Primary Care," *Nurs. Clin. North Am.*, 10:691, (Dec.) 1975.

124. Bowers, John A., and Purcell, E. F. (eds.): *Medicine and Society in China*. Report of a Conference sponsored jointly by National Library of Medicine and Josiah Macy, Jr. Foundation. The Foundation, New York, 1974.

125. Kessen, William (ed.): *Childhood in China*. Yale University Press, New Haven, Conn., 1975.

126. Sidel, Victor W., and Sidel, Ruth: *op. cit.*

127. Maxwell, R.: *Health Care: The Proving Dilemma; Needs Versus Resources in Western Europe, the U.S. and U.S.S.R.* McKinsey & Co., New York, 1974.

128. Quinn, Sheila M.: "Nursing in the Soviet Union," *Int. Nurs. Rev.*, 15:75, (Jan.) 1968.

129. Seldon, Mark: *China: Revolution and Health*. Health Policy Advisory Center, New York, 1972.

130. Simon, Carlton (ed.): *Shobers Directory of Trained Nurses. Being a Selected List of Names and Addresses of Competent Graduated Trained Nurses Practicing in the Cities of Greater New York, Boston, Philadelphia, Baltimore and Washington*. Chober-Cornell Publishing Co., New York, 1902.

131. *Nurses' and Physicians' Director and Health Book of New Haven County*. City Printing Co., New Haven, Conn., 1923.

132. Schutt, Barbara G.: "Spot Check on Primary Care Nursing," *Am. J. Nurs.*, 72:1996, (Nov.) 1972.

133. _____: "Frontier's Family Nurses," *Am. J. Nurs.*, 72:903, (May) 1972.

134. "Frontier Nurses of Kentucky Set an Enviable Record," *Mod. Hosp.*, 39:60, (Sept.) 1932.

135. Djukanovic, V., and Mach, E. P. (eds.): *Alternative Approaches to Meeting Basic Health Needs in Developing Countries. A Joint UNICEF/WHO Study*. World Health Organization, Geneva, 1975.

136. World Health Organization: *The Training and Utilization of Feldshers in the U.S.S.R.* The Organization, Geneva, 1974, p. 7.

ric Services," in *Nursing Personnel for Mental Health Programs*. Report of a Conference sponsored by the Southern Regional Program on Mental Health Training and Research, Wagoner, Okla., Mar. 27–29, 1957, Southern Regional Education Board, Atlanta, Ga., 1958.

171. Tudor, Gwen E.: "A Sociopsychiatric Nursing Approach to Intervention in a Problem of Mutual Withdrawal on a Mental Ward," *Psychiatry, 15*:193, (May) 1952.

172. Ruell, Virginia M.: "Nurse-Managed Care for Psychiatric Patients," *Am. J. Nurs., 75*:1156, (July) 1975.

173. Lewis, C. E., and Resnik, Barbara: "Nurse Clinics and Progressive Ambulatory Care," *N. Engl. J. Med., 277*:1236, (Dec. 7) 1967.

174. _____: "The Nurse Clinic: Dynamics of Ambulatory Care—New Roles for Old Disciplines," *J. Kans. Med. Soc., 68*:123, 1967.

175. Lewis, C. E., et al.: "Activities, Events and Outcomes in Ambulatory Patient Care," *N. Engl. J. Med., 280*:645, (Mar. 20) 1969.

176. Lewis, C. E.: *Dynamics of Nursing in Ambulatory Care*. (Final Report of Study under USPHS Grand NU–00145). US Government Printing Office, Washington, D.C., 1968.

177. Noonan, Barbara R.: "Eight Years in a Medical Nurse Clinic," *Am. J. Nurs., 72*:1128, (June) 1972.

178. Browning, Mary H., and Lewis, Edith P. (comps.): *The Expanded Role of the Nurse*. American Journal of Nursing Co., New York, 1973 (Contemporary Nursing Series).

179. Sadler, Alfred M., Jr., et al.: *The Physician's Assistant Today and Tomorrow: Issues Confronting New Health Practitioners*, 2nd ed. Ballinger Publishing Co., Cambridge, Mass., 1975.

180. National Commission for the Study of Nursing and Nursing Education: *Abstract for Action*. (Report prepared by Jerome P. Lysaught.) McGraw-Hill Book Co., New York, 1970.

181. "AMA Endorses Expanded Role for Nurses. Seeks Study of R.N. and P.A. Functions" (news), *Am. J. Nurs., 72*:1365, (Aug.) 1972.

182. Storey, Patrick B.: *The Soviet Feldsher as a Physician's Assistant*. National Institutes of Health, Bethesda, Md., 1972 (DHEW Pub. No. [NIH] 72–58).

183. World Health Organization: *The Training and Utilization of Feldshers in the U.S.S.R.* The Organization, Geneva, 1974.

184. Quinn, Sheila M.: *op. cit.*

185. International Labour Office: *Employment and Conditions of Work and Life of Nursing Personnel*. International Labour Conference, 1976, 61st Session, Report VII (1). The Office, Geneva, 1976, p. 72.

186. Andreoli, K. G., and Stead, Eugene A.: "Training Physician's Assistants at Duke," *Am. J. Nurs., 67*:1442, (July) 1967.

187. Ingles, Thelma: "A New Health Worker," *Am. J. Nurs., 68*:1059, (May) 1968.

188. "AMA Unveils Surprise Plan to Convert R.N. into Medic" (news), *Am. J. Nurs., 70*:691, (Apr.) 1970.

189. Sadler, Alfred M., Jr., et al.: *The Physician's Assistant Today and Tomorrow: Issues Confronting New Health Practitioners*, 2nd ed. Ballinger Publishing Co., Cambridge, Mass., 1975, p. 153.

190. Sadler, Alfred M., Jr., et al.: *op. cit.*, p. 106.

191. Lambertson, Eleanor C. "Perspective on the Physician's Assistant," *Nurs. Outlook, 20*:32, (Jan.) 1972.

192. Bergman, A.: "Physician's Assistants Belong in the Nursing Profession," *Am. J. Nurs., 71*:975 (May) 1971.

193. deTornyay, R.: "Expanding the Nurse's Role Does Not Make Her a Physician's Assistant," *Am. J. Nurs., 71*:974, (Sept.) 1971.

194. "Nurse Groups Ask R.N.–M.D. Dialogue, Some Get It," *Am. J. Nurs., 70*:953, (May) 1970.

195. Sadler, Alfred M., Jr., et al.: *op. cit.*, p. 106.

196. Lipkin, Mack: *The Care of Patients, Concepts and Tactics*. Oxford University Press, New York, 1974.

197. Rakel, Robert E.: "Primary Care–Whose Responsibility?" *J. Fam. Pract., 2*:429, (Dec.) 1975.

198. Smoyak, Shirley A.: "Origin, Purpose and Thrust of the National Joint Practice Commission," in *Building for the Future*. Papers presented at ANA Conference, Sept., 1974. The Association, Kansas City, Mo., 1975.

199. Ford, Loretta: "Interdisciplinary Education for Nurses in the Expanded Role: The Way of the Future," in *Building for the Future*. Papers presented at ANA Conference, Sept., 1974. The Association, Kansas City, Mo., 1975.

200. Hall, Virginia: *Statutory Regulation of the Scope of Nursing Practice—A Critical Survey*. National Joint Practice Commission, Chicago, 1975.

201. Devlin, M. M.: *Selected Bibliography with Abstracts on Joint Practice*. National Joint Practice Commission, Chicago, 1975.

202. World Health Organization: *Development of Educational Programmes for the Health Professions*. (Prepared by Center for Educational Development, University of Illinois College of Medicine.) The Organization, Geneva, 1973 (Public Health Papers No. 52).

Chapter 20

Nursing as a Constant Factor in Health Services

In most countries it is rare to find a health service that doesn't involve the *nurse*. Care of the sick, the injured, and the helpless has always involved *nursing*, although families, friends, religious or military personnel, and physicians may have given this care. In 1900 physicians outnumbered "trained" nurses and were the most constant factor in health service; now nurses and midwives outnumber them in most countries. E. D. Acheson, speaking for Great Britain, said:

> It is a fact . . . that doctors now constitute only a small minority of the skilled personnel who work together in the health service. Medical and dental staff are small fry, numerically, compared with nurses, midwives, and the professional and technical health service staff; they account for approximately 15 per cent of the total. . . . If such an analysis had been carried out in 1858, the year of the first medical act that delineated the roles, responsibilities, and education of the "smaller medical profession," doctors and dentists, with the help of a few apothecaries, would have been shown to be virtually alone in the field.[a]

Figures for other European countries, especially Scandinavia, the United States and Canada, Australia, and New Zealand now show a comparable preponderance of nurses among health workers. Feldshers in the USSR are also very numerous, as are barefoot and Red Guard doctors in China. They are to be found in these countries in some positions that would be filled by nurses elsewhere.

Settings in Which Nurses Are Employed

Nurses are employed almost anywhere that a health service exists, and it is difficult to make an exhaustive list of settings. Full statistical data in the American Nurses' Association's *Facts About Nursing*[1,2] are available for eight "fields"; other data come under "other specified field" or "field not stated." The specified fields or settings for the United States are hospital, nursing home, school of nursing, private duty, public health, school nurse, industrial nurse, and office nurse. For Canada the fields are hospital/other institutions (which includes nursing homes), public health agency, occupational health, home care/visiting care agency, community health centre, physicians'/dentists' offices, educational institution, and private practice.[3] While complete data are available only in these fields, nursing takes place in the following additional fields: hospices; community health centers and health maintenance type organizations; offices of the private practitioner of nursing; college health services; and jails, prisons, and other correctional institutions. Nursing can also take place in ships, planes, and space transport operations and in health agencies and organizations. Another way to classify nursing is according to functions nurses perform, or positions they hold.[b]

Specialization of Nursing According to Function or Position

After graduation from a school of nursing and taking a licensing examination, nurses may elect to (1) practice nursing; (2) administer a nursing service, agency, or organization; (3) teach nursing, (4) act as a consultant, which is perhaps a form of teaching; (5) conduct research; or (6) write about nursing. Many nurses go beyond the basic program in preparation for any of these functions. It is not feasible in this book to give data on the numbers of nurses according to function or position. As might be expected, registered nurses in practice far exceed those performing any other function.

Specialization According to Clinical Entity

Either by study, years of experience, or both, nurses specialize in the care of age groups, as, for example, child care (pediatrics) or care of the aged (geriatrics). Even with such specialties, there may be subspecialties such as the care of infants or adolescents. Nurses specialize in maternal care, becoming obstetrical nursing specialists or assuming more responsibility and becoming nurse-midwives; others elect to specialize in the care of patients treated medically or surgically or combine these to become medical-surgical nursing specialists. Within surgery and medicine there are many subspecialties. Nurses, for example, become neurosurgical, orthopedic, urologic or gynecologic, ocular, otologic, or dermatologic nurses; they may specialize in the care of patients with one type of surgery and be, for example, an "ostomy nurse"; they may elect to care for patients with a disease, as, for example, cancer (oncologic nursing), heart disease (cardiac nursing), arthritis, tuberculosis, or a group of related diseases such as infections (communicable disease) or metabolic disorders. Surgical nursing can be divided into subspecialties according to the stage of surgery—some nurses electing to care for patients before and during recovery from surgery, others to work with surgeons during the operation, and still others to care for patients in the immediate postanesthesia period in the "recovery room." Surgical nurses may study anesthesia and become nurse anesthetists. Medical nursing could be divided into almost the same subspecialties. Many nurses elect to work in intensive care units, others in short-term acute care hospital units, and others in ambulatory and long-term care institutions and health agencies.

Nursing care of those with behavior disorders comprises one of the major clinical specialties—psychiatric nursing. Nursing the mentally defective is a related (and neglected) specialty. Psychiatric nurse specialists may be divided into those who care for children and those who care for adults and, as in obstetric nursing, some psychiatric nurses elect to assume more responsibility and after certain programs of graduate study call themselves "nurse therapists." Psychiatric nurses in some institutions and agencies spend their time working with other nurses on behavioral problems of patients in nonpsychiatric settings. They are often called "liaison nurses." Lisa Robinson entitles a 1974 text *Liaison Nursing: Psychological Approach to Patient Care.* (F. A. Davis Company, Philadelphia, 1974).

Notes

---

[a]Acheson, E. D.: "Educational Consequences. In Great Britain," in the Royal Society of Medicine, and the Josiah Macy, Jr. Foundation: *The Greater Medical Profession.* The Foundation, New York, 1973, p. 192.

[b]It will be noted that much information on nurses and nursing has been at-

tributed to either the ANA publication *Facts About Nursing 72-73* or *Facts About Nursing 74-75*. The reason for this is that the 74-75 publication does not in every case give or update the information in the 72-73 edition. *Countdown 1974* was the last compendium on Canadian nursing available to the writer in 1976. However, the Canadian Nurses' Association staff has given us late data in some cases.

References

1. American Nurses' Association: *Facts About Nursing* 72–73. The Association, Kansas City, Mo., 1974.

2. American Nurses' Association: *Facts About Nursing* 74–75. The Association, Kansas City, Mo., 1976.

3. Canadian Nurses' Association: personal communication, Aug. 25, 1976.

Chapter 21

The Nurse's Role in Promoting Health Programs

Many useful types of service are given by persons who work from day to day without much thought of anything except what lies immediately before them. Some nurses, who are good technicians, work in this way, doing little to stimulate their imaginations or to broaden their concepts of nursing. Not seeing the larger problems, however, they may waste their energies worrying over trifles, and, like Chicken Little, run around crying that the skies are falling; or, if they are of a carefree disposition, they may be unconcerned when serious issues are at stake that will affect not only themselves but also the profession as a whole and the public at large. Needless to say, those nurses, doctors, dentists, or medical social workers who recognize and live up to the responsibilities of their professions have the widest influence and probably derive the greatest satisfaction from their work. With the close cooperation among welfare groups that exists today and the promise of still greater unification of medical services, it does not seem possible for members of any of these professions to work with maximal effectiveness without knowing a good deal about the community. Nancy Milio's[1] work in a ghetto community demonstrated how influential one nurse can be. She is an ardent spokeswoman for the involvement of nurses in social change essential to health.

In order to be a well-informed medical and health worker, it is desirable to have some knowledge along the following lines: (1) the nationalities, races, and religions represented by the people of the community and the characteristic ways of living among these different groups; (2) the general level of intelligence and the interest of people in, and their knowledge of, laws governing healthful living; (3) the economic status of persons living in different districts of the community; (4) the social agencies and the health facilities available to the people; (5) the local health government and its relationship to the state and national government; and (6) the machinery for the passage of health legislation and the ways in which the individuals in the community may make their influence felt when questions affecting the health and welfare of the community are up for discussion before bodies of lawmakers. Nurses should welcome opportunities to keep up, through the daily newspapers and through regular reference to nursing journals and other professional journals, with what is going on locally and nationally; to observe the work of other health workers and agencies; to take part in discussions of current health problems; to work on coordinating committees and in agencies; to participate in professional and other health-related meetings; to initiate or participate in research on health care; and to write about their activities in professional and other publications. The patterns of nursing practice are constantly changing. The well-informed nurse who is professionally active or inactive is always in a position to promote the health of the population wherever he or she lives and works.

In estimating the resources of a nation, human life and the health of the people are said to exceed all other economic resources. While a growing health consciousness is apparent in the United States and in many other countries, our knowledge of how to prevent and control disease far exceeds its application. The average life span has been increased by more than 20 years since 1900, and the incidence of many diseases has been materially reduced, but conditions for which the means of early detection and treatment are well known still rank high among the common causes of death. Health care costs have markedly increased in the 1960s and 1970s, and our expenditures for better health care have proportionately increased. In order to raise health standards, however, the main problems seem to be the establishment of an economic status that provides people with the necessities of life, a general education that will stimulate a desire for and knowledge of health, and the provision of adequate medical service and other health facilities. Some countries have national health schemes that make health care universally available, just as is education. In the United States, universal coverage has not been effected, but new programs have provided many groups of people with health care or with the opportunity to have it.

An important aspect of health programs has been the improvement and extension of all kinds of nursing service. The part that nursing care plays in raising health standards is recognized and has added not only to the dignity but to the interest of the nurse's work. Some of the changes in nursing that have enhanced the profession are the growth of nurse-midwifery and the enlarged role of nurse practitioners and clinical nurse specialists. Nurses in all specialties today are credited in many circles with being sensitive to the social causes of disease and to the possibilities of prevention and treatment with a comprehensive approach to health. This may be the single most significant development in nursing.

Some outstanding accomplishments in disease control and the promotion of health through scientific and technical advances in medicine that have brought progress in raising health standards are the control of infectious diseases, modern obstetrical and surgical care, an increase in nutritional knowledge, and the changes brought about in psychiatric care. Social scientists working with health professionals have helped improve the psychological and sociological components of health care.

The importance of organization in health care is reflected in the numbers of official and voluntary health agencies. International, national, state, and local health agencies are organized to carry on a variety of programs that are interrelated in their work. The differing functions of tax-supported and voluntary agencies provide services to expand the availability of health care to large numbers of people.

The government's responsibilities in health work have grown since the early 1900s. Some countries have developed a national health service that provides universal coverage. The service, though nationalized, may be administered through smaller geographic units, as in Canada through provincial governments. The United States has not developed a national health service but has created services that provide health care to certain groups, as, for example, the aged, indigent children, Indians, the military, veterans, and certain government employees. The United States government's interest in health care has greatly increased. Proposals for national health insurance have made the public aware that "socialized medicine" or tax-funded medical care is believed by most of the world to be a human right. Current plans embody such concepts as Health Maintenance Organizations, comprehensive health planning, consumer participation in health affairs, and the regionalization of medical care.

The hospital's role in the community health program is an important and crucial one, and most persons see hospitals as part of a regional plan for health care rather than as autonomous, isolated institutions. Systems for preventing hospitalization, such as prepaid group practice plans, screening and diagnostic centers, and health education centers, are taking on added importance as the care provided in most hospitals is economically unsupportable. Extended care and nursing care facilities must be considered part of the health care system also. It is hoped that their services will be more effectively integrated and the quality more adequately ensured than they are presently. As they are developed, hospices will also be a part of the system.

All types of agencies are recognizing their interdependence and the importance of a more unified family health service. Health workers are urged to study the people, the conditions, and the health facilities within their communities in order that they may give the best possible service to persons in their care. In almost every community, better planning, closer coordination, and simplification of health services are needed.

There are few, if any, public or private agencies that do not consider nurses essential members of their staffs. They have taken an active part in all health programs and in all aspects of research. It is significant that the period of time in which professional nursing has existed is also the period in which greatest advances have been made in medical science.

Nurses are credited by many observers as being especially sensitive to human needs. Wolstenholme suggests that "at this moment of human tumult, lost faith, and economic bewilderment, the greater medical profession, the doctors and nurses and all who share their care, concern, and curiosity in the relief of unnecessary suffering could inspire a critical mass of mankind with the determination to give every one in the world an opportunity to enjoy a life worth living."[a]

Notes

[a]Wolstenholme, G. E. W. *Outline of a World Health Service as a step towards men's well being and towards a world society.* In Ciba Foundation Symposium Health of Mankind. J & A Churchill, London, 1969.

References

1. Milio, Nancy: *9226 Kercheval. The Storefront That Did Not Burn.* University of Michigan Press, Ann Arbor, 1971.

Chapter 22

Some Observations on the Health Care "Industry"

F or nursing this is "the best of times and the worst of times." It is the best of times because the World Health Organization and other influential bodies have given global recognition to nurses as providers of primary health care. This presupposes that nurses have an independent as well as an interdependent function.

The WHO goal of "health care for all by 2000" can only be reached if nurses—the largest body of health care providers—are allowed to realize their full potential. This supposition leads, in turn, to the conclusion that nurses, like other "professional" health workers, should be prepared in national, provincial, or state systems of higher education—now a well-established trend world-wide.

Ours is "the worst of times" for nurses because it is a period of accelerated, technological change in health care and nurses (who are with the sick, the handicapped, and the dying more hours of the day than any other category of health worker), bear the brunt of helping to make these changes constructive rather than destructive. Nurses everywhere are frustrated because within existing systems they are so often unable to give the supportive care that they believe would enable people to recover from disease, cope with a handicap or die peacefully when death is inevitable. Most especially, for various reasons, nurses are unable to make health prevention a priority in their practice. If the goal of "health care for all by 2000" is to be realized, the following are some of the important objectives involved:

1. health education to make citizens aware of the conditions that promote well-being and/or those that increase morbidity;
2. acceptance by individuals and organized society of the obligation to adopt a healthful life style; and
3. allocation of adequate funds and the equitable distribution of monies and other resources to promote health and combat disease.

It is generally conceded that the human desire to help others dominates the social services (as for instance education) and that the profit motive dominates industry. "Professionals" are said to be effective when their clients learn enough from them to make their help unnecessary. Industrialists are successful to the extent that they promote dependence of the public on their products and create escalating needs or desires for more and more possessions.

Health care systems in some countries are unabashedly industries, directed by industrialists rather than by experts in the service they offer. They use the depersonalized methods of "scientific management" (as for example, job rather than patient assignment) and tend to compete rather than cooperate. Conferences of health workers may be developed around the concepts of pricing, marketing and power (as opposed to influence).

With more and more health agencies and institutions coming under the dominion of corporate industrialized management it is increasingly difficult to preserve the humane values in health care. Citizens, but especially health care workers, should judge, and, when possible, measure the effect of such management on the welfare of clients and workers. Assessments will be most effective if health care professionals cooperate with other informed persons in society in making them.

Nothing seems more important to me in this era than the provision of universal health education through the curricula of grade schools, high schools, colleges, and universities; and through the channels of communication—radio and television—that reach all ages. An effective programme of health education also implies opening health science libraries to the public. But most particularly, I believe universal ability to deal effectively with health problems is promoted by giving all citizens copies of their health (medical) records.

There is legislation in some countries, provinces or states making health records (like education records) available to adults, parents or guardians. However, health, or medical, records are unintelligible to many who would like to be informed by them. Realizing this, some health agencies provide even their professional workers with glossaries or guides so that they can understand and use the abbreviations and jargon in the particular agency.

I believe that nothing could be more timely than a study by international health organizations of the essentials of an effective health record. This might result in the publication of a universal model that identifies the essential content, the terminology, and the conditions controlling its usefulness to the individual who is the subject of the record and also the usefulness of the record to the public at large—as for instance in litigation, health education, control and treatment of disease.

Nursing, fortunately, has an increasing number of journals, such as the *Journal of Advanced Nursing*, with editorial policies permitting the presentation of controversial ideas and practices. Giving citizens copies of their health records has been, and still is controversial. In the 1978 edition of the text *Principles and Practice of Nursing* (Henderson & Nite, 1978) the authors quote Dr. Lawrence Weed (1975) addressing the public on health management as follows:

> There are those who fear the patient will panic if he owns and understands his own record. But what of the confusion, bad medicine and suffering that results directly from the present practice of keeping source oriented records unavailable to patients and families just when they need them most. . . It [making the record accessible] may be the most effective weapon we have against over-utilization of medical care. . . If you [the public] want to develop a mature and helpful philosophy about maintaining your health, you need to understand the means by which physicians' clinical judgments are made and tested.

Individual health records are the ultimate source of information for patients and their families but they also provide data for evaluation of health care, the incidence of disease, methods of treatment, and any number of questions related to social welfare. Appropriate use by health workers and concerned citizens is almost essential to the improvement of what some critics call our 'ailing health care systems' whether they be health services or health industries.

References

Henderson V., & Nite, G. (1978). *The Principles and Practice of Nursing.* Macmillan, New York.

Weed, L. (1975). *Your Health Care and How to Manage It.* Promis Laboratory, University of Vermont, Vermont.

Index